Lecture Notes in Computer

Commenced Publication in 1973
Founding and Former Series Editors:
Gerhard Goos, Juris Hartmanis, and Jan van Leeuwen

Reinhard R. Beichel Milan Sonka (Eds.)

Computer Vision Approaches to Medical Image Analysis

Second International ECCV Workshop,
CVAMIA 2006
Graz, Austria, May 12, 2006
Revised Papers

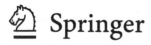 Springer

Volume Editors

Reinhard R. Beichel
Graz University of Technology
Institute for Computer Graphics and Vision
Inffeldgasse 16/2, 8010 Graz, Austria
E-mail: beichel@icg.tu-graz.ac.at

Milan Sonka
University of Iowa
Department of Electrical and Computer Engineering
Iowa City, IA 52242, USA
E-mail: milan-sonka@uiowa.edu

Library of Congress Control Number: 2006933642

CR Subject Classification (1998): I.4, I.2.10, I.3.5, I.5, J.3

LNCS Sublibrary: SL 6 – Image Processing, Computer Vision, Pattern Recognition, and Graphics

ISSN   0302-9743
ISBN-10   3-540-46257-0 Springer Berlin Heidelberg New York
ISBN-13   978-3-540-46257-6 Springer Berlin Heidelberg New York

Springer is a part of Springer Science+Business Media

springer.com

© Springer-Verlag Berlin Heidelberg 2006
Printed in Germany

Typesetting: Camera-ready by author, data conversion by Scientific Publishing Services, Chennai, India
Printed on acid-free paper   SPIN: 11889762   06/3142   5 4 3 2 1 0

Preface

Medical imaging and medical image analysis are developing rapidly. While medical imaging has already become a standard of modern medical care, medical image analysis is still mostly performed visually and qualitatively. The ever-increasing volume of acquired data makes it impossible to utilize them in full. Equally important, the visual approaches to medical image analysis are known to suffer from a lack of reproducibility. A significant research effort is devoted to developing algorithms for processing the wealth of data available and extracting the relevant information in a computerized and quantitative fashion.

Medical imaging and image analysis are interdisciplinary areas combining electrical, computer, and biomedical engineering; computer science; mathematics; physics; statistics; biology; medicine; and other fields. Medical imaging and computer vision, interestingly enough, have developed and continue developing somewhat independently. Nevertheless, bringing them together promises to benefit both of these fields.

This was the second time that a satellite workshop, solely devoted to medical image analysis issues, was held in conjunction with the European Conference on Computer Vision (ECCV), and we are optimistic that this will become a tradition at ECCV. We received 38 full-length paper submissions to the second Computer Vision Approaches to Medical Image Analysis (CVAMIA) Workshop, out of which 10 were accepted for oral and 11 for poster presentation after a rigorous peer-review process. In addition, the workshop included three invited talks. The first was given by Maryellen Giger from the University of Chicago, USA — titled "Multi-Modality Breast CADx". The second invited talk dealt with "Quantification of Growth and Motion Using Non-Rigid Registration" and was presented by Daniel Rueckert, Imperial College London, UK. The third invited talk was entitled "Trends and Challenges in Medical Image Analysis" and was presented by Ravikanth Malladi, GE Global Research, India.

The workshop logistics were handled by the organizers of ECCV 2006, associated with the Institute of Electrical Measurement and Measurement Signal Processing of Graz University of Technology, the Institute for Computer Graphics and Vision of Graz University of Technology, and the Visual Cognitive Systems Laboratory at the University of Ljubljana. We thank all members of these institutions who were involved in the organization of the workshop for their support. We are grateful to the Styrian Government for the generous financial support of the CVAMIA 2006 Workshop. Finally, we extend our sincere thanks to the Program Committee members and to everyone else who made this workshop possible.

May 2006   Reinhard R. Beichel
                                                                  Milan Sonka

Organization

The 2006 Computer Vision Approaches to Medical Image Analysis (CVAMIA) Workshop was held in conjunction with the 9th European Conference on Computer Vision (ECCV) in Graz, Austria, on May 12, 2006. The ECCV conference was organized by the Institute of Electrical Measurement and Measurement Signal Processing and the Institute for Computer Graphics and Vision, both located at the Graz University of Technology, and the Visual Cognitive Systems Laboratory at the University of Ljubljana.

Executive Committee

Reinhard R. Beichel   Graz University of Technology, Austria
Milan Sonka   University of Iowa, USA

Program Committee

Amir Amini   Washington University in St. Louis, USA
Christian Barillot   IRISA, France
Faisal Beg   Simon Fraser University, Canada
Djamal Boukerroui   Université de Technologie de Compiègne, France
Marleen de Bruijne   IT University of Copenhagen, Denmark
Gary Christensen   University of Iowa, USA
Ela Claridge   University of Birmingham, UK
Tim Cootes   University of Manchester, UK
Herve Delingette   INRIA, France
Bram van Ginneken   University Medical Center Utrecht, The Netherlands
Dmitry Goldgof   University of South Florida, USA
Michael Goris   Stanford University School of Medicine, USA
Tomas Gustavsson   Chalmers University of Technology, Sweden
Ghassan Hamarneh   Simon Fraser University, Canada
Kenneth Hoffmann   State University of New York at Buffalo, USA
Ioannis A. Kakadiaris   University of Houston, USA
Ron Kikinis   Harvard Medical School, USA
Ben Kimia   Brown University, USA
Attila Kuba   University of Szeged, Hungary
Jan Kybic   Czech Technical University, Czech Republic
Rasmus Larsen   Technical University of Denmark, Denmark
Boudewijn Lelieveldt   Leiden University Medical Center, The Netherlands
Bostjan Likar   University of Ljubljana, Slovenia
Gabriele Lohmann   Max Planck Institute of Cognitive Neuroscience, Germany

Sponsoring Institutions

Das Land Steiermark - Abteilung 3: Wissenschaft und Forschung

Table of Contents

Clinical Applications

Image Registration

Image Segmentation and Analysis

Poster Session

Melanoma Recognition Using Representative and Discriminative Kernel Classifiers

Tatiana Tommasi[1], Elisabetta La Torre[1], and Barbara Caputo[2]

[1] University of Rome La Sapienza, P.le A. Moro 5, 00185, Rome, Italy
{tatiana.tommasi, elisabetta.latorre}@uniroma1.it
[2] NADA/CVAP, KTH, SE-100 44, Stockholm, Sweden
caputo@nada.kth.se

Abstract. Malignant melanoma is the most deadly form of skin lesion. Early diagnosis is of critical importance to patient survival. Existent visual recognition algorithms for skin lesions classification focus mostly on segmentation and feature extraction. In this paper instead we put the emphasis on the learning process by using two kernel-based classifiers. We chose a discriminative approach using support vector machines, and a probabilistic approach using spin glass-Markov random fields. We benchmarked these algorithms against the (to our knowledge) state-of-the-art method on melanoma recognition, exploring how performance changes by using color or textural features, and how it is affected by the quality of the segmentation mask. We show with extensive experiments that the support vector machine approach outperforms the existing method and, on two classes out of three, it achieves performances comparable to those obtained by expert clinicians.

1 Introduction

Malignant melanoma is a spreading disease in the western world. Its incidence has been increasing over the past decades; currently 132,000 melanoma skin cancer occurs globally each year. One in every three cancers diagnosed is a skin cancer and, according to Skin Cancer Foundation Statistics, one in every five Americans will develop this kind of tumor in their lifetime [15]. Management of melanoma is a complex issue requiring a multidisciplinary approach. The most effective method of protection against the development of skin cancer is minimization of ultraviolet exposure from sunlight. Since advanced melanoma is still practically incurable, early detection and treatment are critical steps towards a reduction in mortality. Surgical excision remains the mainstay of treatment [9]. In northern Europe a deceleration in the incidence and mortality trends occurred recently in persons aged under 70, whereas in southern Europe both incidence and mortality rates are still increasing [4]. The most plausible explanations for the deceleration in these trends in northern Europe are earlier detection, more frequent excision of pigmented lesions and a growing public awareness of the dangers of excessive sunbathing [4].

Epiluminescence Microscopy (ELM or dermoscopy) is the most used diagnostic technique used by clinicians to reveal malignant melanoma. It is non-invasive

R.R. Beichel and M. Sonka (Eds.): CVAMIA 2006, LNCS 4241, pp. 1–12, 2006.

and allows for a detailed surface analysis of a suspicious skin lesion by using hand-held device emitting incident light from a light source penetrating the epidermal skin layer. Physicians visually inspect dermoscopic images for abnormal morphologic and chromatic features that indicate malignancy. They commonly use the ABCD (Asymmetry, Border, Color, Dimension and Dermoscopic structures) method as guideline. Due to the subjective nature of examination the accuracy of diagnosis is highly dependent upon physician's expertise.

There is a growing awareness that one of the weakest links in the biomedical interpretation process is the perception of details and the recognition of their meaning by the dermatologists. An automatic system for melanoma recognition would constitute a valuable support for physicians in every day clinical practice. Such a system should reproduce the perceptual and cognitive strategy followed by doctors, and should allow the dermatologist to trace each step of the process which led to a given diagnosis, so to leave space for exploring multiple interpretations. Recently numerous research on this topic have been proposed (for a more comprehensive discussion of the most significant literature we refer the reader to section 2); a key factor for the development and evaluation of these systems is the availability of a statistically significant database. One of the largest databases of melanoma images available to the research community was contributed by H. Ganster et al. [5]. That paper presented a database of 5363 images, accompanied by: (a) a segmentation algorithm for isolating the potential melanoma from the surrounding skin, determined by several basic segmentation algorithms combined together with a fusion strategy [5]; (b) a set of features containing shape and radiometric features as well as local and global parameters, calculated to describe the malignancy of a lesion, from which significant features are selected by application of statistical feature subset selection methods [5]; (c) a nearest neighbor classification algorithm [5]. In that work the authors concentrated particularly on the segmentation technique and the features selection process, obtaining results that, to the best of our knowledge, represent the state-of-the-art on this topic. Here we focus instead on the classification algorithm, proposing to use kernel methods for classification of skin lesion images. Specifically, we selected a discriminative method and a probabilistic one. As discriminative method we chose Support Vector Machines (SVM, [12]), a state-of-the-art large margin classifier, where the optimal separating surface is defined by a linear combination of scalar products between the view to be classified and some support vectors [11][12]. By introducing a Mercer kernel, a non-linear SVM can be constructed replacing the scalar products in the linear SVM via the kernel function. SVMs have demonstrated remarkable performance on object recognition and categorization [13] and biomedical imaging [14]. As probabilistic method we chose Spin Glass-Markov Random Fields (SG-MRF, [2]), a fully connected MRF which integrates results of statistical mechanics with Gibbs probability distributions via non linear kernel mapping [2]. Experiments have shown the robustness and categorization capabilities of this algorithm for object recognition [2] and its applicability for biomedical applications [3]. We conducted an experimental evaluation of these two techniques on the Ganster's database[1], which allows for a straightforward benchmarking of our algorithms against theirs. We tested out two methods on two different types of features, Color Histograms (CH) and Multidimansional receptive Fields Histograms (MFH, [10]). These features reproduce two of the criteria followed by dermatologists for diagnosis, respectively "C" for color variegation and "D" for differential local structures. Several series of experiments were performed for selecting optimal feature descriptors. We also evaluated the influence of the segmentation method by running two series of experiments: the first using the segmentation masks obtained by Ganster, the second using an hand-made rectangular mask which roughly contains the whole lesion while minimizing the amount of surrounding skin in the image. In order to have a fair comparison, we replicated the experimental setup used in [5] for a benchmark evaluation. Our results show that SVM obtains remarkably better performances than SG-MRF and Ganster's method with both feature types and regardless of the segmentation method. More important, on two classes out of three, SVM achieves recognition results comparable to those obtained by skilled clinicians.

The rest of the paper is organized as follows: section 2 reviews the state of the art in computer-assisted melanoma recognition. Then we briefly review the theory behind SG-MRF (section 3) and SVMs (section 4). Section 5 describes the experimental setup and reports on our findings. The paper concludes with a summary discussion and some possible directions for future research.

2   Related Work

Recently there has been an increasing interest in developing algorithms for melanoma classification. Grana et al. [6] provided mathematical descriptors for the border of pigmented skin lesion images and assessed their efficacy for distinction among different lesion groups. They introduced new descriptors such as lesion slope and lesion slope regularity and define them mathematically, then they employed a new algorithm based on the Catmull Rom spline method and the computation of the gray-level gradient of points extracted by interpolation of normal direction on spline points [6]. The efficacy of these descriptors was tested on a data set of 510 pigmented skin lesions, composed by 85 melanomas and 425 nevi, by employing statistical methods for discrimination between the two populations [6]. Grzymala-Busse et al. [7] used discretization based on cluster analysis, LEM2 algorithm for rule induction, and standard LERS classification scheme to check whether the ABCD formula is optimal [7]. The data consisted in total of 276 cases of benign nevus, blue nevus, suspicious nevus, and malignant melanoma [7]. Lefevre et al. [8] proposed a theory used in different fields such as data fusion, regression or classification: the Dempster-Shafer's theory, or evidence theory [8]. They applied the classification process on a training set of 81 lesions: 61 benign lesions (nevi) and 20 malignant lesions (melanoma) and a test set of 209 lesions: 191 nevi and 18 melanoma [8].

---

[1] We gratefully thank H. Ganster and A. Pinz for making the database and their segmentation masks available to us.

Ganster et al. [5] presented a system where as initial step the binary mask of the skin lesion was determined by several basic segmentation algorithms combined together with a fusion strategy [5]. The algorithms used to segment the lesion are: global thresholding, dynamic thresholding, and a 3-D color clustering concept [5]. A set of features was then calculated to describe the malignancy of a lesion: global features (size and shape descriptors), color features and local features [5]. Significant features were then selected from this set by application of statistical feature subset selection methods [5]. The classification experiments were performed with a 24-NN classifier based on the derived features [5]. A notable characteristic of this work is the large dimension of the database. They had at their disposal overall 5363 skin lesion images, categorized into three classes. The three classes are: clearly benign lesions, dysplastic lesions and malignant lesions [5]. The training set for the classifier was a set of 270 lesions (90 images for each class). The test set was the entire database of 5363 lesions in three categories [5]. They obtained a mean recognition rate of 61%. To the best of our knowledge, this is the largest existing database on skin lesions, and these results constitute the state of the art in the field. This is the database on which we ran our experiments, and the results with which we compare our performance.

3   Spin Glass - Markov Random Fields

Consider a visual class Ω_j and a set of k observations $\{x^1 \ldots x^k\}, x \in \Re^m$, that we consider random samples from the underlying, unknown, probability distribution $P(x)$ defined on $\Re^m$. Consider also $\mathcal{K}$ different visual classes $\Omega_j, j = \{1, \ldots \mathcal{K}\}$ (here, $\mathcal{K}$ will be 3, corresponding to the visual labels "benign", "dysplastic" and "malignant"). Given an observation $\hat{x}$, our goal is to classify $\hat{x}$ as a sample from Ω_{j*}, one of the Ω_j visual classes. Using a Maximum A Posteriori (MAP) criterion we have

$$j^* = \underset{j}{\operatorname{argmax}} P(\Omega_\kappa | x) = \underset{j}{\operatorname{argmax}} \{P(x|\Omega_j)P(\Omega_j)\}$$

using Bayes rule, where $P(x|\Omega_j)$ are the Likelihood Functions (LFs) and $P(\Omega_j)$ are the prior probabilities of the classes. Assuming that $P(\Omega_j)$ are constant, the Bayes classifier simplifies to

$$j^* = \underset{j}{\operatorname{argmax}} P(x|\Omega_j) \ . \tag{1}$$

Spin Glass-Markov Random Fields (SG-MRFs) [2] are a new class of MRFs which connect SG-like energy functions (mainly the Hopfield one [1]) with Gibbs distributions via a non linear kernel mapping. The resulting model overcomes many difficulties related to the design of fully connected MRFs, and enables to use the power of kernels in a probabilistic framework. The SG-MRF probability distribution is given by

$$P_{SG-MRF}(x|\Omega_j) = \frac{1}{Z} \exp\left[-E_{SG-MRF}(x|\Omega_j)\right] \ , \tag{2}$$

$$Z = \sum_{\{\boldsymbol{x}\}} \exp\left[-E_{SG-MRF}(\boldsymbol{x}|\Omega_j)\right] , \tag{3}$$

with

$$E_{SG-MRF} = -\sum_{\mu=1}^{p_j} \left[K(\boldsymbol{x}, \tilde{\boldsymbol{x}}^{(\mu)})\right]^2 , \tag{4}$$

where the function $K(\boldsymbol{x}, \tilde{\boldsymbol{x}}^\mu)$ is a Generalized Gaussian kernel [11]:

$$K(\boldsymbol{x}, \boldsymbol{y}) = \exp\{-\rho d_{a,b}(\boldsymbol{x}, \boldsymbol{y})\} , \quad d_{a,b}(\boldsymbol{x}, \boldsymbol{y}) = \sum_i |x_i^a - y_i^a|^b$$

and $\{\tilde{\boldsymbol{x}}^\mu\}_{\mu=1}^{p_j}, j \in [1, \mathcal{K}]$ are a set of vectors selected (according to a chosen ansatz, [2]) from the training data that we call *prototypes*. The number of prototypes per class must be finite, and they must satisfy the condition:

$$K(\tilde{\boldsymbol{x}}^i, \tilde{\boldsymbol{x}}^k) = 0 , \tag{5}$$

for all $i, k = 1, \ldots p_j, i \neq k$ and $j = 0, \ldots \mathcal{K}$ (the interested reader can find a detailed discussion regarding the derivation and properties of SG-MRF in [2]). Thus, the Bayes classifier (1) will become

$$j^* = \operatorname*{argmin}_j E_{SG-MRF}(\boldsymbol{x}|\Omega_j) . \tag{6}$$

4   Support Vector Machines

Support Vector Machines are state-of-the-art large margin classifiers which have gained popularity within visual pattern recognition. Here we provide a brief review of the theory behind this type of algorithm. For a more detailed treatment, we refer to [12].

Suppose we are in the two class case. Consider the feature vector $\boldsymbol{x} \in \Re^N$ and its class label $y \in \{-1, +1\}$. Let $(\boldsymbol{x}_1, y_1), (\boldsymbol{x}_2, y_2), \ldots, (\boldsymbol{x}_m, y_m)$ denote a given set of m training examples. If we assume that the two classes are linearly separable, there exists a linear function

$$f(\boldsymbol{x}) = \boldsymbol{w} \cdot \boldsymbol{x} + b \tag{7}$$

such that for each training example $\boldsymbol{x}_i$, it yields $f(\boldsymbol{x}_i) \geq 0$ for $y_i = +1$ and $f(\boldsymbol{x}_i \mathrm{x}) \leq 0$ for $y_i = -1$. The optimal separating hyperplane is the one which has maximum distance to the closest points in the training set. Mathematically this hyperplane can be found by solving a constrained minimization problem using Lagrange multipliers α_i $(i = 1, \ldots, m)$. It results in a classification function

$$f(\boldsymbol{x}) = \operatorname{sgn}\left(\sum_{i=1}^{i=m} \alpha_i y_i \boldsymbol{w} \cdot \boldsymbol{x} + b\right) , \tag{8}$$

where α_i and b are found by using an SVC learning algorithm [12]. It turns out that a small number of the α_is are different from zero; their corresponding data x_i are called support vectors [12].

SVM can be extended to non-linear problems by using a non-linear operator $\Phi(\cdot)$ to map the input feature vectors x_i from the original $\Re^N$ into a higher dimensional feature space $\mathcal{H}$ by $x \rightarrow \Phi(x) \in \mathcal{H}$. Here the mapped data points of the two classes become linearly separable. Assuming there exists a kernel function K associated with the inner product of the desired nonlinear mapping such that $K(x,y) = \Phi(x) \cdot \Phi(y)$, then a non linear SVM can be obtained by replacing $x \cdot y$ by the kernel $K(x,y)$ in the decision function, obtaining then

$$f(x) = \text{sgn}\left(\sum_{i=1}^{i=m} \alpha_i y_i K(x_i, x) + b\right). \tag{9}$$

This corresponds to constructing an optimal separating hyperplane in the feature space. In this paper we consider four kernel types:

Polynomial kernel ("poly")	$K(x, y) = (\gamma * x \cdot y)^d$
Generalized Gaussian kernel ("gengauss")	$K(x, y) = \exp\{-\gamma * |x^a - y^a|^b\}$
Gaussian kernel ("gauss")	$K(x, y) = \exp\{-\gamma * |x - y|^2\}$
Chi-squared kernel ("chi")	$K(x, y) = \exp\{-\gamma * \chi^2(x, y)\}$.

5   Experiments

In this section we present experiments that show the effectiveness of kernel methods for melanoma recognition. To this purpose, in a preliminary step, we ran a first series of experiments for feature selection. Then we used the selected features for an extensive set of classification experiments. In the rest of the section we describe the database used (section 5.1), the experimental setup (section 5.2) and our experimental findings (section 5.3).

5.1   Database

We performed our experiments on the database created by the Department of Dermatology of the Vienna General Hospital [5]. The whole database consists of 5380 skin lesion images, divided into three classes: 4277 of these lesions are classified as clearly benign lesions (Class 1), 1002 are classified as dysplastic lesions (Class 2) and 101 lesions are classified as malignant melanomas (Class 3).[2] The lesions of the classes 2 and 3 were all surgically excised and the ground truth was generated by means of histological diagnosis [5]. In order to have statistically significant results, we ran experiments with five different partitions, then we calculated the mean and the standard deviation of the obtained recognition rates. This procedure has been adopted for all the experiments reported here.

---

[2] These numbers are not perfectly coincident with those reported in [5], where the database is said to be of 5363 images, but this difference should not affect the comparison between the two algorithms.

5.2   Experimental Setup

The three key components for an automated melanoma recognition algorithm are: segmentation/preprocessing, features extraction and classification. We describe below the general approach followed in this paper for each of these steps:

Segmentation/preprocessing: Following the approach proposed in [5], we didn't implement any preprocessing step such as color normalization or hair removal. As for the segmentation procedure, we used two different methods. The first consists in simply cutting all the images with the help of a common image editor software, selecting for each image the smallest rectangle containing the lesion and keeping out as much skin as possible. We call the resulting images "hand-segmented". The second method is the one developed by Ganster et al. [5]. It consists of a binary mask determined by several segmentation algorithms combined together with a fusion strategy. We call the resulting images "mask--segmented". An example of the images obtained by these two segmentation techniques is in Fig.1. Running experiments on these two types of images allows us to explore how the classification performance is affected by the quality of the segmentation process.

Feature Extraction: In the ABCD rule, the color variegation and the dermoscopic structures in the skin lesion are two of the discriminant characteristics for clinical melanoma recognition, thus we decided to use CH and MFH as features able to retain chromatic and textural information respectively. The color histogram was computed by discretizing the colors within the image and counting the number of pixels for each color. We ran several experiments for selecting the best features, namely using hue, rg, RG, RB and GB color histograms. The resolution of the bin axes was varied for each representation consisting of 8, 16, 32, 64 (for bidimensional histograms we chose the resolution of each axis with the same bin value). We found that the GB representation obtained the best results for all the bin values, thus we used it in all the following experiments.

The main idea of MFH is to calculate multidimensional histograms of the response of a vector of receptive fields. A MFH is determined once we chose the local property measurements (i.e., the receptive field functions), which determine the dimensions of the histogram, and the resolution of each axis. We converted originally RGB images to gray-scale and then we used two different kinds of MFH representation: the first consisted in Gaussian derivatives along x and y directions and with $\sigma = 1.0$ $(D_x D_y)$; the second consisted in Laplacian Gaussian operator with $\sigma_1 = 1.0, 1.5, 3.0$, and $\sigma_2 = 2.0, 3.0, 6.0$ respectively $(Lp2\sigma)$. The bin axes' resolution was varied for each representation consisting of 8, 16, 32, 64 for Gaussian-filter MFH and 16, 32 for Laplacian-filter MFH.

Classification: We used SG-MRF and SVM algorithms (see section 3 and 4 respectively). For SG-MRF we learned the kernel parameters during the training stage using a leave-one-out strategy. For SVM we used the four kernel types described in section 4. The kernel parameters were chosen via cross validation.

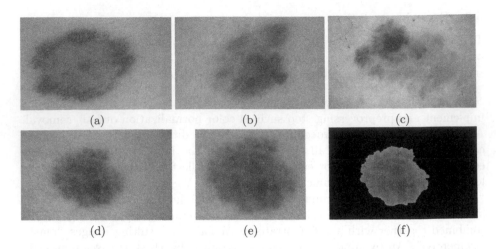

Fig. 1. Examples of skin lesion's images used: (a) image of a benign lesion, (b) image of a dysplastic lesion,(c) image of a malignant lesion. (d) shows an example of an entire image, (e) the same image hand-segmented, (f) the same image mask-segmented.

All the experiments were performed respecting the procedure reported by Ganster et al. [5]. The training set consisted of 270 images (90 for each class); the test set consisted of the whole database [5]. Note that training and test set are not disjoint; once again we underline that this follows the procedure proposed in [5] which allows for benchmarking.

5.3   Experimental Results

A first set of experiments was ran using CH with GB. A second set of experiments was ran with MFH with D_xD_y and $Lp2\sigma$ representations as features. The obtained recognition rates for hand-segmented and mask-segmented images using SG-MRF and SVM, with both features types are reported in Table 1. Results for each class are averaged on five partitions. We also report the average of the recognition rate obtained class by class ("Mean Class"), and the overall recognition rate ("Overall"). For sake of clarity we report the results obtained in [5] too; note that these results were obtained on a single run.

A first comment is that SVM obtains the best result with respect to Ganster's method and SG-MRF, for both feature types and for both segmentation strategies. The best result, in terms of overall recognition rate, is of 82.5%, obtained using the generalized Gaussian kernel, MFH features and mask-segmented images; comparable results are obtained with color features, selected kernels and on hand-segmented images. The best result obtained by using SG-MRF is of 49.5%, obtained using mask-segmented images and MFH features; finally, the best performance obtained by using the Ganster's method is of 58%. These results clearly show the effectiveness of SVMs for melanoma recognition. A second comment is that SVM performance varies considerably depending on the kernel type used. For instance, using color features and hand-segmented images, the overall recognition rate goes from a minimum of 59.0% for the Gaussian kernel to a maximum of 76.0% for chi-squared kernel. A similar behavior is observed by using mask-segmented images, and on textural features. It is also interesting to note that with both segmentation techniques and feature types, for the overall recognition rate, the kernels which obtains the worst performances tend to have the highest standard deviations, while the kernel with the best performance has the smallest one. This illustrates the importance of doing kernel selection in the training phase; the low standard deviation of the SVM's best results also shows the stability of our findings. By comparing the hand-segmented overall best result with the mask-segmented one, we can see an improvement in recognition rate and stability passing from the first to the second, for both feature types. This is an experimental proof of the importance of using a sophisticated segmentation method. A final remark should be made on the poor performance

Table 1. Recognition results obtained by Ganster et al [5], with SG-MRF and SVM methods using different kernels, for hand-segmented and mask-segmented images and using CH and MFH as features. We report the recognition rates for the three classes, the mean and the overall recognition rates. Results obtained with SG-MRF and SVM are mean values from five different runs with their standard deviations. Class 1, Class 2, Class 3 correspond to the benign, dysplastic and malignant lesions respectively.

			Class 1	Class 2	Class 3	Mean Class	Overall
Ganster et al. [5] (%)			59	53	73	61	58
CH features							
hand	SG-MRF (%)		43.2 ± 4.5	41.2 ± 2.1	95.1 ± 1.6	59.8 ± 17.6	46.1 ± 5.6
	SVM (%)	poly	91.7 ± 4.9	9.8 ± 7.3	5.5 ± 0.5	35.7 ± 28.0	74.9 ± 2.8
		gauss	65.7 ± 17.1	31.6 ± 16.0	49.5 ± 26.0	48.9 ± 9.8	59.0 ± 10.3
		gengauss	89.8 ± 20.4	15.6 ± 13.6	82.6 ± 14.6	62.7 ± 23.6	75.9 ± 14.0
		chi	90.0 ± 20.2	15.0 ± 12.3	89.1 ± 0.0	64.7 ± 24.9	$\textbf{76.0} \pm \textbf{13.7}$
mask	SG-MRF (%)		48.6 ± 4.2	38.8 ± 3.4	94.1 ± 3.4	60.5 ± 17.0	47.7 ± 2.9
	SVM (%)	poly	80.1 ± 13.0	15.7 ± 13.7	29.5 ± 20.4	41.8 ± 19.6	67.1 ± 7.8
		gauss	71.9 ± 11.1	24.8 ± 12.7	45.0 ± 28.5	47.2 ± 13.6	62.6 ± 6.2
		gengauss	96.2 ± 4.0	11.0 ± 1.8	89.5 ± 0.9	65.6 ± 27.4	$\textbf{80.2} \pm \textbf{2.8}$
		chi	68.6 ± 17.7	22.4 ± 7.5	62.6 ± 19.7	51.2 ± 14.5	59.9 ± 12.9
MFH features							
hand	SG-MRF (%)		39.2 ± 4.1	42.2 ± 3.1	94.5 ± 2.9	58.6 ± 18.0	40.8 ± 2.8
	SVM (%)	poly	85.3 ± 18.3	9.7 ± 8.5	19.8 ± 22.9	38.3 ± 23.7	66.9 ± 13.1
		gauss	55.7 ± 13.9	31.6 ± 17.1	54.1 ± 19.4	47.1 ± 7.8	51.1 ± 8.6
		gengauss	96.7 ± 2.8	11.7 ± 3.0	89.7 ± 0.9	66.0 ± 27.2	$\textbf{80.7} \pm \textbf{1.7}$
		chi	80.8 ± 2.3	23.1 ± 4.0	93.1 ± 1.4	65.7 ± 21.6	70.3 ± 1.5
mask	SG-MRF (%)		49.3 ± 5.1	45.4 ± 4.0	94.5 ± 1.8	63.1 ± 15.7	49.5 ± 3.9
	SVM (%)	poly	80.5 ± 4.2	28.5 ± 14.9	22.0 ± 19.1	43.7 ± 18.5	69.7 ± 3.8
		gauss	80.9 ± 3.6	27.2 ± 13.5	25.3 ± 23.0	44.5 ± 18.2	69.8 ± 3.7
		gengauss	99.4 ± 0.1	9.6 ± 0.4	89.3 ± 0.4	66.1 ± 28.4	$\textbf{82.5} \pm \textbf{0.1}$
		chi	96.7 ± 0.4	13.0 ± 1.6	90.5 ± 0.5	66.7 ± 26.9	81.0 ± 0.2

Table 2. Confusion matrices for different classification methods. Top left, Ganster's method [5]; top right, clinical diagnosis performed from expert dermatologists of the Department of Dermatology at the Vienna General Hospital [5] . Middle left, SVM results with the "chi" kernel and GB CH feature for hand-segmented images; middle right, SVM results with the "gengauss" kernel and GB CH feature for mask-segmented images. Bottom left, SVM results with the "gengauss" kernel and MFH feature for hand-segmented images; bottom right, SVM results with the "gengauss" kernel and MFH feature for mask-segmented images. The number of images reported are mean value of the number obtained from five different partitions. Class 1, class 2 and class 3 identify the three classes corresponding to benign, dysplastic and malignant lesions respectively.

Ganster et al [5]				Clinicians		
	Assigned				Assigned	
True	class 1	class 2	class 3	True	class 1	class 2	class 3
class 1	2500	1347	410	class 1	4161	94	9
class 2	324	531	155	class 2	42	960	8
class 3	14	12	70	class 3	6	19	78

CH hand				CH mask		
	Assigned				Assigned	
True	class 1	class 2	class 3	True	class 1	class 2	class 3
class 1	3850.6	259.4	167.0	class 1	4112.6	112.6	50.8
class 2	798.2	150.4	53.4	class 2	874.8	110.0	17.2
class 3	9.8	1.2	90.0	class 3	10.4	0.2	90.4

MFH hand				MFH mask		
	Assigned				Assigned	
True	class 1	class 2	class 3	True	class 1	class 2	class 3
class 1	4184.8	45.5	45.8	class 1	4251.8	4.2	20.0
class 2	861.6	116.8	23.6	class 2	901.0	95.8	5.2
class 3	9.8	0.6	90.6	class 3	10.4	0.4	90.2

of SG-MRF. This might be due to the dimension of the training set for each class; it could be possible that the probabilistic method needs a higher statistic in order to estimate properly the energy function.

Table 2 reports the confusion matrices for the best results obtained by each possible combination of (segmentation mask, feature type) and SVMs, plus the confusion matrix obtain by Ganster and that relative to clinicians' performance on the database [5].[3] For both segmentatation techniques and feature types, we see that SVM outperforms Ganster's method for class 1 and class 3 and it is comparable with the dermatologists' performances. It is very interesting to note that, in contrast, SVM performs poorly on class 2, which corresponds to dysplastic lesions. This might be explained considering that here we are using only one feature type for each set of experiments, while Ganster used a selection of

---

[3] For more details on the number of images used in the these last two confusion matrices we refer the reader to [5].

different features and dermatologists used the ABCD rule. It is thus possible that just color/textural information is not discriminant enough in order to recognize correctly dysplastic lesions, while both feature types seem to be effective for separating benign and malignant lesions.

6 Conclusions

In this paper we presented a learning approach to melanoma recognition. To this purpose, we proposed two kernel-based classification algorithms: a probabilistic one, spin glass-Markov random fields, and a discriminative one, support vector machines. Both methods have proved successful on visual recognition problems like object recognition. The two classifiers were tested on a database of more than 5000 images, using two feature types and two segmentation methods. Our results show that SVM obtains an improvement in recognition rate of more than 20% compared to what reported in [5], which to our knowledge constitutes the state of the art in the field. Moreover, on two classes out of three, SVM achieves recognition results comparable to those obtained by skilled clinicians.

This work can be extended in many ways: first, we plan to repeat the experiments presented here on different partitions of the Ganster's database (disjoint training and test set, several partitions, varying number of images in training and test set), so to assess better our method's performance and the database at the same time. Second, we plan to conduct similar experiments using shape descriptors, and finally to experiment with cue integration schemes, in order to test the effectiveness of different types of information and eventually to reproduce the ABCD method followed by the dermatologists in every day clinical practice.

References

1. D. J. Amit: Modeling Brain Function. Cambridge University Press, Cambridge, USA, 1989.
2. B. Caputo: A new kernel method for object recognition: spin glass Markov random fields. PhD thesis, Stockholm, November 2004. Available at http://www.nada.kth.se/~caputo
3. B. Caputo, E. La Torre, S. Bouattour, G.E. Gigante: A New Kernel Method for Microcalcification Detection: Spin Glass- Markov Random Fields. Proc. of MIE02, Budapest, August 2002.
4. E. De Vries, F. I. Bray, J. W. W. Coebergh and D. M. Parkin: Changing Epidemiology of Malignant Cutaneous Melanoma in Europe 1953-1997: Rising Trends in Incidence and Mortality but Recent Stabilizations in Western Europe and Decreases in Scandinavia. Int. J. Cancer 107: 119-126; 2003 Wiley-Liss, Inc..
5. H. Ganster, A. Pinz, R. Rhrer, E. Wildling, M. Binder and H. Kittler: Automated Melanoma Recognition. IEEE Trans on MI, 20, 3, march 2001.
6. C. Grana, G. Pellacani, R. Cucchiara, and S. Seidenari: A New Algorithm for Border Description of Polarized Light Surface Microscopic Images of Pigmented Skin Lesions. IEEE Trans on MI, 22, 8, August 2003.
7. J. P. Grzymala-Busse, J. W. Grzymala-Busse and Z. S. Hippe: Melanoma Prediction Using Data Mining System LERS. Proc COMPSAC 2001, pp 615-620.

8. E. Lefevre, O. Colot , P. Vannoorenberghe, D. de Brucq: Knowledge modeling methods in the framework of Evidence Theory An experimental comparison for melanoma detection. Proc of Int Conf on Systems, Man, and Cybernetics, 4, pp 2806-2811.
9. D. S. Rigel and J. A. Carucci: Malignant Melanoma: Prevention, Early Detection, and Treatment in the 21st Century. CA Cancer J Clin 2000; 50:215-236.
10. B. Schiele, J. L. Crowley: Recognition without correspondence using Multidimensional Receptive Field Hisograms. IJCV, 36(1), 2000, pp 31-52.
11. B. Scholkopf, A. J. Smola: Learning with kernels. 2001, the MIT Press.
12. V. Vapnik: Statistical learning theory. Wiley and Son, 1998.
13. C. Wallraven, B. Caputo, A. Graf: Recognition with Local features: the kernel recipe. Proc. ICCV03.
14. L. Wei, Y Yang, R. M. Nishikawa and Y Jiang: A Study on Several Machine-Learning Methods for Classification od Malignant and Benign Clustered Microcalcifications. IEEE Trans. On MI, 24, 3, march 2005.
15. Informations available at the World Healt Organization website: http://www.who.int

Detection of Connective Tissue Disorders from 3D Aortic MR Images Using Independent Component Analysis

Michael Sass Hansen[1,4], Fei Zhao[1], Honghai Zhang[1], Nicholas E. Walker[2], Andreas Wahle[1], Thomas Scholz[3], and Milan Sonka[1]

[1] Department of Electrical and Computer Engineering, University of Iowa,
Iowa City, IA 52242, USA
[2] Department of Internal Medicine, University of Iowa, Iowa City, IA 52242, USA
[3] Department of Pediatrics, University of Iowa, Iowa City, IA 52242, USA
[4] Department of Informatics and Mathematical Modelling,
Technical University of Denmark, 2800 Lyngby, Denmark

Abstract. A computer-aided diagnosis (CAD) method is reported that allows the objective identification of subjects with connective tissue disorders from 3D aortic MR images using segmentation and independent component analysis (ICA). The first step to extend the model to 4D (3D + time) has also been taken. ICA is an effective tool for connective tissue disease detection in the presence of sparse data using prior knowledge to order the components, and the components can be inspected visually.

3D+time MR image data sets acquired from 31 normal and connective tissue disorder subjects at end-diastole (R-wave peak) and at 45% of the R-R interval were used to evaluate the performance of our method. The automated 3D segmentation result produced accurate aortic surfaces covering the aorta. The CAD method distinguished between normal and connective tissue disorder subjects with a classification accuracy of 93.5 %.

1 Introduction

Aortic aneurysms and dissections are the 15th leading cause of death in the the U.S., representing 0.7 % of all deaths in 2004 [1]. Persons with certain connective tissue disorders, such as Marfan's syndrome and Familial Thoracic Aortic Aneurysm syndrome are at increased risk of developing aortic aneurysm and dissection, which makes an early detection very important .

This study is approaching cardiovascular disease diagnosis using magnetic resonance (MR) imaging. Producing manual outlining of the aorta in 3D images requires expert knowledge and is a tedious and time-consuming task. Detection of connective tissue disorder is based on a crude diameter measure of the ascending aorta from a single 2D MR-slice. Figure 1 shows three 2D slices of a typical 3D cardiac MR images with manually traced aorta contours.

The aortic segmentation of computed tomography (CT) and MR images has already undergone a lot of research. Rueckert [2] used Geometric Deformable Models (GDM) to track the ascending and descending aorta. Behrens [3] obtained a coarse segmentation using a Randomized Hough Transform (RHT).

R.R. Beichel and M. Sonka (Eds.): CVAMIA 2006, LNCS 4241, pp. 13–24, 2006.

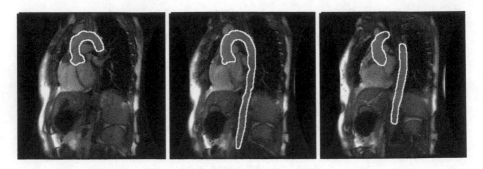

Fig. 1. Three sample 2D slices of a typical aorta candy-cane MR image with manually traced contours outlining aortic lumen

Bruijne [4] introduced Adapting Active Shape Models (ASM) for tubular structure segmentation. Subasic [5] utilized the level-set algorithm for segmentation of abdominal aortic aneurysm (AAA). Though aortic segmentation has been repeatedly attempted in the past, we believe this is the first study investigating its use for connective tissue detection. We report a computer-aided diagnosis (CAD) method for objective identification of subjects with connective tissue disorders from 16-phase 3D+time aortic MR images using independent component analysis (ICA).

2   Methods

Our CAD method consists of three main stages – aortic segmentation, landmarking of the aortic shape and connective tissue disorder diagnosis using ICA. This paper focuses on the ICA-based diagnosis process. The results of the 3D image segmentation were reported previously [6] and are provided here for completeness. The surface segmentation of the aortic lumen is obtained with an automatic 3D segmentation method described in Sect. 2.1. ICA is performed on the aortic 3D shape to provide better descriptors that are visually inspectable, for use in the disease classification step.

2.1   Segmentation

The 3D segmentation algorithm consists of the following three stages:

1. *Aortic surface presegmentation.* A fast marching level set method yields an approximate spatial segmentation of the aorta.
2. *Centerline extraction.* Aortic centerline is obtained by skeletonization.
3. *Accurate aortic surface segmentation.* Accurate aorta surface results from the application of a 2D optimal border detection method.

Aortic Surface Presegmentation. A 3D fast marching segmentation method was used to obtain an approximate aortic surface [7]. Starting with a small

number of interactively identified seed points within the aorta, the initial surface
Γ propagates in an outward direction with the speed F. The fast marching
segmentation algorithm stops the surface in the vicinity of object boundaries
yielding an approximate object surface.

In order to achieve an accurate segmentation, a skeletonization algorithm [8]
is applied to the result of the approximate segmentation to extract the aortic
centerline. As a last segmentation step, a cylindrical surface graph search method
is used to accurately determine the final luminal surface.

Accurate Aortic Surface Segmentation. Optimal surface detection [9] is
an efficient segmentation algorithm applicable to tubular surfaces such as blood
vessel. The method consists of 1) a coordinate transformation, 2) surface detection using dynamic programming, 3) mapping of the segmentation result back
onto the original image. This method has been utilized in the reported work.

2.2   Point Distribution Model

A Point Distribution Model (PDM) was built on which independent components
suitable for discrimination were estimated.

The Point Distribution Model of the aorta population was obtained using the
segmentation results. Building the PDM consists of two stages: 1) Automatic
generation of aortic landmarks on the 3D segmentation result, using a generated
template shape with landmarks and a subsequent landmark mapping. A marching cubes algorithm [10] was used to generate triangular meshes, and vertices of
these triangular meshes were used as landmarks.. 2) Capturing the shape variation by performing independent component analysis on the shape vectors of
the individual aortic instances. After landmarking each resulting shape sample
was represented by a shape vector $x = (x_1, y_1, z_1, ..., x_m, y_m, z_m)$, consisting of
m sets of (x, y, z) coordinates of the landmark points.

2.3   Independent Component Analysis

The ICA approach in this study was based on the assumption that the observed
signal vector x can be described as a vector of n linear mixtures of p independent non-gaussian source signals represented by the random vector s. The signal
vector contains the landmarks of an instance of the aorta. The source signals are
assumed centered and of unit variance. The mixture process, performed by the
unknown mixing matrix $A_{n \times p}$ is governed by

$$x = A \cdot s \tag{1}$$

To calculate the original sources a de-mixing matrix $W_{p \times n}$ is introduced by the
following equation.

$$y = W \cdot x \tag{2}$$

Estimating the de-mixing matrix W is done by maximizing the belief that the
estimated sources Y are independent sources. The different existing methods find

projections that maximize some independence measure of the distributions of the estimated sources. The central limit theorem states that a mixture of signals is more gaussian distributed than the individual parts. The original sources s can be recovered except for a scaling factor, if the number of observed signals n are at least as big as the number of sources p.

Kurtosis. The Kurtosis K of the distribution of a random variable is one measure of Gaussianity. Kurtosis is included it in this paper because it has some simple analytical properties. The Kurtosis is defined by

$$K(x) = \frac{E\{x^4\}}{E\{x^2\}^2} - 3, \tag{3}$$

where x is a random variable. It can be shown that the Kurtosis is 0 for a Gaussian distribution. For practical estimation Kurtosis is far from the optimal measure due to sensitivity to outliers [11]. For theoretical considerations this does not pose a problem, and for two random independent variables x and y it holds that

$$K(x+y) = K(x) + K(y), \tag{4}$$
$$K(cx) = c^4 K(x), \tag{5}$$

where c is an arbitrary constant. Let the row vector w be a projection wx on the input data x, and let the projection vector be bounded by $E\{(wx)^2\} = 1$. As stated earlier x is assumed to be generated by the model $x = As$ (1). Let z be defined by $z = wA$ and observe that $E\{(wx)^2\} = wAE\{s^2\}(wA)^T = \|z\|^2 = 1$, since the sources are independent and assumed of unit variance.

$$K(wx) = K(wAs) = K(zs) = \sum_{i=1}^{p} z_i^4 K(s_i). \tag{6}$$

To find distributions diverging from the Gaussian distribution, the numerical value of the Kurtosis can be maximized under the constraint $\|z\|^2 = 1$. This can be shown to be the canonical base vectors $\pm e_i$, projections on only one independent source. Intuitively, remembering the constraint $\|z\|^2 = 1$, it is also expected that maximizing Kurtosis corresponds to distributing the variance over fewer components, as values smaller than one raised to the power of four are reduced even more.

The Number of Source Signals. Maximizing the absolute value of the Kurtosis can be interpreted as recovering a projection, that is only directed along a single of several independent components. Now examining $w^T x = w^T As$ the normal assumption in ICA is that $A_{n \times p}$ satisfies $n >= p$ because in this way no constraints are imposed on z given by $z = wA$. Assuming that $n < p$ gives that wA is only spanning a subspace of $\mathbb{R}^n$, the space of z. This could mean that some of the minima are not described in this subspace. Denote the subspace of

z's space not spanned by wA by $\hat{V}_{p-n \times p}$. The additional constraints on z are given by (7), where $0_{1 \times p-n}$ is a vector of zeros due to the orthogonality.

$$z\hat{V}^T = 0_{1 \times p-n} \tag{7}$$

The number of constraints under the maximization is bigger than the number of parameters and thus the earlier described minima can not be reached. The Kurtosis measure is still favoring distributing the z_i's on as few components as possible though, and though recovering a true independent component is not to be expected, the maxima will by this measure be more independent than an arbitrary linear mixture of the source signals.

To illustrate the properties of maximizing the Kurtosis, an example of a randomly selected mixing matrix $A_{2 \times 3}$ is chosen. This corresponds to 3 sources but only two observables. The Kurtosis of the three distributions are also randomly chosen (8).

$$A = \begin{bmatrix} 0.6136 & 1.0320 & 0.7604 \\ -0.8242 & -0.4344 & 1.2546 \end{bmatrix} \quad K_1 = 0.118 \quad K_2 = 0.7005 \quad K_3 = 2.133. \tag{8}$$

The projection vector w is rotated from 0 to π and the size is set to match the constraint $E\{(wx)^2\} = 1$, z is still defined by $z = wA$. The result is seen in Fig. 2. The rotation of w giving the maximum Kurtosis is seen to include mainly one of the three independent components, whereas the two eigenvectors, defined by the maximum and the minimum of the dash-dotted curve, are mixtures of comparable fractions of all three independent components. This illustrates the tendency, that the Kurtosis measure under constraints as without constraints is better than the PCA measure at isolating a few independent components.

The Algorithm. For recovering the independent components the *FastICA* algorithm is applied due to its fast convergence and robustness [11]. As mentioned in Sect. 2.3 the Kurtosis is not very well suited in practical implementations with only a limited number of samples. The *FastICA* algorithm is iterative and finds the components sequentially. The weight vector w is randomly initialized which influences the obtained solution due to multiple local maxima. Several w's were initialized in order to be able to select the one giving the source with the most desirable properties, namely the best separation between diseased and normal subjects. The multiple initialization scheme is crucial in finding components well suited for discrimination.

Ordering Measures. Two different ordering measures are introduced in this paper. An ordering measure for extraction of the component that separates the diseased and normals, and an ordering measure that maximizes localization, which is preferable in the interpretation of the extracted components.

The Fisher discriminant. The hypothesis of this study is that connective tissue disorder is one of the sources shaping the aorta. Having no exact knowledge

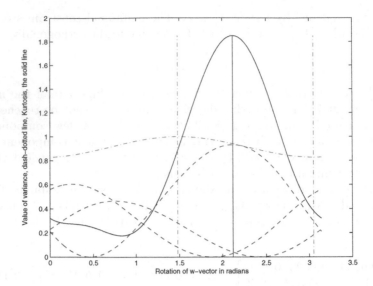

Fig. 2. w-projections in an over-constrained independent component system. The x-axis is the rotation of w in radians. The solid line is the calculated Kurtosis with the maximum illustrated. The dashed lines are representing the fraction of variance contributed from each independent component. The dash-dotted line is the variance of the projection along the w-direction.

of the distribution of such a component, it is modeled to be composed of two normal distributions, one representing the normals and one the diseased offset by the difference between being diseased and having a normal aorta. As an ordering measure the Fisher discriminant, evaluating the projection separation the two populations, is expected to have its maximum at the true source.

The localization of the components. The true sources are believed to be localized in the sense that the effect of being diseased for instance is expected not to influence the entire shape of the aorta, but only a part of it close to the heart. A measure is defined, that focuses on the peaks of the variance, extending a measure defined in [12] to 3D. The variation of the shape by a given projection is mapped onto the normals of the mean surface. Peaks with a peak value of over 50% of the maximum peak value are counted and the average volume of these peaks taken as a measure of how the component has centered its changes to the shape in these large peaks. The principal components represent global variations which can be seen in Fig. 3.

Independent Component Analysis on the Aorta. The data is describing the shape of the aorta and therefore the number of independent source signals is expected to be rather high. The physical shape of the subject, the gender of the subject, the height and the age of the subject just to mention a few, could all be

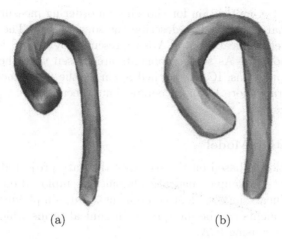

(a)   (b)

Fig. 3. (a) Aortic shape variations captured by the first PCA mode. (b) Shape variations captured by the second PCA mode. Variance from the mean shape is represented by colors from blue to red. Notice the big variance in color over the whole aortic surface.

independent sources shaping the aorta. One of our interest divides the subjects in two groups with or without connective tissue disorder.

The number of dimensions is an important factor because the data is very sparse. The observed data X in this study have $n_{landmarks} \cdot 3 = 248 \cdot 3 = 744$ dimensions when using one phase and 1581 when using two phases of the cardiac cycle. The number of samples is only 31, 21 normals and 10 diseased. For computational convenience and because the data is only distributed along these directions, the data is projected onto the principal components. To reduce the number of free parameters a constraint is introduced, that only a certain number of the parameters are allowed to change at a time, during the estimation of the independent components. 22 principal components were retained explaining 97.5 % of the variance. The subspace was divided in 5 ($\approx \sqrt{22}$) subspaces each containing $\approx 20\%$ of the variance. Each subspace was initially searched for independent components. Subsequently independent combinations of the found projections were found and combined to form the actual independent components. This approach proved necessary to avoid overfitting due to the high number of free paramters compared to the number of samples. In this work this way of constraining different elements is found to give much more robust results than just reducing the search space by only retaining a few principal components. Setting the 16 least-variance principal components to zero, were originally chosen as the constraints on the ICA, which gave a good separation, but a poor ability to generalize.

Due to the reduced number of free dimensions and complex shaping of an aorta there are probably more sources than dimensions of the observed signal. Several locally stable projections are found, depending on the initialization of the algorithm, and it is assumed, based on the discussion in Sect. 2.3, that the different projections favor different source signals. None of them may fully describe a true source signal, but it will be more or less represented in every projection. This is the motivation for choosing an ordering measure that favors the components that is believed to describe the sources well. The aortic shape of each subject after application of ICA is represented by the projection on the independent components. As the components are chosen with the property to divide the two populations, ICA is applied again on the (two) most significant projections to extract more localized components, because we a priori believe the sources are localized.

2.4   Discrimination Model

The disease detection is based on the scores of the data projected on the independent components. A simple quadratic classifier is employed on the scores of the two most significant independent components. This simple form is reinforcing that the components can be interpreted in clinical terms which has been a strong motivation for using ICA.

3   Results

3.1   Segmentation Result

3D candy-cane view and outflow tract MR images were acquired and merged to form a 3D image at the R-wave peak and at the time point of 45% R-R interval from 31 subjects (21 normal, 10 diseased) with image resolution ranging from $1.5 \times 1.5 \times 3.0$ mm^3 to $2.0 \times 2.0 \times 6.0$ mm^3. To assess the accuracy of the automated 3D segmentation, the aortic surfaces were compared with the expert tracing outlines. The positioning errors were defined as the shortest distances between the manually traced surfaces and the computer-determined surfaces in the 3D aortic images.

The developed segmentation method produced aortic surfaces with subvoxel accuracy as judged by the signed surface positioning errors of -0.09±1.21 voxel (-0.15 ± 2.11 mm) and unsigned positioning errors of 0.93±0.76 voxel (1.62 ± 1.25 mm). An example of a typical segmentation result is shown in Fig. 4. The segmentation result is shown in transverse and coronal views. For each view shown in the figure, 4 slices were randomly selected from the 3D image. The volumetric representation of segmentation is shown in Fig. 5.

3.2   Disease Detection Results

To assess the performance of the diagnostic model, two different classification tasks were performed: 1) Disease status prediction using features generated from single-phase MR images. 2) Disease status prediction using features generated from two cardiac phases. Features generated by the ICA were used as input while expert-defined disease status formed the binary prediction output (normal/diseased). A leave-one-out validation method was used to evaluate the predictive classifier performance. Performance was assessed in terms of the sensitivity, the fraction of correctly identified diseased and the specificity, the fraction of correctly classified normals.

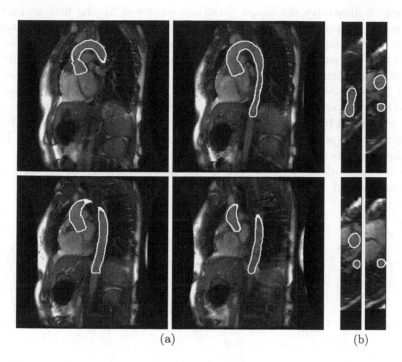

(a) (b)

Fig. 4. Automated segmentation result in 4 randomly selected slices; the segmentation outlines are shown in green. (a) Transverse view. (b) Coronal view.

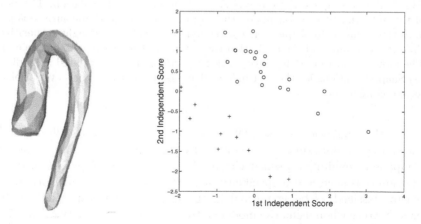

Fig. 5. Volumetric representation of the segmentation result

Fig. 6. Projection of data along the two first independent components. Diseased subjects are marked with '+' and healthy subjects with 'o'. A clear separation is observed.

Figure   7 illustrates the shape variations captured by the first and second independent components applying ICA on the first phase. The analysis suggests that the independent components mainly represents the variation along the aortic arch and the ascending aorta. Together they describe a dilation for diseased subjects which corresponds to the clinical observation that the effect is centered around the ascending aorta. The distribution of the projection of the data on the two first independent components, Fig. 6, illustrates that the separation task can be performed by a simple classifier. Though it always seems possible to find estimates of independent components dividing the two populations, it is not guaranteed to generalize to the unseen sample.

The two first independent components for the second phase of the aortic cycle are more localized, but show similar results.

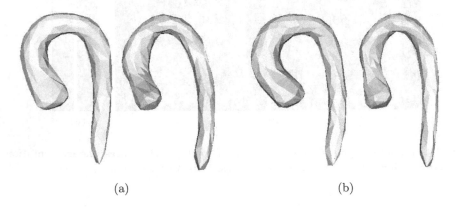

(a)   (b)

Fig. 7. Aortic shape variations observed in the analyzed population. The projection of the independent components on the normal of the mean shape surface is projected onto the mean aorta shape. Left corresponds to negative and right to positive variation. Positive values of the projection correspond to higher likelihood of being healthy. The diseased subjects (left) have a thicker aortic arch and a dilated ascending aorta. (a) Shape variations for the first independent component. (b) Shape variations for the second component.

For the single-phase case, 248 landmarks were automatically generated on each aortic luminal surface. The quadratic classifier working on two independent components exhibited a sensitivity of 80%, meaning that 80% of diseased were diagnosed as such and a specificity of 100%, meaning that all normal subjects where classified as being normal in the leave-one-out test. The classification proved worse when using the model on two phases, a sensitivity of only 70%.The localization ordering measure was designed for only one object and not two phases and this may have affected the outcome, but tests on more subjects are required to see if this difference is significant.

The overall results are summarized in Table 1 and Table 2, showing the confusion matrices of the single-phase model and the two-phase model.

The single-phase model applied to either one of the two phases gives the same confusion table, but one of the errors in classifying the diseased was for different subjects, so a combination of the one phase models might actually give an even better classification. The very encouraging results obtained analyzing a single phase is the motivation for further exploration analyzing 2 phases and later also 16 phases. An issue that may also make the sensitivity worse than the specificity could be that the number of diseased is only 10 compared to 21 normals. Though more laborious, ICA can also be a more specific tool than PCA, when reducing dimensionality as only two components are needed to feature the classification. With a prior knowledge of desired features of the component, more task-specific information can be contained in the independent components than in the variance ordered principal components by applying a suitable ordering measure.

Table 1. Classification results of the single-phase model

	Predicted	
Disease Status	Diseased	Normal
Diseased	8	2
Normal	0	21

Table 2. Classification results of the two-phase model

	Predicted	
Disease Status	Diseased	Normal
Diseased	7	3
Normal	0	21

4 Discussion and Conclusion

In this study, a computer-aided diagnostic method using ICA to identify subjects with connective tissue disorders from 3D aortic MR images was presented. Accurate and reliable aortic surfaces were provided by an automated 3D segmentation algorithm which combines a fast marching level set segmentation with an optimal graph-based border detection.

Independent component analysis in a high-dimensional space with sparse data was applied to landmarked 3D shapes resulting from the aortic segmentation and formed a very efficient approach for capturing the structure's shape variation important to the classification task. A simple quadratic classifier was efficient for the simple classification task in the 2D space spanned by the two first independent components. ICA is well suited for assisting in the disease diagnostic task at hand, as it assists in an easily interpretable classification. It is shown that ICA is a well suited tool for dimensionality reduction, when prior information about the desired features exist for ordering the components. Two examples of ordering measures are introduced.

Using 3D MR image data of a single cardiac phase per subject, the classification accuracy using a basis of two independent components was 93.5%. The independent components showed a more localized behavior than the principal components and could be easier interpreted in terms of shape variation. Earlier results using a support vector machine for classification demonstrated the importance of utilizing functional information about the aortic motion for the connective tissue disease diagnosis using shape modeling, and our continued effort will be put into benifitt from the second available cardiac phase. For improved classification accuracy we will also explore the utility of full 4D information (3D + 16 cardiac phases) in the near future.

References

1. *The Centers for Disease Control and Prevention (CDC)*. http://www.cdc.gov/.
2. D. Rueckert, P. Burger, S. Forbat, R. Mohiaddin, and G. Yang, "Automatic tracking of the aorta in cardiovascular MR images using deformable models," *IEEE Trans. on Medical Imaging* **16(5)**, pp. 581–590, 1997.
3. T. Behrens, K. Rohr, and H. Stiehl, "Robust segmentation of tubular structures in 3D medical images by parametric object detection and tracking," *IEEE Trans. on Systems, Man, and Cybernetics* **33(4)**, pp. 554–561, 2003.
4. M. de Bruijne, B. van Ginneken, M. A. Viergever, and W. J. Niessen, "Adapting active shape models for 3D segmentation of tubular structures in medical images," in *Proceedings of IPMI'03*, pp. 136–147, 2003.
5. M. Subasic, S. Loncaric, and E. Sorantin, "3D image analysis of abdominal aortic aneurysm," in *Proceedings of SPIE'02*, pp. 1681–1689, 2002.
6. F. Zhao, H. Zhang, N. E. Walker, F. Yang, M. E. Olszewski, A. Wahle, T. Scholz, and M. Sonka, "Quantitative analysis of two-phase 3D+time aortic MR images," *SPIE 2006* **Image Processing**, p. not published yet, 2006.
7. R. Malladi and J. A. Sethian, "A real-time algorithm for medical shape recovery," in *Proceedings of ICCV '98*, pp. 304–310, 1998.
8. K. Palagyi, E. Sorantin, E. Balogh, A. Kuba, C. Halmai, B. Erdhelyi, and K. Hausegger, "A sequential 3D thinning algorithm and its medical applications," in *Proceedings of IPMI'01*, pp. 409 – 415, 2001.
9. K. Li, X. Wu, D. Z.Chen, and M. Sonka, "Efficient optimal surface detection: Theory,implementation and experimental validation," *Proceddings of SPIE'04* **5370(48)**, pp. 620–627, 2004.
10. W. E. Lorensen and H. E. Cline, "Marching cubes: A high resolution 3D surface construction algorithm," in *Proceedings of SIGGRAPH '87*, **21(4)**, pp. 163–169, 1987.
11. A. Hyvärinen, "Survey on independent component analysis," *www.cis.hut.fi/ aapo/* **1**, pp. 1–35, 2001.
12. M. Üzümcü, A. F. Frangi, J. H. Reiber, and B. P. Lelieveldt, "Independent component analysis in statistical shape models," *Proceeding of SPIE* **5032**, pp. 375–383, 2003.

Comparing Ensembles of Learners: Detecting Prostate Cancer from High Resolution MRI

Anant Madabhushi[1], Jianbo Shi[2], Michael Feldman[2],
Mark Rosen[2], and John Tomaszewski[2]

[1] Rutgers The State University of New Jersey, Piscataway, NJ 08854
[2] University of Pennsylvania, Philadelphia, PA 19104
anantm@rci.rutgers.edu

Abstract. While learning ensembles have been widely used for various pattern recognition tasks, surprisingly, they have found limited application in problems related to medical image analysis and computer-aided diagnosis (CAD). In this paper we investigate the performance of several state-of-the-art machine-learning methods on a CAD method for detecting prostatic adenocarcinoma from high resolution (4 Tesla) *ex vivo* MRI studies. A total of 14 different feature ensemble methods from 4 different families of ensemble methods were compared: Bayesian learning, Boosting, Bagging, and the k-Nearest Neighbor (kNN) classifier. Quantitative comparison of the methods was done on a total of 33 2D sections obtained from 5 different 3D MRI prostate studies. The tumor ground truth was determined on histologic sections and the regions manually mapped onto the corresponding individual MRI slices. All methods considered were found to be robust to changes in parameter settings and showed significantly less classification variability compared to inter-observer agreement among 5 experts. The kNN classifier was the best in terms of accuracy and ease of training, thus validating the principle of *Occam's Razor*[1]. The success of a simple non-parametric classifier requiring minimal training is significant for medical image analysis applications where large amounts of training data are usually unavailable.

1 Introduction

Learning ensembles (Bagging [2], Boosting [3], and Bayesian averaging [4]) are methods for improving classification accuracy through aggregation of several similar classifiers' predictions and thereby reducing either the bias or variance of the individual classifiers [1]. In Adaptive Boosting (AdaBoost) proposed by Freund and Schapire [3] sequential classifiers are generated for a certain number of trials and at each iteration the weights of the training dataset are changed based on the classifiers that were previously built. The final classifier is formed using a weighted voting scheme. With the Bagging [2] algorithm proposed by Brieman, many samples are generated from the original data set via *bootstrap sampling*

---

[1] One should not increase, beyond what is necessary, the number of entities required to explain anything.

R.R. Beichel and M. Sonka (Eds.): CVAMIA 2006, LNCS 4241, pp. 25–36, 2006.

and then a component learner is trained from each of these samples. The predictions from each of these learners is then combined via *majority voting*. Another popular method of generating ensembles is by combining simple Bayesian classifiers [5]. The class conditional probabilities for different attributes or features can be combined using various different rules (e.g., median, max, min, majority vote, average, product, and weighted average). The drawback of Boosting, Bagging, and Bayesian learners, however, is that they require training using labeled class instances. This is an issue in most medical image analysis applications where training data is usually limited. Consequently there still remains considerable interest in simple fusion methods such as the k-Nearest Neighbor (kNN) classifier for performing general, non-parametric classification [5] which have the advantages of (1) being fast, (2) having the ability to learn from a small set of examples, and (3) can give competitive performance compared to more sophisticated methods requiring training.

While several researchers have compared machine learning methods on real world and synthetic data sets [1,7,8,9,10], these comparison studies have usually not involved medical imaging data [11]. Warfield *et al.* proposed STAPLE [6] to determine a better ground truth estimate for evaluating segmentation algorithms by combining weighted estimates of multiple expert (human or machine learners) segmentations. Other researchers have attempted to combine multiple classifiers with a view to improving classification accuracy. Attempts to compare learning ensembles have often lead to contradictory results, partly due to the fact that the data sets used in these comparisons tend to be application specific. For instance Wei *et al.* [11] found that Support Vector Machines (SVMs) outperformed Boosting in distinguishing between malignant and benign microcalcifications on digitized mammograms. Martin *et al.* [10], however, found that Boosting significantly outperformed SVMs in detecting edges in natural images. Similarly, while Quinlan [1] found that Boosting outperformed Bagging, Bauer and Kohavi [8] found that in several instances the converse was true.

In [4] we presented a computer-aided diagnosis (CAD) method for identifying lesions on high-resolution (4 Tesla (T)) *ex vivo* MRI studies of the prostate. Our methodology comprised of (i) extracting several different 3D texture features at multiple scales and orientations, (ii) estimating posterior conditional Bayesian probabilities of malignancy at every spatial location in the image, and (iii) combining the individual posterior conditional probabilities using a weighted linear combination scheme. In this paper we investigate the performance of 14 different ensembles from 4 families of machine learning methods, Bagging, Boosting, Bayesian learning, and kNN classifiers for this important CAD application. The motivations for this work were (1) to improve the performance of our CAD algorithm, (2) to investigate whether trends and behaviors of different classifiers reported in the literature [1,7,8] hold for medical imaging data sets, and (3) to analyze the weaknesses and strengths of known classifiers to this CAD problem, not only in terms of their accuracy but also in terms of training and testing speed, feature selection methods, and sensitivity to system parameters. These issues are important for (i) getting an understanding of the classification process and (ii) because the trends observed for this CAD application may be applicable to other CAD applications as well.

This paper is organized as follows. Section 2 briefly describes the different classification methods investigated in this paper. In Section 3 we describe the experimental setup, while in Section 4 we present and discuss our main results. Concluding remarks and future directions are presented in Section 5.

2   Description of Feature Ensemble Methods

2.1   Notation

Let $D=\{(\mathbf{x}_i,\omega_i) \mid \omega_i \in \{\omega_T, \omega_{NT}\}, i\in\{1,..,N\}\}$ be a set of objects (in our case image voxels) $\mathbf{x}$ that need to be classified into either the tumor class ω_T or the non-tumor class ω_{NT}. Each object is also associated with a set of K features f_j, for $j \in \{1,..,K\}$. Using Bayes rule [5] a set of posterior conditional probabilities $P(\omega_T|\mathbf{x}, f_j)$, for $j\in\{1,..,K\}$, that object $\mathbf{x}$ belongs to class ω_T are generated. A feature ensemble $\mathbf{f}(\mathbf{x})$ assigns to $\mathbf{x}$ a combined posterior probability of belonging to ω_T, by combining either (i) the individual features $f_1, f_2, ..., f_K$, or (ii) the associated posterior conditional probabilities $P(\omega_T|\mathbf{x}, f_1)$, $P(\omega_T|\mathbf{x}, f_2)$,..., $P(\omega_T|\mathbf{x}, f_K)$ associated with $\mathbf{x}$, or (iii) other feature ensembles.

2.2   Bayesian Learners

Employing Bayes rule [5], the posterior conditional probability $P(\omega_T|\mathbf{x}, f)$ that an object $\mathbf{x}$ belongs to class ω_T given the associated feature f is given as

$$P(\omega_T|\mathbf{x}, f) = \frac{P(\omega_T)p(\mathbf{x}, f|\omega_T)}{P(\omega_T)p(\mathbf{x}, f|\omega_T) + P(\omega_{NT})p(\mathbf{x}, f|\omega_{NT})}, \tag{1}$$

where $p(\mathbf{x}, f|\omega_T)$, $p(\mathbf{x}, f|\omega_{NT})$ are the *a-priori* conditional densities (obtained via training) associated with feature f for the two classes ω_T, ω_{NT} and $P(\omega_T)$, $P(\omega_{NT})$ are the prior probabilities of observing the two classes. Owing to a limited number of training instances and due to the *minority class problem*[2] we assume $P(\omega_T)=P(\omega_{NT})$. Further since the denominator in Equation 1 is only a normalizing factor, the posterior conditional probabilities $P(\omega_T|\mathbf{x}, f_1)$, $P(\omega_T|\mathbf{x}, f_2)$,..., $P(\omega_T|\mathbf{x}, f_K)$ can be directly estimated from the corresponding prior conditional densities $p(\mathbf{x}, f_1|\omega_T)$, $p(\mathbf{x}, f_2|\omega_T)$,..., $p(\mathbf{x}, f_K|\omega_T)$. The individual posterior conditional probabilities $P(\omega_T|\mathbf{x}, f_j)$, for $j \in \{1,2,..,K\}$, can then be combined as an ensemble $(\mathbf{f}(\mathbf{x})=P(\omega_T|\mathbf{x}, f_1, f_2, ..., f_K))$ using the rules described below.

A. Sum Rule or General Ensemble Method (GEM): The ensemble $\mathbf{f}^{GEM}(\mathbf{x})$ is a weighted linear combination of the individual posterior conditional probabilities

$$\mathbf{f}^{GEM}(\mathbf{x}) = \sum_{j=1}^{K} \lambda_j P(\omega_T|\mathbf{x}, f_j), \tag{2}$$

---

[2] An issue where the instances belonging to the target class are a minority in the data set considered.

where λ_j, for $j \in \{1, 2, .., K\}$, corresponds to the individual feature weights. In [4] we estimated λ_j by optimizing a cost function so as to maximize the true positive area and minimize the false positive area detected as cancer by the base classifiers f_j. Bayesian Averaging ($\mathbf{f}^{AVG}$) is a special case of GEM, in which all the feature weights (λ_j) are equal.

B. *Product rule or Naive Bayes:* This assumes independence of the base classifiers and hence sometimes called *Naive Bayes* on account of the unrealistic assumption. For independent classifiers $P(\omega_T | \mathbf{x}, f_j)$, for $1 \leq j \leq K$, the probability of the joint decision rule is given as

$$\mathbf{f}^{PROD}(\mathbf{x}) = \prod_{j=1}^{K} P(\omega_T | \mathbf{x}, f_j). \tag{3}$$

C. *Majority Voting:* If for a majority of the base classifiers, $P(\omega_T | \mathbf{x}, f_j) > \theta$, where θ is a pre-determined threshold, $\mathbf{x}$ is assigned to class ω_T.

D. *Median, Min, Max:* According to these rules the combined likelihood that $\mathbf{x}$ belongs to ω_T are given by the median ($\mathbf{f}^{MEDIAN}(\mathbf{x})$), maximum ($\mathbf{f}^{MAX}(\mathbf{x})$), and minimum ($\mathbf{f}^{MIN}(\mathbf{x})$) of the posterior conditional probabilities $P(\omega_T | \mathbf{x}, f_j)$, for $1 \leq j \leq K$.

2.3 k-Nearest Neighbor

For a set of training samples $S = \{(\mathbf{x}_\alpha, \omega_\alpha) \mid \omega_\alpha \in \{\omega_T, \omega_{NT}\}, \alpha \in \{1, .., A\}\}$ the k-Nearest Neighbor (kNN) [5] decision rule requires selection from the set S of k samples which are nearest to $\mathbf{x}$ in either the feature space or the combined posterior conditional probability space. The final decision for the class label of $\mathbf{x}$ is to choose among the class label that appears most frequently among the k nearest neighbors of $\mathbf{x}$. Instead of making a hard (in our case binary) decision with respect to $\mathbf{x}$, as in the traditional kNN approach [5], we instead assign a soft likelihood that $\mathbf{x}$ belongs to class ω_T. Hence we define the classifier as

$$\mathbf{f}^{NN}(\mathbf{x}) = \frac{1}{k} \sum_{\gamma=1}^{k} e^{\frac{-||\Phi(\mathbf{x}) - \Phi(\mathbf{x}_\gamma)||}{\sigma}}, \tag{4}$$

where $\Phi(\mathbf{x})$ could be the feature vector $[f_1(\mathbf{x}), f_2(\mathbf{x}), ..., f_K(\mathbf{x})]$ or posterior conditional probability vector $[P(\omega_T | \mathbf{x}, f_1), P(\omega_T | \mathbf{x}, f_2), ..., P(\omega_T | \mathbf{x}, f_K)]$ associated with $\mathbf{x}$, $||\cdot||$ is the L_2 norm or Euclidean distance, and σ is a scale parameter that ensures that $0 \leq \mathbf{f}^{NN}(\mathbf{x}) \leq 1$.

2.4 Bagging

The Bagging algorithm (**Bootstrap aggregation**) [2] votes classifiers generated by different bootstrap samples (replicates). For each trial $t \in \{1, 2, .., T\}$, a training set $S^t \subset D$ of size A is sampled with replacement. For each bootstrap training set S^t a classifier $\mathbf{f}^t$ is generated and the final classifier $\mathbf{f}^{BAG}$ is formed by aggregating the T classifiers from these trials. To classify new instance $\mathbf{x}$, a vote for each class (ω_T, ω_{NT}) is recorded by every classifier $\mathbf{f}^t$ and $\mathbf{x}$ is then assigned to the class with most votes. Bagging however improves accuracy only if perturbing the training sets can cause significant changes in the predictor constructed [2]. In this paper Bagging is employed on the following base classifiers.

A. Bayes: For each training set S^t the *a-priori* conditional density $p^t(\mathbf{x}, f_j | \omega_T)$, for $j \in \{1, 2, .., K\}$, is estimated and the corresponding posterior conditional probabilities $P^t(\omega_T | \mathbf{x}, f_j)$ using Bayes rule (Equation 1) calculated. $P^t(\omega_T | \mathbf{x}, f_j)$, for $j \in \{1, 2, .., K\}$, can then be combined to obtain $\mathbf{f}^t(\mathbf{x})$ using any of the fusion rules described in Section 2.2. The *Bagged* Bayes classifier is then obtained as,

$$\mathbf{f}^{BAG,BAYES}(\mathbf{x}) = \frac{1}{T} \sum_{t=1}^{T} (\mathbf{f}^t(\mathbf{x}) > \theta), \qquad (5)$$

where θ is a predetermined threshold, and $\mathbf{f}^{BAG,BAYES}(\mathbf{x})$ is the likelihood that the object belongs to class ω_T. Note that, for class assignment based on $\mathbf{f}^{BAG,BAYES}(\mathbf{x}) > 0.5$ we obtain the original Bagging classifier [2].

B. kNN: The stability of kNN classifiers to variations in training set makes ensemble methods obtained by bootstrapping the data ineffective [2]. In order to generate a diverse set of kNN classifiers with (possibly) uncorrelated errors we sample the feature space $\mathcal{F} = \{f_1, f_2, ..., f_K\}$ to which the kNN method is highly sensitive [12]. For each trial $t = \{1,2,..,T\}$, a bootstrapped feature set $F^t \subset \mathcal{F}$ of size $B \leq K$ is sampled with replacement. For each bootstrap feature set F^t a kNN classifier $\mathbf{f}^{t,NN}$ is generated (Equation 4). The final bagged kNN classifier $\mathbf{f}^{BAG,kNN}$ is formed by aggregating $\mathbf{f}^{t,NN}$, for $1 \leq t \leq T$, using Equation 5.

2.5 Adaptive Boosting

Adaptive Boosting (AdaBoost) [3] has been shown to significantly reduce the learning error of any algorithm that consistently generates classifiers whose performance is a little better than random guessing. Unlike Bagging [2], Boosting maintains a weight for each instance - the higher the weight, the more the instance influences the classifier learned. At each trial the vector of weights is adjusted to reflect the performance of the corresponding classifier. Hence the weight of misclassified instances is increased. The final classifier is obtained as a weighted combination of the individual classifiers votes, the weight of each classifier's vote being determined as a function of its accuracy.

Let $w_{\mathbf{x}_\gamma}^t$ denote the weight of instance $\mathbf{x}_\gamma \in S$, where $S \subset D$, at trial t. Initially for every $\mathbf{x}_\gamma$, we set $w_{\mathbf{x}_\gamma}^1 = \frac{1}{A}$, where A is the number of training instances. At each trial $t \in \{1, 2, .., T\}$, a classifier $\mathbf{f}^t$ is constructed from the given instances under the distribution $w_{\mathbf{x}_\gamma}^t$. The error ϵ^t of this classifier is also measured with respect to the weights, and is the sum of the weights of the instances that it mis-classifies. If $\epsilon^t \geq 0.5$, the trials are terminated. Otherwise, the weight vector for the next trial $(t+1)$ is generated by multiplying the weights of instances that $\mathbf{f}^t$ classifies correctly by the factor $\beta^t = \frac{\epsilon^t}{1-\epsilon^t}$ and then re-normalizing so that $\sum_{\mathbf{x}_\gamma} w_{\mathbf{x}_\gamma}^{t+1} = 1$. The Boosted classifier $\mathbf{f}^{BOOST}$ is obtained as

$$\mathbf{f}^{BOOST}(\mathbf{x}) = \sum_{t=1}^{T} \mathbf{f}^t \log(\frac{1}{\beta^t}) \tag{6}$$

In this paper the performance of Boosting was investigated using the following base learners.

A. Feature Space: At each iteration t, a classifier $\mathbf{f}^t$ is generated by selecting the feature f_j, for $1 \leq j \leq K$, which produces the minimum error with respect to the ground truth over all training instances for class ω_T.

B. Bayes: At each iteration t, classifier $\mathbf{f}^t$ is chosen as the posterior conditional probability $P^t(\omega_T|\mathbf{x}, f_j)$, for $j \in \{1, 2, .., K\}$, for which $P^t(\omega_T|\mathbf{x}, f_j) \leq \theta$ results in the least error with respect to the ground truth, where θ is a predetermined threshold which.

C. kNN: Since kNN classifiers are robust to variations of the training set, we employ Boosting on the bootstrap kNN classifiers $\mathbf{f}^{t,NN}$ generated by varying the feature set as described in Section 2.4. At each iteration t the kNN classifier with the least error with respect to the ground truth is chosen and after T iterations the selected $\mathbf{f}^{t,NN}$ are combined using Equation 6.

3 Experimental Setup

3.1 Data Description and Feature Extraction

Prostate glands obtained via radical prostatectomy were imaged using a 4 T Magnetic Resonance (MR) imager using 2D fast spin echo at the Hospital at the University of Pennsylvania. MR and histologic slices were maintained in the same plane of section. Serial sections of the gland were obtained by cutting with a rotary knife. Each histologic section corresponds roughly to 2 MR slices. The ground truth labels for tumor on the MR sections were manually generated by an expert by visually registering the MR with the histology on a per-slice basis. Our database comprised of a total of 5 prostate studies, with each MR image volume comprising between 50-64 2D image slices. Ground truth for the cancer on MR was only available on 33 2D slices from the 5 3D MR studies. Hence quantitative evaluation was only possible on these 33 2D MR sections.

After correcting for MR specific intensity artifacts [4], a total of 35 3D texture features at different scales and orientations and at every spatial location in the 3D MRI scene were extracted. The 3D texture features included: first-order statistics (intensity, median, standard and average deviation), second order Haralick features (energy, entropy, contrast, homogeneity and correlation), gradient (directional gradient and gradient magnitude), and a total of 18 Gabor features corresponding to 6 different scales and 3 different orientations. Additional details on the feature extraction are available in [4].

3.2 Machine Training and Parameter Selection

Each of the classifiers described in Section 2 are associated with a few model parameters that need to be fine-tuned during training for best performance. For the methods based on Bayesian learning we need to estimate the prior conditional densities $p(\mathbf{x}, f_j \mid \omega_T)$, for $1 \leq j \leq K$, by using labeled training instances. Changes in the number of training instances (A) can significantly affect the prior conditional densities. Other algorithmic parameters include (1) an optimal number of nearest neighbors (k) for the kNN classifier, (2) an optimal number of iterations (T) for the Bagging and Boosting methods, and (3) optimal values for the feature weights for the GEM technique which depends on the number of training samples used (A). These parameters were estimated via a *leave-one-out* cross validation procedure. Except for the Bagging and Boosting methods on the kNN classifiers where each kNN classifier was trained on $\frac{1}{6}^{\text{th}}$ (6) and $\frac{1}{3}^{\text{rd}}$ (12) of the total number of extracted features (35), all other classifiers were trained on the entire feature set. The Bayesian conditional densities were estimated using 5 training samples from the set of 33 2D MR slices for which ground truth was available. In Table 1 are listed the values of the parameters used for training the 14 different ensemble methods. The numbers in the parenthesis in Table 1 indicate the number of ensembles employed for each of the 4 families of learning methods.

Table 1. Values of parameters used for training the different ensemble methods and estimated via the *leave-one-out* cross validation procedure

Method	kNN (2)		Bayes	Bagging (2)		Boosting (3)		
	Features	Bayes	(7)	kNN	Bayes	kNN	Features	Bayes
Parameter	$k=8$	$k=8$	-	$T=50,k=8$	$T=10$	$T=50,k=8$	$T=50$	$T=50$
No. of features	35	35	35	6,12	35	6,12	35	35

3.3 Performance Evaluation

The different ensemble methods were compared in terms of accuracy, execution time, and parameter sensitivity. Varying the threshold θ such that an instance $\mathbf{x}$ will be classified into the target class if $\mathbf{f}(\mathbf{x}) \geq \theta$ leads to a trade-off between sensitivity and specificity. Receiver operating characteristic (ROC) curves (plot of sensitivity versus 100-specificity), were used to compare classification accuracy of the different ensembles using the 33 MR images for which ground truth was available. A larger area under the ROC curve implies higher accuracy of the classification method. The methods were also compared in terms of time required for classification and training. Precision analysis was also performed to assess possible *over-fitting* and parameter sensitivity of the methods compared against the inter-observer agreement of 5 human experts.

4   Results and Discussion

4.1   Accuracy

In Figure 1(a) are superposed the ROC curves for Boosting using (i) all 35 features, (ii) the posterior conditional probabilities associated with the features in (i), and (iii) the kNN classifiers trained on subsets of 6 and 12 features. Boosting all 35 features and the associated Bayesian learners results in significantly higher accuracy compared to Boosting the kNN classifiers. No significant difference was observed between Boosting the features and Boosting the Bayesian learners (Figure 1(b)), appearing to confirm previously reported results [8] that Boosting does not improve Bayesian learners.

Figure 2(a) reveals that Bagging Bayes learners performs better compared to Bagging kNN classifiers trained on reduced feature subsets. Figure 2(b), the ROC plot of 50 kNN classifiers trained on a subset of 6 features, with the corresponding Bagged and Boosted results overlaid, indicates that Bagging and

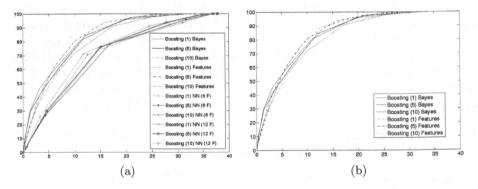

(a)   (b)

Fig. 1. ROC plots of (a) Boosting features, Bayesian learners, and kNN classifiers, (b) Boosting features and Bayesian learners. The first set of numbers (1,5,10) in the parenthesis in the figure legends indicate the number of training samples and the second set of numbers (6,12) shows the number of features used to form the kNN classifiers.

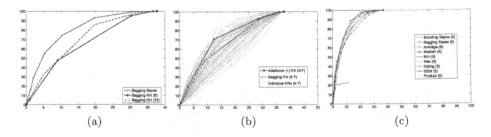

(a)   (b)   (c)

Fig. 2. ROC plots of (a) all Bagging methods, (b) 50 individual kNN classifiers trained using 6 features with the corresponding Bagged and Boosted results overlaid, and (c) different rules for combining the Bayesian learners

Boosting still perform worse than the best base kNN classifier. Figure 2(c) shows the ROC curves for the different rules for combining the Bayesian learners trained using 5 samples. Excluding the product, min, and max rules which make unrealistic assumptions about the base classifiers, all the other methods have comparable performance, with the weighted linear combination (GEM) and Boosting methods performing the best. Further, both methods outperformed Bagging. Figures 2(b), (c) suggest that on average Boosting outperforms Bagging, confirming similar trends observed by other researchers [1]. Figure 3(a) which shows kNN classifiers built using Bayesian learners perform the best, followed by kNN classifiers built using all features, followed by Boosting, and lastly Bagging. In fact Figure 3(b) which shows the ROC curves for the best ensembles from each family of methods (Bagging, Boosting, Bayes, and kNN) reveals that the kNN classifier built using Bayesian learners yields the best overall performance. This is an extremely significant result since it suggests that a simple non-parametric classifier requiring minimal training can outperform more sophisticated parametric methods that require extensive training. This is especially pertinent for CAD applications where large amounts of training data are usually unavailable. Table 2 shows A_z values (area under ROC curve) for the different ensembles.

Table 2. A_z values for different ensembles from the 4 families of learning methods

Method	kNN		Bayes	Bagging			Boosting	
	Features	Bayes	(GEM)	kNN	Bayes	kNN	Features	Bayes
A_z	.943	.957	.937	.887	.925	.899	.939	.936

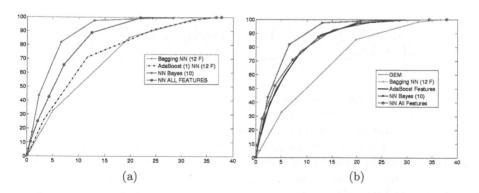

(a)   (b)

Fig. 3. ROC curves for (a) ensembles of kNN classifiers, and (b) the best ensemble methods from each of the 4 families of classifiers: Bagging, Boosting, Bayes, and kNN

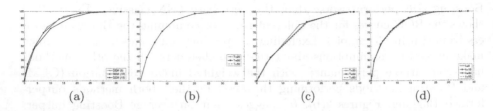

Fig. 4. ROC curves for (a) GEM for 3 sets of training data (5, 10, 15 samples), (b) Boosting on the feature space ($T \in \{20,30,50\}$), (c) Bagging on kNN classifiers ($T \in \{20,30,50\}$, number of features=12), and (d) kNN on feature space ($k \in \{8,10,50,100\}$)

4.2   Parameter Sensitivity

The following parameter values were used for the different ensembles: (a) kNN - $k \in \{8,10,50,100\}$, (b) Bayes - 4 different training sets comprising 1, 5, 10, and 15 images from the set of 33 2D image slices for which ground truth was available, and (c) Boosting/Bagging - $T \in \{20,30,50\}$ trials. The results in Table 3 which list the standard deviation in A_z values for the 4 families of methods for different parameter settings and the plots in Figure 4 suggest that all ensembles considered are robust to changes in parameter settings, and to training. Table 3 and Figure 5 further reveal the high levels of disagreement among five human experts who independently segmented tumor on the MR slices without the aid of the corresponding histology.

Table 3. Columns 2-5 correspond to standard deviation in A_z values for the different ensembles for different parameter settings, while column 6 corresponds to the average standard deviation (%) in manual segmentation sensitivity for 5 human experts

Method	kNN	Bayes	Bagging	Boosting	Experts
Std. Deviation	1.3×10^{-3}	6.1×10^{-3}	2.7×10^{-3}	7.1×10^{-6}	20.55

Figures 5(a) corresponds to slice of a prostate MRI study and 5(b corresponds to ground truth for tumor in (a) slices obtained via histology. Figures 5(c) which represents the overlay of 5 human expert segmentations for tumor on 5(a) clearly demonstrate (i) high levels of disagreement among the experts (only the bright regions correspond to unanimous agreement), and (ii) the difficulty of the problem since all the expert segmentations had significant false negative errors. The bright areas in Figure 5(d) which represents the overlay of the kNN classification on the feature space for $k \in \{10,50,100\}$ (θ=0.5) reveals the precision of the ensemble for changes in parameter settings.

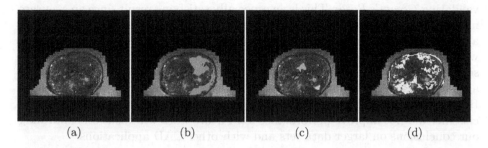

(a)   (b)   (c)   (d)

Fig. 5. Slices from (a) a 4 T MRI study, (b) tumor ground truth on (a) determined from histology, (c) 5 expert segmentations of cancer superposed on (a), (d) result of kNN classifier for $k \in \{10,50,100\}$ (θ=0.5) superposed on (a). Note (i) lower parameter sensitivity of ensemble methods compared to inter-expert variability and (ii) higher accuracy in terms of the crucial false negative errors.

4.3 Execution Times

Table 4 shows average execution times for the ensembles for a 2D image slice from a 3D MRI volume of dimensions $256 \times 256 \times 50$. Feature extraction times are not included. The parameter values used were: k=10, number of features K=35, training samples for Bayesian learners (A=5), and number of iterations for Bagging and Boosting T=30. All computations were performed on a 3.2 GHz Pentium IV Dell desktop computer (2 GB RAM). The kNN methods required no training, while Boosting Bayesian learners required the most amount of time to train. In terms of testing, the Boosting and kNN methods were the fastest while the Bayesian methods were the slowest. Note however that the time required to estimate the Bayesian posterior class conditional probabilities is a function of the dynamic intensity range of the different features employed, which in our case was 0-4095. Note also that columns 3, 6, and 9 do not include the time for computing the posterior class conditional probabilities.

Table 4. Execution times (training and classification) for the different ensemble methods. For brevity only one of the Bayesian methods (GEM) has been shown.

Method	kNN		Bayes	Bagging		Boosting		
	Features	Bayes	(GEM)	kNN	Bayes	kNN	Features	Bayes
Training	-	-	0.86	18.15	25.65	18.15	35.33	77.82
Classification	0.98	1.59	131.21	16.71	34.99	1.59	1.09	0.60

5 Concluding Remarks

In this paper we compared the performance of 14 ensembles from 4 families of machine learning methods: Bagging, Boosting, Bayesian learning, and kNN, for detecting prostate cancer from 4 T *ex vivo* MRI prostate studies. The kNN classifier performed the best, both in terms of accuracy and ease of training, thus validating *Occam's Razor*. This is an especially satisfying result since an accurate non-parametric classifier requiring minimal training is ideally suited to CAD applications where large amounts of data are usually unavailable. All classifiers were found to be robust with respect to training and changes in parameter settings. By comparison the human experts had a low degree of inter-observer agreement. We also confirmed two trends previously reported in the literature, (i) Boosting consistently outperformed Bagging [1] and (ii) Boosting the Bayesian classifier did not improve performance [8]. Future work will focus on confirming our conclusions on larger data sets and with other CAD applications.

References

1. J. R. Quilan Bagging, Boosting, and C4.5 *AAAI/IAAI*, 1996, vol. 1, pp. 725-30.
2. L. Breiman, "Bagging Predictors", *Machine Learning*, vol. 24[2], pp. 123-40, 1996.
3. Y. Freund, R. Schapire, "Experiments with a new Boosting Algorithm", *National Conference on Machine Learning*, 1996, pp. 148-156.
4. A. Madabhushi, M. Feldman, D. Metaxas, J. Tomasezweski, D. Chute, "Automated Detection of Prostatic Adenocarcinoma from High Resolution Ex Vivo MRI", *IEEE Transactions on Medical Imaging*, vol. 24[12], pp. 1611-25, 2005.
5. R. Duda, P. Hart, *Pattern Classification and Scene Analysis*, New York Wiley, 1973.
6. Simon K. Warfield, Kelly H. Zou, William M. Wells "Simultaneous Truth and Performance Level Estimation (STAPLE): An Algorithm for the Validation of Image Segmentation", *IEEE Trans. on Med. Imag.*, 2004, vol. 23[7], pp. 903-21.
7. T. Dietterich, "Ensemble Methods in Machine Learning", *Workshop on Multiple Classifier Systems*, pp. 1-15, 2000.
8. E. Bauer, R. Kohavi, "An empirical comparison of voting classification algorithms: Bagging, Boosting, and Variants", *Machine Learning*, vol. 36, pp. 105-42, 1999.
9. Q-L Tran, K-A Toh, D. Srinivasan, K-L Wong, S Q-C Low, "An empirical comparison of nine pattern classifiers", *IEEE Trans. on Systems, Man, and Cybernetics*, vol. 35[5], pp. 1079-91, 2005.
10. D. Martin, C. Fowlkes, J. Malik "Learning to detect natural image boundaries using local brightness, color, and texture cues", *IEEE Trans. on Pattern Anal. & Machine Intel.*, 2004, vol. 26[5], pp. 530-49.
11. L. Wei, Y. Yuang, R. M. Nishikawa, Y. Jiang, "A study on several machine-learning methods for classification of malignant and benign clustered micro-calcifications", *IEEE Trans. on Medical Imag.*, 2005, vol. 24[3], pp. 371-80.
12. S. Bay "Nearest neighbor classification from multiple feature subsets", *Intelligent Data Analysis*, vol. 3(3), pp. 191-209, 1999.

Accurate Measurement of Cartilage Morphology Using a 3D Laser Scanner

Nhon H. Trinh[1], Jonathan Lester[2], Braden C. Fleming[1,2,3],
Glenn Tung[2,3], and Benjamin B. Kimia[1]

[1] Division of Engineering, Brown University, Providence RI 02912, USA
[2] Department of Orthopaedics, Brown Medical School, Providence RI 02903, USA
[3] Department of Diagnostic Imaging, Brown Medical School, Providence
RI 02903, USA
[4] Rhode Island Hospital, Providence, RI 02903, USA

Abstract. We describe a method to accurately assess articular cartilage morphology using the three-dimensional laser scanning technology. Traditional methods to obtain ground truth for validating the assessment of cartilage morphology from MR images have relied on water displacement, anatomical sections obtained with a high precision band saw, stereophotogrammetry, manual segmentation, and phantoms of known geometry. However, these methods are either limited to overall measurements such as volume and area, require an extensive setup and a highly skilled operator, or are prone to artifacts due to tissue sectioning. Alternatively, 3D laser scanning is an established technology that can provide high resolution range images of cartilage and bone surfaces. We present a method to extract these surfaces from scanned range images, register them spatially, and combine them into a single surface representing the articular cartilage from which volume, area, and thickness can be computed. We validated the laser scanning approach using a knee model which was covered with a synthetic articular cartilage model and compared the computed volume against water displacement measurements. Using this method, the volume of articular cartilage in five sets of cadaver knees was compared to volume estimates obtained from segmentation of MR images.

1 Introduction

Osteoarthritis (OA) is associated with degeneration of cartilage in articulating joints. It is the most common form of arthritis and a leading cause of disability in elderly people [1]. Of significant interest in OA research is the accurate assessment of articular cartilage morphology, which includes overall measurements such as total volume and average thickness and more localized ones such as local thickness and surface curvature, because it is central to monitoring the progression of OA, assessing the effectiveness of treatments, and to the development of computer models for stress-strain analysis of joint motion [2,3].

The challenge in measuring the morphology of articular cartilage arises due to its thinness, the complexity of its shape, and the spatial variability of its

R.R. Beichel and M. Sonka (Eds.): CVAMIA 2006, LNCS 4241, pp. 37–48, 2006.

thickness. The voxel size in the most predominant imaging modality, MR [1], is typically 0.3-1.0 mm while the average thickness of knee articular cartilage is only about 1.3-2.5 mm [2]. Thus, typical and otherwise negligible errors in delineating this thin structure in the presence of low signal to noise ratio, low contrast to noise ratio, MR artifacts, especially those caused by screws in OA patients under treatment [2,4], translate to significant relative errors, *i.e.* a one pixel error could lead to a 25% change in the measured thickness of the cartilage. This level of relative error could prevent the use of these measurements for monitoring OA since changes due to the progression of the disease could potentially be overcome by the relative error. Therefore, it is imperative to measure the true accuracy of assessing cartilage morphology so as to correctly interpret the measurements made from MR imagery.

Traditional techniques for obtaining ground truth to validate the accuracy of articular cartilage measurements have included *(i)* water displacement of surgically removed cartilage tissue, *(ii)* manual segmentation, *(iii)* microscopic examination of high resolution scans of anatomical sections obtained with high precision saws, *(iv)* computed tomography (CT) arthrography, *(v)* stereophotogrammetry, and *(vi)* the use of phantoms with known geometry [2]. Some of these techniques can only measure a restricted set of overall quantities, *e.g.*, water displacement of surgically removed tissue can only measure total cartilage volume. However, recent studies have suggested that total cartilage volume is not an accurate metric of cartilage degeneration in OA and that other factors such as focal volume areas and thickness mapping should also be included in the assessment [5]. In addition to being limited to volume measurements, the water displacement method is highly prone to error and requires a highly skilled technician. Manual segmentation, on the other hand, allows for a variety of morphological measurements, but is limited by the resolution of MR imaging, and is subject-dependent with non-negligible inter-observer and intra-observer variations. CT arthrography suffers the same resolution problem as with MRI images. Stereophotogrammetry uses multiple cameras and a projected pattern to retrieve the 3D geometry of surfaces, such as the cartilage [6,3]. However, in addition to requiring extensive setup to calibrate the cameras, this method also requires that the specimen be attached to an alignment frame, thus limiting the number of viewing angles that images can be taken from, possibly missing the high curvature surface of the femoral cartilage.

We propose to use a 3D laser scanner to interrogate the surface geometry of knee articular cartilage. A 3D laser scanner, such as the one shown in Figure 1 and used in this project, measures depth by shining a laser on the surface of the specimen and using a camera to image the laser dot. The coordinates of the laser dot can be triangulated from its position in the camera's field of view and the known geometry between the camera and the laser emitter. The 3D laser scanning technology is an established technology and has been widely used in many applications, including modeling, industrial inspection, and reverse engi-

---

[1] MR is the most commonly used non-invasive imaging test for quantification of cartilage morphology, mainly due to the superior ability to differentiate soft tissue [4].

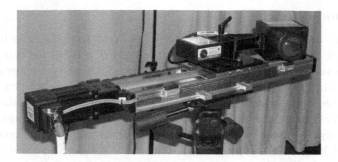

Fig. 1. The ShapeGrabber® PLM300 Laser Scanner System features a linear motion range of 300 *mm* and accuracy of 0.05 *mm*. The scan head, SG-1000, has a depth field of 250-900 *mm* and a depth accuracy of 5.0 *μm* at the farthest point.

neering [7,8]. Its high precision and reliability together with the availability of a wide range of algorithms to work with range images make this technology suitable for determining the morphology of knee cartilage as ground truth for validating segmentations from various imaging modalities.

Our approach is summarized as follows. First, the bone surface is scanned with a laser range scanner both with the articular cartilage in place, and after it has been meticulously removed. The protocol for scanning these surfaces and dissolving the cartilage is discussed in Section 2. Second, the bone surfaces, which are implicit in the laser range images, are explicitly reconstructed and represented as a mesh, Section 3. Third, the top and bottom surfaces of the cartilage are then extracted, aligned, and combined into a complete 3D mesh representing the cartilage. Measurements of cartilage volume, surface area, average thickness, as well as surface curvature, focal thickness, and its spatial variation can be directly computed from this mesh. The accuracy of this methodology has been validated on a synthetic cartilage model. Finally, we use our approach to measure volume of articular cartilage in five sets of cadaver knees and compare to volume estimates obtained from segmentation of MR images.

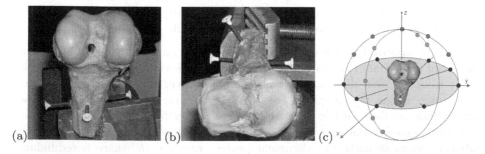

(a)   (b)   (c)

Fig. 2. Photographs of dissected cadaver knee bones. A femur (a) and a tibia (b) are shown with cartilage intact. Each bone is scanned from 20 different viewing directions, each of which is represented as a circular dot on the diagram, (c).

2   Methods

Specimen: 5 intact fresh frozen human cadaver knees from the right limb (mean age: 56 years, range: 51-59, 3 males/2 females) were utilized for this study. By visual inspection there were no indications of ligament injury, meniscal damage, or osteochondral defects. To facilitate the alignment of scans, we placed fiducial markers on the bones which could be easily recognized and did not interfere with the articular cartilage region. Specifically, four dry-wall screws were inserted into the bone body spanning the four disparate views of each bone, Figure 2(a, b). The cadaver knees were imaged using MRI and CT before they were dissected from the surrounding tissue.

Dissolving cartilage off the bone: Knee cartilage was dissolved from the articular surface by immersing the bone in Clorox® bleach 5.25% sodium hypochlorite for 4 to 5 hours. This technique works well for the relatively flat surface of the tibia but requires additional care for the more curved surface of the femur because by the time the cartilage is completely dissolved, a portion of soft tissues on the bone will also be removed. Thus, the femurs were rotated regularly, leaving only the thin articular cartilage layer in the solution. This additional rotation step causes it to take longer to dissolve the femoral cartilage, approximately 8 to 9 hours. With this precaution the technique is reliable and not error-prone, in contrast to the surgical removal of cartilage tissue which requires a highly skilled technician.

3D Laser Range Scanner: We used a ShapeGrabber® PLM series laser scanning system from Vitana Corporation, Ottawa, Ontario, Canada. The scan head, SG-1000, was a high resolution head and had a depth range of 250-900 mm with corresponding field of view 220-750 mm and a depth accuracy of 5 μm at the farthest point. In our experiments, we set the resolution along the scanning direction to 100 μm and place the specimens approximately 50 cm away from the scanner. This setting allowed for taking very high resolution range images, recording about 300,000 points per scan, while keeping the scanning time to a reasonable amount, approximately 2 minutes per scan. Each bone was scanned from 20 views as described below, so that together with the set-up time it took about one hour to scan each bone. Lighting at the scanning site was dimmed to minimize noise due to ambient light. In addition to laser range images, the strength of the returning laser signal provides a "visual" image of the specimen. We use this image to identify hand-marked painted fiducials in the synthetic model.

Scanning protocol: Since each scan of the laser scanner only creates a "point cloud" of the surface portion that is visible under the viewing direction, multiple scans from different directions are necessary to cover the entire bone surface. The range images thus acquired are then aligned and merged to construct the full surface, as described in Section 3. Our strategy for selecting the scanning directions ensures that *(i)* there is sufficient overlap (at least 30%) between adjacent scans to make the alignment process reliable, *(ii)* there is redundant scans of the cartilage portion of the bone surface to minimize chances of having holes on the cartilage when the scans are merged, and *(iii)* the equipment can be set up quickly. Specifically, the viewing directions were rotations around the

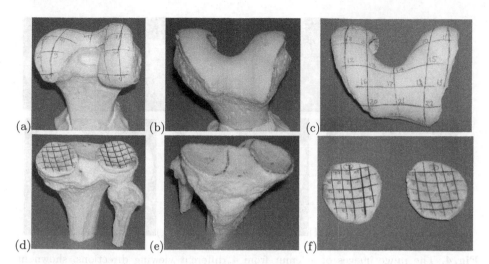

Fig. 3. The synthetic articular cartilage model: (a) Model femur with cartilage, (b) Model femur without cartilage, (c) Femur cartilage, (d) Model tibia with cartilage, (e) Model tibia without cartilage, (f) Tibia cartilage

x, y, and z axis, which are orthogonal to the sagittal, coronal, and transverse planes, respectively, Figure 2(c). Rotations around the z-direction ($-135°$, $-90°$, $-45°$, $0°$, $45°$, $90°$, $135°$, $180°$) covered the bone body, while rotations around the x-direction ($-60°$, $-30°$, $0°$, $30°$, $60°$) and y-direction ($-60°$, $-30°$, $0°$, $30°$, $60°$, $120°$, $150°$) gave redundant coverage of the articular surface. The two scans at $120°$ and $150°$, rotating around the y-direction, are to capture the high curvature portion of the bone surface on the $x - z$ plane. This protocol was used to scan the bones both before and after the dissolution of articular cartilage.

Synthetic knee cartilage: A synthetic cartilage was constructed in our lab using Sculpey® Modelling Compound (Polyform Products Co., Elk Grove Village, IL) covering the surface of a "basic knee model" (Saunders Group, Chaska, MN), simulating the realistic situation as closely as possible, Figure 3. The compound is initially deformable but can become firm and water proof after curing at $130°C$ for 15 minutes per 6 mm. We marked the surface with a grid containing 16 crosses using permanent ink. These fiducials were easily recognizable in the intensity range images and were used to validate the thickness computation.

3   Reconstruction of Cartilage and Bone Surfaces from Range Data

The laser range scan results in an unorganized cloud of points so that the surface on which these points lie on is implicit. Since the point clouds from each view are different, they must be aligned and the aligned points must be connected to form a mesh representing the surface. A rigid transformation is needed to align each pair of range images. We use the Polyworks® IMAlign [9] software to perform

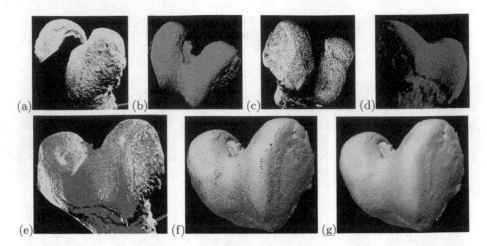

Fig. 4. The range images of a femur from 4 different viewing directions, shown in different colors (a, b, c, d). These point clouds are aligned using the ICP algorithm to bring all the images to one common coordinate system, (e). Next the range images are merged to create a single triangular mesh, which often contains holes, junctions, and disconnected parts, (f). These topological abnormalities are then removed to create a simple manifold surface of the bone, (g).

the alignment. The software requires a user to select a minimum of three pairs of corresponding points between the two scans to determine a rough estimate of the alignment. It then fine-tunes the alignment using a proprietary variant of the Iterative Closest Point (ICP) algorithm [10], which iteratively minimizes the mean distance between the two scans at the overlapping regions. To ensure the ICP algorithm's reliability, we divided each image set into groups of adjacent views and align images in each group separately. The groups are then aligned following the same procedure as aligning the original scanned images. Although this procedure theoretically brings all the range images into one common coordinate system, accumulative error due to the incremental alignment can be significant because the number of images in each set is large. Thus, as a final step the ICP algorithm is applied on all the range images simultaneously to get the optimal global alignment.

Next we use Polyworks® IMMerge to merge the aligned range images into one single triangular mesh representing the surface, Figure 4. The IMMerge software determines and discard the outlier points in the range images and creates a triangular mesh that minimizes the mean distance to the remaining points. To save processing time, we roughly outline the points close to our area of interest, the articular cartilage, and set the program to only merge those points.

Holes, cracks, and imperfections in the topology are common problems in surface construction from range images, particularly for rough surfaces like bones covered with soft tissues, Figure 4(f). Many methods have been proposed to solve such problems [11,12,13]. We used the PolyMender algorithm, which is fast and robust, has efficient memory usage, and is guaranteed to produce a closed surface

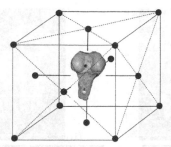

Fig. 5. To eliminate the internal membranes, the object is viewed under 14 different directions, each represented by a blue dot. Any part of the object not visible under any of these views is discarded.

that partitions the space into disjoint internal and external volumes [13,14]. However, the algorithm has several known drawbacks.

First, because of its simplistic approach, the patches used to fill in the holes are not always optimal with respect to the surrounding mesh. Our reconstructed surface does not suffer from this drawback because the cartilage area is smooth and well covered with multiple scans, and thus does not contain big holes.

Second, the reconstructed surface may still contain topological redundancies in the form of cavities, disconnected components, and internal membranes. Since our goal is to reconstruct a simple manifold surface, we need to address these issues in details. The problem of cavities and disconnected components can be solved by discarding all but the largest connected component. To remove the internal membranes, which are completely covered by the outer shell, we put the mesh under multiple viewing directions chosen to maximize the coverage of the surface, Figure 5, and discard triangles that are not visible under any of those views. Originated from range images, any valid triangle on the surface is theoretically visible from some viewing direction and thus not affected by this process. However, because the number of chosen viewing directions is finite, the process occasionally creates small holes on the surface. A second application of Polymender typically fixes all the resulting small holes, Figure 4(g).

4   Constructing the Cartilage Volume from the Cartilage and Bone Surface Meshes

The two surfaces of each knee bone, *i.e.*, with and without cartilage, are aligned using the ICP algorithm, taking only the bone body as input data, as the two surfaces differ at the cartilage area. Ideally, the two surfaces should overlap at all points except for the cartilage area. However, because portions of the surfaces are reconstructed by PolyMender, which does not always generate optimal patches, the two surfaces may differ at these common areas. This means that a simple "volumetric difference" between the two meshes would *not* yield the shape of the cartilage. Instead, we rely on an interactive specification of the cartilage

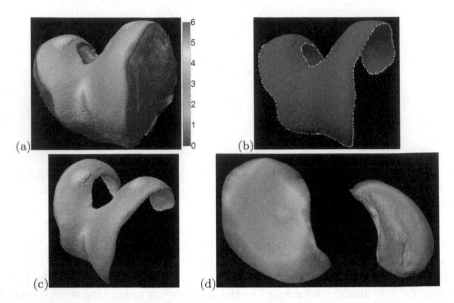

Fig. 6. (a) Articular surface is delineated from the color-coded bone surface by having an expert user manually outline the region. The thickness unit on the color bar is mm. (b) shows the segmentation result for the "outer" surface. (c) and (d) show the reconstructed cartilage surfaces color-coded with thickness measurements for the femoral (c) and tibial (d) cartilage.

boundary by an expert user who is familiar with the anatomy of human knees. Specifically, with the bone's "outer" surface color-coded according to the distance between the two reconstructed surfaces, the user marks the boundary of the articular cartilage as a dense collection of points, which are then interpolated using NURBS curves to get a continuous closed boundary, Figure 6(a). The interpolated curve is projected orthogonally onto both meshes to segment out the top and bottom surface patches that enclose the cartilage of the bone. A band-like mesh is then created to connect the two surface patches and combine all three into a complete closed triangular mesh of the cartilage. Since the knee cartilage is anatomically thickest in the center area and gets thinner as it gets close to the edge, a small error in estimating the boundary of the cartilage would not significantly affect the overall estimate of the shape and volume of the articular cartilage.

5   Morphological Quantifications of the Knee Cartilage

Morphological quantifications of the cartilage triangular mesh can be used as ground truth for validating measurements based on segmentations of MRI images of the knees. First, the volume of this polyhedron mesh can be accurately computed [15]. Let the mesh have vertices $P = \{v_1, v_2, \cdots, v_n\}$, where $v_i = (x_i, y_i, z_i)$ and triangular faces $F = \{f_1, f_2, \cdots, f_m\}$, where $f_i = (v_1^i, v_2^i, v_3^i)$ and assume all the triangular faces are consistently oriented, the volume of the polyhedron mesh is computed as:

$$V = \frac{1}{6} \sum_{f_i \in F} \begin{vmatrix} x_1^i & x_2^i & x_3^i \\ y_1^i & y_2^i & y_3^i \\ z_1^i & z_2^i & z_3^i \end{vmatrix} \qquad \text{where} \qquad \begin{cases} v_1^i = (x_1^i, y_1^i, z_1^i) \\ v_2^i = (x_2^i, y_2^i, z_2^i) \\ v_3^i = (x_3^i, y_3^i, z_3^i) \end{cases}$$

Second, the thickness of the cartilage is the distance between the two reconstructed (top and bottom) surface patches of the cartilage. This distance can be defined *(i)* by using one surface as the reference surface and computing the distance of the closest point or *(ii)* as the distance along the normal at each point of the reference surface or *(iii)* by using the distance in the distance transform of the reference surface [6,16,18]. In this paper we adopt the first approach and use the algorithm in [17]. The triangles of the reference surface are divided spatially into cubical cells to limit the search space in computing the distance between a point and the reference surface. The search is limited to only triangles that belong to the cells in a small neighborhood of the point. This algorithm has been proven in practice to be faster than the brute-force method and allows for computing distances between two very large triangular meshes.

6   Results and Discussion

We treated the synthetic knee and cartilage models as if they were from a real cadaver. The models were scanned, the scans were aligned and merged, a cartilage triangular mesh was constructed, and its volume and thickness were computed. To validate our volume assessment, we measured the volumes of the synthetic cartilage using water displacement method and compare against the computed measurements, Table 1. The average discrepancy between the two measurements is 5.2%. It is not clear to us which method is superior but the volume measurements from the laser scanning method are well within the variability of the water displacement method.

Table 2 compares the volume measurements of the cadaver knees' articular cartilage using the laser scanning method and using manual segmentation of MR images. In the manual segmentation method, volume was computed by simply counting the segmented cartilage voxels, and thus may not be accurate. Nevertheless, the two measurements are of the same order, which signifies the applicability of the laser scanning method on cadavers.

Table 1. Comparison of volume measurements of articular cartilage using 3D laser scanner (LS) and by water displacement (WD). The WD values are the measurements of three trials.

Cartilage type	LS Volume (ml)	WD Volume (ml)	Error (%)
Femoral cartilage	11.8	12.3±0.9	4.0
Tibial cartilage	5.0	4.7±0.2	6.4

Table 2. Comparison of volume measurements of femoral (F) and tibial (T) cartilage using 3D laser scanner and manual segmentation from 3T MR images

Cadaver	971		972		973		974		975	
	F	T	F	T	F	T	F	T	F	T
Volume - Laser scanner(ml)	14.5	4.9	10.7	5.8	9.4	4.6	2.9	1.9	8.8	3.1
Volume - Manual Seg. (ml)	13.1	5.6	9.3	4.2	10.7	4.8	2.2	1.6	7.2	3.2
Err(%)	9.7	14.3	13.1	29.3	13.8	4.3	24.1	15.8	19.3	3.2

As for validating thickness assessment, we measured the thickness of the cartilage model at fiducial points using a caliper and compared against thickness measurements from the laser scanning method, Table 3 and Figure 7. We note that at most points the caliper thickness measurements are slightly larger than those computed from the laser range scans. This is expected because measuring thickness using a caliper requires manually finding the points on the bottom surface of the synthetic cartilage that are closest to the fiducial points. This process is generally difficult, especially when the surface is curvy, and any errors incurred will *only* increase the caliper measurement values. Nevertheless, the average discrepancies between the two measurements for the femoral and tibial cartilage were 4.5% and 3.6 %, respectively. Given the accuracy and reliability of the laser scanner (50 μm) is superior to that of the MR imaging and assuming similar errors in segmentation, computed thickness from laser range scans are expected to provide ground truth data for MR thickness measurements.

In a recent approach [19] a 3D laser scanner is similarly used to scan the femur of three porcine knees, both with the cartilage intact and after it had been dissolved. The result data were then used to validate the B-Spline Snake method used to segment knee cartilage from MR images. This approach and ours are similar in utilizing the 3D laser scanner but differ in the following aspects. First, our method determines a complete 3D mesh of the cartilage instead of just the thickness map. Second, in our approach it is not required to attach the specimen to a frame; this allows for more freedom in choosing the scanning angles and reduces one source of error caused by the physical attachment between the bone and the frame. In addition, we provide validation of our method on a synthetic cartilage model.

We have presented a method to accurately assess articular cartilage morphology using the 3D laser scanning technology. To use these measurements as ground truth for segmentations from MR images, we note that care needs to be taken to preserve the morphological properties of the cartilage between the time of MR scans and the time of laser scans and during laser scans, e.g., regularly bathing the bones with physiological saline solution when they are exposed to the air to prevent the cartilage from drying out. We plan to validate our method for reproducibility (inter-observer and intra-observer) as well as for accuracy with more reliable methods to quantify volume and thickness, e.g., coordinate measuring machine. Segmenting the articular surface is currently done manually, but can be automated by using a marker to outline the cartilage on the bone before it is scanned. This will potentially reduce the human errors in determining the

Table 3. Comparison of thickness measurements of femoral (top, Fn) and tibial (bottom, Tn) cartilage using 3D laser scanner (L) and by caliper (C)

Points	F1	F2	F3	F4	F5	F6	F7	F8	F9	F10	F11	F12	F13	F14	F15	F16
L(mm)	1.51	2.08	3.34	3.81	5.18	3.65	4.24	3.95	5.24	4.22	4.24	1.73	4.64	2.35	3.22	1.79
C(mm)	1.50	2.21	3.70	3.80	5.41	3.76	4.67	4.20	5.70	4.58	4.59	1.72	4.65	2.47	3.07	1.79
Err(%)	0.24	5.92	9.65	0.21	4.32	2.99	9.25	5.98	7.98	7.73	7.75	0.64	0.24	4.90	4.64	0.30
Points	T1	T2	T3	T4	T5	T6	T7	T8	T9	T10	T11	T12	T13	T14	T15	T16
L(mm)	2.39	3.52	4.04	4.66	3.38	4.34	3.89	2.55	4.32	3.87	2.94	3.28	3.08	3.06	2.70	3.24
C(mm)	2.44	3.34	4.09	4.67	3.73	4.19	4.19	2.74	4.53	3.93	3.12	3.36	3.23	3.05	2.72	3.29
Err(%)	2.11	5.50	1.12	0.33	9.52	3.61	7.20	6.80	4.79	1.54	5.86	2.23	4.67	0.33	0.84	1.64

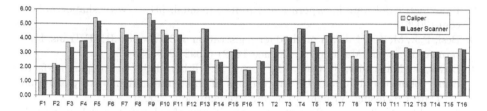

Fig. 7. Comparison of thickness measurements of femoral (Fn) and tibial (Tn) cartilage using 3D laser scanner and by caliper

outline of the cartilage surface. As for surface reconstruction, since the surface patches produced by Polymender are not optimal, we plan to try other alternative methods, e.g., [11]. We expect that the 3D laser technology will become a standard in establishing ground truth data for the comparison of the morphological properties of the cartilage to those obtained from other noninvasive imaging modalities such as MR.

Acknowledgements. This study was supported by the NIH grant AR047910S1 and the NSF grant IIS-0413215. We would like to thank Professor Richard Fishman for his help in constructing the synthetic knee cartilage. We would also like to thank Tao Ju and Nicolas Aspert for sharing their programs on the web.

References

1. Reginster, J.Y.: The prevalence and burden of arthritis. Rheumatology **41**(suppl. 1) (2002) 3–6
2. Eckstein, F., Glaser, C.: Measuring cartilage morphology with quantitative magnetic resonance imaging. Seminars in Musculoskeletal Radiology **8**(4) (2004) 329–53
3. Ateshian, G.A., Soslowsky, L.J., , Mow, V.C.: Quantitation of articular surface topography and cartilage thickness in knee joints using stereophotogrammetry. Journal of Biomechanics **24**(8) (1991) 761–776
4. Berquist, T.H.: Imaging of articular pathology: MRI, CT, arthrography. Clinical Anatomy **10**(1) (1997) 1–13

5. Gandy, S.J., Dieppe, P.A., Keen, M.C., Maciewicz, R.A., Watt, I., Waterton, J.C.: No loss of cartilage volume over three years in patients with knee osteoarthritis as assessed by magnetic resonance imaging. Osteoarthritis and Cartilage **10**(12) (2002) 929–937

6. Cohen, Z.A., McCarthy, D.M., Kwak, S.D., Legrand, P., F., F., Ciaccio, E.J., Ateshian, G.A.: Knee cartilage topography, thickness, and contact areas from mri: in-vitro calibration and in-vivo measurements. Osteoarthritis and Cartilage **7**(1) (1999) 95–109

7. Son, S., Park, H., Lee, K.H.: Automated laser scanning system for reverse engineering and inspection. International Journal of Machine Tools and Manufacture **42**(8) (2002) 889–897

8. Milroy, M.J., Weir, D.J., Bradley, C., Vickers, G.W.: Reverse engineering employing a 3d laser scanner: A case study. The International Journal of Advanced Manufacturing Technology **12**(2) (1996) 111 – 121

9. Innovmetric Software Incorporation: Product manual. http://www.shapegrabber. com (2006)

10. Besl, P.J., McKay, N.D.: A method for registration of 3D shapes. IEEE Trans. Pattern Analysis and Machine Intelligence **14**(2) (1992) 239–256

11. Davis, J., Marschner, S., Garr, M., Levoy, M.: Filling holes in complex surfaces using volumetric diffusion. In: Proceedings of First International Symposium on 3D Data Processing, Visualization, and Transmission. (2002)

12. Nooruddin, F., Turk, G.: Simplification and repair of polygonal models using volumetric techniques. IEEE Transactions on Visualization and Computer Graphics **9**(2) (2003) 191–205

13. Ju, T.: Robust repair of polygonal models. ACM Trans. Graph. **23**(3) (2004) 888–895

14. Ju, T.: Polymender. http://www.cs.rice.edu/ jutao/code/polymender.htm (2006)

15. Gelder, A.V.: Efficient Computation of Polygon Area and Polyhedron Volume. In: Graphics Gems V. AP Professional (1995)

16. Hardy, P.A., Nammalwar, P., Kuo, S.: Measuring the thickness of articular cartilage from mr images. Journal of Magnetic Resonance Imaging **13**(1) (2001) 120–6

17. Aspert, N., Santa-Cruz, D., Ebrahimi, T.: Mesh: Measuring errors between surfaces using the hausdorff distance. In: Proc. of the IEEE International Conference in Multimedia and Expo (ICME). (2002) 705–708

18. Stammberger, T., Eckstein, F., Englmeier, K.H., Reiser, M.: Determination of 3d cartilage thickness data from MR imaging: computational method and reproducibility in the living. Magnetic Resonance in Medicine **41**(3) (1999) 529–36

19. Koo, S., Gold, G.E., Andriacchi, T.P.: Considerations in measuring cartilage thickness using MRI: factors influencing reproducibility and accuracy. Osteoarthritis and Cartilage **13**(9) (2005) 782–9

Quantification of Growth and Motion Using Non-rigid Registration

D. Rueckert, R. Chandrashekara, P. Aljabar, K.K. Bhatia[1], J.P. Boardman[2],
L. Srinivasan[2], M.A. Rutherford[2], L.E. Dyet[2], A.D. Edwards[2],
J.V. Hajnal[2], and R. Mohiaddin[3]

[1] Department of Computing, Imperial College London, UK
[2] Imaging Sciences Department, Hammersmith Hospital,
Imperial College London, UK
[3] Cardiovascular MR Unit, Royal Brompton Hospital,
Imperial College London, UK

Abstract. Three-dimensional (3D) and four-dimensional (4D) imaging
of dynamic structures is a rapidly developing area of research in medical
imaging. Non-rigid registration plays an important role for the analysis
of these datasets. In this paper we will show some of the work of our
group using non-rigid registration techniques for the detection of temporal changes such as growth in brain MR images. We will also show how
non-rigid registration can be used to analyze the motion of the heart
from cardiac MR images.

1   Introduction

The analysis of medical images plays an increasingly important role in many clinical applications. Image registration is a key component in many image analysis
applications. The goal of image registration is to find corresponding anatomical locations in two images. Image registration concerns images from the same
subject acquired by different imaging modalities or at different time points as
well as images acquired from different subjects. To bring images into registration
it is usually necessary to estimate a geometric transformation which aligns the
images. This is typically achieved by minimization of a cost function which measures the degree of (mis-) alignment of the images as a function of the geometric
transformation. Most registration algorithms use a cost function based on image
intensity information to directly to measure the degree of (mis-)alignment of the
images. These methods are called voxel-based registration techniques and are
especially successful since they do not require any feature extraction or segmentation of the images. Comprehensive reviews of image registration techniques
can be found in [26, 21, 47].

A key application of image registration is the alignment of images from the
same subject acquired at different time points. The difference between successive
time points can range from fractions of a second (e.g. in cardiac motion studies)
to several years (e.g. in longitudinal growth or atrophy studies). The comparison
of images across time points enables the quantification of the anatomical differences between time points. These differences can have a number of reasons. The

R.R. Beichel and M. Sonka (Eds.): CVAMIA 2006, LNCS 4241, pp. 49–60, 2006.
© Springer-Verlag Berlin Heidelberg 2006

difference can be caused by patient or organ motion, by growth or atrophy, or by disease progression. In this paper we will concentrate on the application of registration techniques for the quantification of brain growth as well as for the quantification of cardiac motion.

2   Analysis of Brain Growth Using Non-rigid Registration

Image registration has been widely used for the quantification of changes in the human brain using rigid [23, 22] and non-rigid serial registration [19, 36]. For example, growth patterns have been mapped in 4-D (3-D plus time) in older children [33, 40], and clinically useful information has been extracted in conditions such as Alzheimer's Disease [41, 18], and imaginative studies of neurogenetics and development have been undertaken [42]. In many of these studies changes over time are particularly important to answer the scientific questions.

The work in our own group has focused on the analysis of brain growth during the first two years of life in children born prematurely. The first two years constitute a period of significant growth in the developing brain. Preterm birth can have substantial effects in that preterm infants can show neuropsychiatric problems later in childhood [27, 44, 7]. This motivates the need for characterizing structural brain development in the early years.

2.1   Deformation-Based Morphometry

In longitudinal studies images are acquired from the same subject at different time points. To compare the brain structure of the same subject at different times, the registration transformation between the baseline image and the follow-up images of a subject must be computed. The first step of the registration is to compute a global transformation which compensates for pose differences between the images. Since we are interested in estimating local changes in brain volume caused by growth we only want to correct for rigid pose differences. For the rigid registration we are using a registration algorithm which maximizes the normalized mutual information (NMI) [39] between the baseline image and a follow-up image.

The second step of the registration is to compute a non-rigid transformation which compensates for local deformations as the result of growth. We have previously developed a spline-based deformation model [37]. Using this approach, the deformation can be represented as a free-form deformation (FFD) based on B-splines which is a powerful tool for modeling 3D deformations and can be written as the 3D tensor product of the familiar 1D cubic B-splines,

$$\mathbf{u}(\mathbf{x}) = \sum_{l=0}^{3}\sum_{m=0}^{3}\sum_{n=0}^{3} B_l(u)B_m(v)B_n(w)\mathbf{c}_{i+l,j+m,k+n} \tag{1}$$

where $\mathbf{c}$ denotes the control points which parameterize the transformation. The optimal transformation is found by minimizing a cost function associated with the global transformation parameters as well as the local transformation parameters. The cost function comprises two competing goals: The first term represents the cost associated with the voxel-based similarity measure, in this case normalized mutual information [39], while the second term corresponds to a regularization term which constrains the transformation to be smooth [37]. The performance of this registration method is limited by the resolution of the control point mesh, which is linearly related to the computational complexity: more global and intrinsically smooth deformations can only be modeled using a coarse control point spacing, whereas more localized and intrinsically less smooth deformations require a finer spacing. An example of such a registration can be seen in Figure 1.

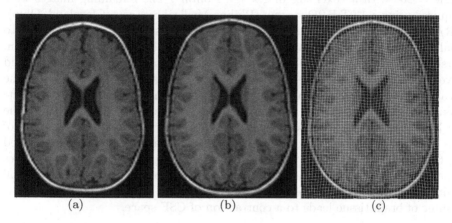

(a)   (b)   (c)

Fig. 1. A brain MRI of a child at the age of (a) one year and (b) two years. (c) shows the non-rigid deformation required to explain the growth between the two time points.

When two images are related to each other by a nonrigid transformation, the target image is subjected to local deformation, which locally changes the volume of regions in the coordinate space. The local volume change in an infinitesimally small neighborhood around any given point is represented by the local Jacobian determinant of the coordinate transformation at that point:

$$|J(x,y,z)| = \det \begin{pmatrix} \frac{\partial u_x}{\partial x} & \frac{\partial u_x}{\partial y} & \frac{\partial u_x}{\partial z} \\ \frac{\partial u_y}{\partial x} & \frac{\partial u_y}{\partial y} & \frac{\partial u_y}{\partial z} \\ \frac{\partial u_z}{\partial x} & \frac{\partial u_z}{\partial y} & \frac{\partial u_z}{\partial z} \end{pmatrix} \tag{2}$$

If there is no local volume change, the Jacobian determinant is 1. If there is a local volume decrease, it is smaller than 1, and larger than 1 if there is a local volume increase. Thus, local volume change (e.g. growth or atrophy) can be directly estimated from the deformation field which aligns the baseline and follow-up images [19].

In crosssectional studies a similar approach can be used to compare the brain structure of subjects within a population with those of a reference subject. In this case the registration transformation between the reference subject and all other subjects in the population must be computed. Again, a similar approach based on global registration, followed by local registration is often used for this purpose. By combining longitudinal and crosssectional registration the images of all subjects can be mapped into a common coordinate system and we can perform any morphometric analysis in this standardized coordinate system [38].

2.2   Deformation-Based Morphometry Applied to Brain Growth

The data used for this study consists of T1 weighted MR volumes of 22 preterm born children who were all scanned at one and two years. Seven subjects' images were acquired using a Marconi 0.5 T Apollo scanner, TR/TE = 23ms/6ms, flip angle = 30° with a voxel size of $1 \times 1 \times 1.6mm^3$. The remaining images were acquired using a 1.0T HPQ system (Philips Medical Systems, Cleveland, Ohio), TR/TE = 23ms/6ms, flip angle = 35° with a voxel size of $1 \times 1 \times 1.6mm^3$. To analyze these datasets we combine longitudinal and crosssectional registration. First, we compute for each subject the registration transformation between 1 and 2 years. In the next step we compute growth as local volume change, e.g. the local Jacobian determinant of the non-rigid transformation. In the final step the volume change maps are then mapped into average anatomical space of all the subjects at the age of 2 years using an approach described in [1]. An overview of this is shown in Figure 2 and an example of an average growth map calculated by this method is shown in Figure 3. In this example the red color indicates expansion and blue color shows contraction. It can be clearly seen that frontal white matter show the highest levels of growth while the general increase in the volume of brain tissue leads to a contraction of CSF space.

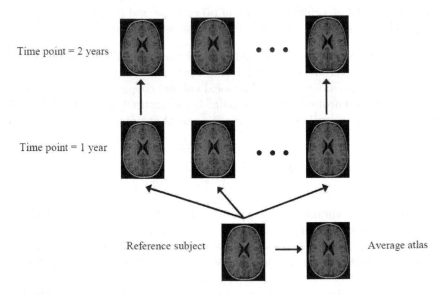

Fig. 2. Deformation-based morphometry for brain development using longitudinal and crosssectional registration [1]

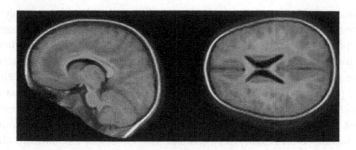

Fig. 3. An average growth map showing areas of expansion (red color) and contraction (blue color)

3   Analysis of Cardiac Motion Using Non-rigid Registration

With the development of new imaging and surgical techniques, the care and treatment of patients with cardiovascular diseases (CVDs) has steadily improved over the last 50 years, but they are still the leading cause of death in the western world [16]. Using magnetic resonance imaging (MRI) it is possible to obtain high resolution cine-images of cardiac motion noninvasively enabling global functional parameters such as *left ventricular volume* (LVV), *left ventricular mass* (LVM), *stroke volume* (SV), *ejection fraction* (EF), and *cardiac output* (CO) to be measured once suitable pre-processing has been applied on the acquired images and the left ventricle (LV) has been segmented out.

Although global functional parameters are useful indicators of cardiovascular diseases they do not indicate which regions of the heart have reduced contractile function, and it is even possible that for some patients global functional parameters fall within normal limits even though regional wall motion may be abnormal [24, 31]. MRI combined with tissue tagging [46, 6, 5] is an important imaging technique for the noninvasive measurement of three dimensional (3D) motion and strain patterns within the walls of the heart. Radio-frequency (RF) pulses applied at the start of the cardiac cycle produce planes of saturated magnetization in the muscle walls which appear as dark stripes when imaged immediately afterwards, and can be tracked to reconstruct dense deformation fields within the myocardium.

Since the introduction of tissue tagging by Zerhouni *et al.* [46] and Axel and Dougherty [6, 5] in the late 1980's, a tremendous amount of effort has been expended in developing methods for extracting deformation fields from tagged MR images efficiently. Among these methods optical flow [20, 35, 15], active contour models [4, 2, 3, 45, 28], and harmonic phase MRI (HARP) [29, 30, 32] have yielded moderately successful results although none have proved to meet all requirements in terms of accuracy and efficiency to come to dominate clinical practice. Among the main difficulties encountered is the need to estimate through-plane motion: As the tag pattern produced during image acquisition is two dimensional, multiple sets of short-axis (SA) and long-axis (LA) images are needed to estimate the 3D motion of the heart over time (see Figure 4). Another problem is patient and respiratory motion: The time required to acquire these images varies between typically 40 mins to 1 hour and although breath-hold sequences are used to minimize respiratory motion while scanning a single image plane, little can be done to compensate for whole body motion. Finally, the intensity of the tag pattern produced during scanning is time varying and the contrast between the tags fades during the cycle. Tag fading complicates motion field estimation as this must be taken account of. Although complementary spatial modulation of magnetization (C-SPAMM) [17] reduces the effects of tag fading, the image acquisition time is increased.

3.1   Motion Tracking by Image Registration

In recent years image registration techniques have also been successfully applied to cardiac motion tracking [9, 11, 34, 43]. Image registration offers a number of advantages over other cardiac motion tracking techniques. First, no assumptions need to be made about the nature of the tag pattern and so image registration based motion tracking is applicable to images with parallel tag patterns as well as grid tag patterns. It also means that the configuration of imaging planes chosen can be arbitrary (the tag planes in the long-axis direction do not need to be aligned with the tag planes in the short-axis direction). Second, using a statistical measure of image similarity (normalized mutual information) we do not need to make any assumptions about the variation of intensity in the sequence of images and so the effects of tag fading can be accounted for.

In our own group we have developed methods for cardiac motion tracking based on the volumetric image registration algorithm of Rueckert *et al* [37] described earlier. The deformation of the myocardium is estimated by registering simultaneously sequences of SA and LA images taken during the cardiac cycle to the corresponding sets of segmented images of the myocardium taken at end-diastole. We have also investigated the use of cylindrical deformation models [10], statistical deformation models [13], and 4D B-spline models for cardiac motion [12] tracking.

Our most recent work has focused on using subdivision lattices [25] for motion tracking. Subdivision lattices are volumetric extensions of subdivision surfaces [8, 14] and are used to define a region of volume through recursive refinement of an initial base lattice. They have the advantage that cells defining the lattices can have an arbitrary topology and that it is possible to use a base lattice with a relatively small number of control vertices to describe the volume of the LV.

Lattice Creation

To aid in the construction of the subdivision lattice representing the LV a graphical user interface (GUI) tool has been created. To create the LV lattice a semi-automatic procedure is used to first create surface models of the endocardium and epicardium. A user places point markers delineating the endocardial surface and a template surface is then registered to the point markers to define the endocardial surface. The epicardial surface is defined in the same manner. Once

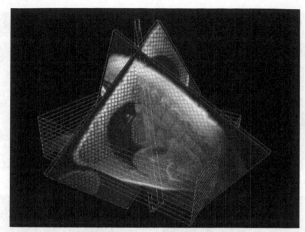

(a) Non-contiguous LA images

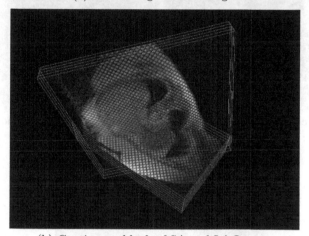

(b) Contiguous block of SA and LA Images

Fig. 4. Multiple sets of short-axis (SA) and long-axis (LA) images need to be acquired to reconstruct the motion of the heart

the two surface models have been created the base polygon meshes defining the endocardial and epicardial surfaces are connected vertex to vertex to define the base lattice of the LV. In Figure 5 (e) 50 vertices are required to model the LV. As can also be seen in the figure the boundary faces of the subdivision lattice conform exactly with the endocardial and epicardial surfaces. This is because the subdivision rules for lattices at the boundary faces are precisely those of the subdivision rules for surfaces.

Motion Tracking

To reconstruct the deformation field within the myocardium sequences of SA and LA images taken during the cardiac cycle are simultaneously registered to corresponding sets of images of the myocardium taken at end-diastole. The esti-

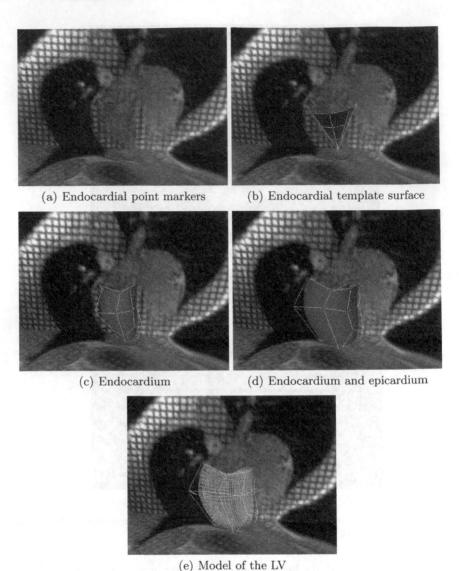

(a) Endocardial point markers   (b) Endocardial template surface

(c) Endocardium   (d) Endocardium and epicardium

(e) Model of the LV

Fig. 5. These figure shows how a subdivision lattice representing the LV is constructed: (a) Using LA and SA views of the LV a user places point markers delineating the endocardial border. (b) The approximate positions of the apex, base, and septum are then specified by the user to align a template surface of the LV with the point set. (c) The template surface is then registered to the point set to define the endocardial surface. (d) Steps (a), (b), and (c) are repeated for the epicardial surface. (e) Finally, the vertices of the base polygon meshes defining the endocardial and epicardial surfaces are connected together to define the base lattice representing the LV (shown in thick yellow lines). The edges of the cells of the subdivided LV lattice are shown in blue.

mation of the motion field proceeds in a sequence of registration steps: Initially, we register the SA and LA images taken at time $t = 1$ to the the SA and LA images taken at time $t = 0$ (end-diastole). We do this by optimizing a cost function which is based on the sum of the normalized mutual information [39] of the images being registered. The motion field for time frame 2 is obtained by registering the images taken at time $t = 2$ to $t = 0$ using the transformation obtained for $t = 1$ as an input. Similarly, the motion field for all other time frames is obtained by registering the images taken at that time frame to the image at time $t = 0$ using the transformation from the previous time frame as an input. In our current implementation it is possible to register a single frame in about 2 minutes using a Pentium IV 3.2 GHz machine with 2 GB of memory.

4 Discussion and Conclusion

In this paper we have shown that non-rigid registration is a powerful tool for estimating local deformations. These local deformations can be either the result of a growth or disease process or a result of organ motion. In both case generic non-rigid registration algorithms can be used successfully to quantify growth or motion. It should be pointed out that non-rigid registration is very much an area of on-going research and most algorithms are still in the stage of development and evaluation. The lack of a generic gold standard for assessing and evaluating the success of non-rigid registration algorithms is one of their most significant drawbacks. In the absence of any such gold standard, it is necessary to compare any non-rigid registration algorithm to other established techniques.

References

1. P. Aljabar, K. K. Bhatia, J. V. Hajnal, J. Boardman, L. Srinivasan, M. Rutherford, L. Dyet, D. Edwards, and D. Rueckert. Analysis of growth in the developing brain using non-rigid registration. In *IEEE International Symposium on Biomedical Imaging*, page in press, 2006.
2. A. A. Amini, Y. Chen, R. W. Curwen, V. Mani, and J. Sun. Coupled B-snake grids and constrained thin-plate splines for analysis of 2D tissue deformations from tagged MRI. *IEEE Transactions on Medical Imaging*, 17(3):344–356, June 1998.
3. A. A. Amini, Y. Chen, M. Elayyadi, and P. Radeva. Tag surface reconstruction and tracking of myocardial beads from SPAMM-MRI with parametric B-spline surfaces. *IEEE Transactions on Medical Imaging*, 20(2):94–103, February 2001.
4. A. A. Amini, R. W. Curwen, and J. C. Gore. Snakes and splines for tracking non-rigid heart motion. In Bernard Buxton and Roberto Cipolla, editors, *Proceedings of the Fourth European Conference on Computer Vision*, volume 1065 of *Lecture Notes in Computer Science*, pages 251–261, Cambridge, UK, April 1996. Springer.
5. L. Axel and L. Dougherty. Heart wall motion: Improved method of spatial modulation of magnetization for MR imaging. *Radiology*, 172(2):349–360, 1989.
6. L. Axel and L. Dougherty. MR imaging of motion with spatial modulation of magnetization. *Radiology*, 171(3):841–845, 1989.
7. N.F. Botting. *Psychological and educational outcome of very low birthweight children at 12 years*. PhD thesis, University of Liverpool, 1997.

8. E. Catmull and J. Clark. Recursively generated B-spline surfaces on arbitrary topological meshes. *Computer Aided Design*, 10(6):350–355, 1978.

9. R. Chandrashekara, R. H. Mohiaddin, and D. Rueckert. Analysis of myocardial motion in tagged MR images using nonrigid image registration. In *Proceedings of the SPIE International Symposium on Medical Imaging: Image Processing*, pages 1168–1179, 2002.

10. R. Chandrashekara, R. H. Mohiaddin, and D. Rueckert. Analysis of myocardial motion and strain patterns using a cylindrical B-spline transformation model. In *Surgery Simulation and Soft Tissue Modeling*, pages 88–99, 2003.

11. R. Chandrashekara, R. H. Mohiaddin, and D. Rueckert. Analysis of 3-D myocardial motion in tagged MR images using nonrigid image registration. *IEEE Transactions on Medical Imaging*, 23(10):1245–1250, October 2004.

12. R. Chandrashekara, R. H. Mohiaddin, and D. Rueckert. Cardiac motion tracking in tagged MR images using a 4D B-spline motion model and nonrigid image registration. In *isbi*, Arlington, VA, USA, April 2004. IEEE.

13. R. Chandrashekara, A. Rao, G. I. Sanchez-Ortiz, R. H. Mohiaddin, and D. Rueckert. Construction of a statistical model for cardiac motion analysis using nonrigid image registration. In *Information Processing in Medical Imaging*, pages 599–610, 2003.

14. D. Doo and M. A. Sabin. Behaviour of recursive subdivision surfaces near extraordinary points. *Computer Aided Design*, 10(6):356–360, 1978.

15. L. Dougherty, J. C. Asmuth, A. S. Blom, L. Axel, and R. Kumar. Validation of an optical flow method for tag displacement estimation. *IEEE Transactions on Medical Imaging*, 18(4):359–363, April 1999.

16. T. Thom et al. Heart disease and stroke statistics – 2006 update: A report from the american heart association statistics committee and stroke statistics subcommittee. *Circulation*, 113:e85–e151, February 2006.

17. S. E. Fishcer, G. C. McKinnon, S. E. Maier, and P. Boesiger. Improved myocardial tagging contrast. *Magnetic Resonance in Medicine*, 30(2):191–200, August 1993.

18. N. C. Fox, W. R. Crum, R. I. Scahill, J. M. Stevens, J. C. Janssen, and M. N. Rossor. Imaging of onset and progression of Alzheimer's disease with voxel-compression mapping of serial magnetic resonance images. *Lancet*, 358:201–205, 2001.

19. P. A. Freeborough and N. C. Fox. Modeling brain deformations in Alzheimer disease by fluid registration of serial 3D MR images. *Journal of Computer Assisted Tomography*, 22(5):838–843, 1998.

20. S. N. Gupta and J. L. Prince. On variable brightness optical flow for tagged MRI. In *Information Processing in Medical Imaging*, pages 323–334. Kluwer, June 1995.

21. J. V. Hajnal, D. L. G. Hill, and D. J. Hawkes, editors. *Medical Image Registration*. CRC Press, 2001.

22. J. V. Hajnal, N. Saeed, , E. J. Soar, A. Oatridge, I. R. Young, and G. M. Bydder. A registration and interpolation procedure for subvoxel matching of serially acquired MR images. *Journal of Computer Assisted Tomography*, 19(2):289–296, 1995.

23. J. V. Hajnal, N. Saeed, A. Oatridge, E. J. Williams, I. R. Young, and G. M. Bydder. Detection of subtle brain changes using subvoxel registration and subtraction of serial MR images. *Journal of Computer Assisted Tomography*, 19(5):677–691, 1995.

24. C. M. Kramer, N. Reichek, V. A. Ferrari, T. Theobald, J. Dawson, and L. Axel. Regional heterogeneity of function in hypertrophic cardiomyopathy. *Circulation*, 90(1):186–194, July 1994.

25. R. MacCracken and K. I. Joy. Free-form deformations with lattices of arbitrary topology. In *Proceedings of the 23rd Annual Conference on Computer Graphics and Interactive Techniques*, pages 181–188. ACM, 1996.

26. J. B. A. Maintz and M. A. Viergever. A survey of medical image registration. *Medical Image Analysis*, 2(1):1–36, 1998.

27. N. Marlow, D. Wolke, M.A. Bracewell, and M. Samara. Neurologic and developmental disability at six years of age after extremely preterm birth. *New England Journal of Medicine*, 352(1):9–19, 2005.

28. W. G. O'Dell, C. C. Moore, W. C. Hunter, E. A. Zerhouni, and E. R. McVeigh. Three-dimensional myocardial deformations: Calculation with displacement field fitting to tagged MR images. *Radiology*, 195(3):829–835, June 1995.

29. N. F. Osman, W. S. Kerwin, E. R. McVeigh, and J. L. Prince. Cardiac motion tracking using cine harmonic phase (HARP) magnetic resonance imaging. *Magnetic Resonance in Medicine*, 42:1048–1060, 1999.

30. N. F. Osman, E. R. McVeigh, and J. L. Prince. Imaging heart motion using harmonic phase MRI. *IEEE Transactions on Medical Imaging*, 19(3):186–202, March 2000.

31. L. C. Palmon, N. Reichek, S. B. Yeon, N. R. Clark, D. Brownson, E. Hoffman, and L. Axel. Intramural myocardial shortening in hypertensive left ventricular hypertrophy with normal pump function. *Circulation*, 89(1):122–131, January 1994.

32. L. Pan, J. A. C. Lima, and N. F. Osman. Fast tracking of cardiac motion using 3D-HARP. In *Proceedings of the 18th International Conference on Information Processing in Medical Imaging*, pages 611–622, Ambleside, UK, July 2003.

33. T. Paus, A. Zijdenbos, K. Worsley, D. L. Collins, J. Blumenthal, J. N. Giedd, J. L. Rapoport, and A. C. Evans. Structural maturation of neural pathways in children and adolescents: In vivo study. *Science*, 283:1908–1911, 1999.

34. C. Petitjean, N. Rougon, F. Preteux, P. Cluzel, and P. Grenier. Measuring myocardial deformation from MR data using information-theoretic nonrigid registration. In *Proceedings of the Second International Workshop on Functional Imaging and Modeling of the Heart*, pages 162–172, Lyon, France, June 2003.

35. J. L. Prince and E. R. McVeigh. Optical flow for tagged MR images. In *Proceedings of the 1991 International Conference on Acoustics, Speech, and Signal Processing*, pages 2441–2444, 1991.

36. D. Rey, G. Subsol, H. Delingette, and N. Ayache. Automatic detection and segmentation of evolving processes in 3D medical images: Application to multiple sclerosis. In *Information Processing in Medical Imaging: Proc. 16th International Conference (IPMI'99)*, pages 154–167, 1999.

37. D. Rueckert, L. I. Sonoda, C. Hayes, D. L. G. Hill, M. O. Leach, and D. J. Hawkes. Nonrigid registration using free-form deformations: Application to breast MR images. *IEEE Transactions on Medical Imaging*, 18(8):712–721, August 1999.

38. C. Studholme, V. Cardenas, N. Schuff, H. Rosen, Miller B, and M. Weiner. Detecting spatially consitent structural differences in alzheimer's and fronto temporal dementia using deformation morphometry. In *Fourth Int. Conf. on Medical Image Computing and Computer-Assisted Intervention (MICCAI '01)*, pages 41–48, 2001.

39. C. Studholme, D. L. G. Hill, and D. J. Hawkes. An overlap invariant entropy measure of 3D medical image alignment. *Pattern Recognition*, 32(1):71–86, 1998.

40. P. M. Thompson, J. N. Giedd, R. P. Woods, D. MacDonald, A. C. Evans, and A. W. Toga. Growth patterns in the developing brain detected by continuum mechanical tensor maps. *Nature*, 404:190–193, March 2000.

41. P. M. Thompson, C. Vidal, J. N. Giedd, P. Gochman, J. Blumenthal, R. Nicholson, A. W. Toga, and J. L. Rapoport. Mapping adolenscent brain change reveals dynamic wave of accelerated grey matter loss in very early-onset schizophrenia. *Nature*, 98(20):11650–11655, 2001.
42. P. M. Thomson, T. D. Cannon, K. L. Narr, T. van Erp, V.-P. Poutanen, M. Huttunen, J. Lönnqvist, Standertskjöld-Nordenstam C.-G, J. Kaprio, M. Khaledy, R. Dali, C. I. Zoumalan, and A. W. Toga. Genetic influences on brain structure. *Nature Neuroscience*, 4(12):1–6, 2001.
43. N. J. Tustison and A. A. Amini. Biventricular myocardial strains via nonrigid registration of anfigatomical NURBS models. *IEEE Transactions on Medical Imaging*, 25(1):94–112, January 2006.
44. N. S. Wood, N. Marlow, K. Costeloe, A. T. Gibson, and W. R. Wilkinson. Neurologic and developmental disability after extremely preterm birth. *New England Journal of Medicine*, 343(6):429–430, 2000.
45. A. A. Young, D. L. Kraitchman, L. Dougherty, and L. Axel. Tracking and finite element analysis of stripe deformation in magnetic resonance tagging. *IEEE Transactions on Medical Imaging*, 14(3):413–421, September 1995.
46. E. A. Zerhouni, D. M. Parish, W. J. Rogers, A. Yang, and E. P. Shapiro. Human heart: Tagging with MR imaging — a method for noninvasive assessment of myocardial motion. *Radiology*, 169(1):59–63, 1988.
47. Barbara Zitová and Jan Flusser. Image registration methods: a survey. *Image Vision Comput.*, 21(11):977–1000, 2003.

Image Registration Accuracy Estimation Without Ground Truth Using Bootstrap

Jan Kybic[1] and Daniel Smutek[2]

[1] Center for Machine Perception, Czech Technical University,
Prague, Czech Republic
kybic@fel.cvut.cz
http://cmp.felk.cvut.cz/~kybic
[2] Faculty of Medicine I, Charles University, Prague, Czech Republic

Abstract. We consider the problem of estimating the local accuracy of image registration when no ground truth data is available. The technique is based on a statistical resampling technique called bootstrap. Only the two input images are used, no other data are needed. The general bootstrap uncertainty estimation framework described here is in principle applicable to most of the existing pixel based registration techniques. In practice, a large computing power is required. We present experimental results for a block matching method on an ultrasound image sequence for elastography with both known and unknown deformation field.

1   Introduction

Image registration algorithms [1,2,3,4,5,6] estimate a displacement field aligning corresponding features in two given input images. The common feature of most of these algorithms is that they provide a single-valued, deterministic answer. For each point from one image, the algorithm calculates the coordinates of one corresponding point from the other image. However, in practice, the estimate is always known only with limited accuracy; there is always an uncertainty associated with it.

Here we shall consider the problem of estimating this uncertainty in the case when no ground truth or a priori information is available, using only the two input images. The bootstrap method [7,8,9] will permit us to use the same data for estimation of both the deformation and the accuracy of this estimation.

1.1   Motivation

Knowing the accuracy of the registration result is always useful. The accuracy information permits us to judge whether and to what extent can the registration be trusted. It can be also used to identify optimal registration parameters and as a weighting factor for information fusion. It can also help us to determine the quality of the input data, so that we can discard or repeat unsuitable experiments.

In many cases the displacement field is an input to subsequent analysis. We are especially interested by the problem of elastography [10,11,12], specifically the

R.R. Beichel and M. Sonka (Eds.): CVAMIA 2006, LNCS 4241, pp. 61–72, 2006.

estimation of the elastic properties of tissues from ultrasound sequences [13,14]. Knowing the uncertainty of the motion estimation will permit us to give more weight to reliably estimated points for the inverse problem solution.

1.2   Previous Work

The precision of the estimated displacement has been studied experimentally using ground truth data, for computer vision [15,16,17,18] as well as for medical applications [19,20,21]. A 'bronze standard' [22] uses combined results of several distinct registration algorithms as a reference. Statistical properties of the estimation errors have been studied theoretically for rotations [23,24]. Heuristic or Gaussian noise based uncertainty measures have been introduced for block matching [25] and optical flow estimation [26,27]. Finally, for low-rank transformations (such as rigid motion), the covariance can be estimated a posteriori from a sufficiently high number of corresponding features [28].

1.3   Proposed Approach

We shall describe a general procedure applicable to a large class of image registration algorithms so that they provide not only the point (crisp) estimate of the displacement field but also an estimate of the accuracy of this displacement. In contrast to the prior work we shall neither require additional test or ground truth data, nor restrict the allowed motion.

We consider images to be random processes and the input images as realizations of these random processes. If we had more acquisitions of the same scene under identical conditions, we could regard them as independent realizations of the random image processes. We could run our registration algorithm of choice on each realization and the statistical distribution of the results would give us an information about the accuracy of the registration.

Since we only have a single pair of images (one realization), we need to use a trick called bootstrap resampling (Section 1.4). More specifically, we shall randomly draw pixels from some neighborhood in the input images and treat them as if they came from independent realizations of the image processes (see Section 2.2 for more details). Then we can continue as above.

1.4   Bootstrap

Let us have N samples $X = \{x_1, \ldots, x_N\}$ of a random variable $\mathcal{X}$. A bootstrap [7,8,9] data set (resample) $B_X^{(\cdot)} = \{y_1, \ldots, y_N\}$ is constructed by randomly selecting N points from X, with replacement. Note that $B_X^{(\cdot)}$ is a multiset (also known as a collection or a bag), which is unordered like a set but in which each element can have a multiplicity greater than 1. The multiset $B_X^{(\cdot)}$ is constructed from the same elements as X, but it contains some of them more than once, some not at all. In bootstrap estimation, the resampling is repeated M times, yielding M data sets $B_X^{(b)}$, which we shall treat as independent.

Let ϑ be some statistic of the random variable $\mathcal{X}$ (such as its mean or variance). We can calculate the estimate $\hat{\vartheta}(\mathsf{X})$ of ϑ from the samples X. Now, we might be interested in the distribution of $\hat{\vartheta}$, for example to check its accuracy or bias. To do this, we calculate $\hat{\vartheta}^{(b)} = \hat{\vartheta}(B_{\mathsf{X}}^{(b)})$ for each bootstrap set $B_{\mathsf{X}}^{(b)}$; the distribution $p_{\hat{\vartheta}}$ of $\hat{\vartheta}$ can then be approximated by an empirical bootstrap distribution $p_{\hat{\vartheta}}^{(*)}$, constructed from the samples $\hat{\vartheta}^{(1)}, \dots, \hat{\vartheta}^{(M)}$.

2   Image Registration

We shall define the registration problem more precisely and show how the bootstrap uncertainty estimation can be performed. We shall use a block matching algorithm as an example.

2.1   Problem Formulation

Let us have two images $f, g : \mathbb{R}^m \to \mathbb{R}^n$. Let $\Omega \in \mathbb{Z}^m$ be a set of pixels from the image f. We assume that the two images are related by a transformation $T_\theta : \mathbb{R}^m \to \mathbb{R}^m$ described by a parameter vector $\theta \in \Theta \subseteq \mathbb{R}^d$. In other words, the point of coordinates $\mathbf{x}$ in image f and the point of coordinates $T_\theta(\mathbf{x})$ in image g correspond to the same physical point and as such are related by a statistical dependence. We assemble the pairs of corresponding pixels into a set S_θ:

$$S_\theta = \left\{ \left(f(\mathbf{x}), g(T_\theta(\mathbf{x}))\right) ; \; \mathbf{x} \in \Omega \right\}$$

and define a scalar similarity criterion J measuring the dependence between $f(\mathbf{x})$ and $g(T_\theta(\mathbf{x}))$ on Ω. This leads to the following estimate of the transformation parameters θ:

$$\hat{\theta} = \arg\min_{\theta \in \Theta} J(S_\theta) \tag{1}$$

The only restriction with respect to the usual formulation is that J operates on a multiset. Most existing pixel based image registration methods [29], [30,31,32,33,34] can be expressed in this form directly, whether the similarity criterion is the sum of square differences, correlation coefficient, or mutual information. The feature space can be extended (so that the elements of S are more than just pairs of pixel values) to accommodate methods that need information from a small pixel neighborhood [35], such as the image gradient [36]. The optical flow [37] and fluid registration methods [38] can also be cast into this framework.

2.2   Uncertainty Estimation

Following the general bootstrap strategy, we make M bootstrap data (multi)sets $\Omega^{(b)}$ by resampling Ω. For each $\Omega^{(b)}$ we perform the minimization (1) yielding an estimate

$$\hat{\theta}^{(b)} = \arg\min_{\theta \in \Theta} J(S_\theta^{(b)}) \quad \text{with} \quad S_\theta^{(b)} = \left\{ \left(f(\mathbf{x}), g(T_\theta(\mathbf{x}))\right) ; \; \mathbf{x} \in \Omega^{(b)} \right\}$$

The probability distribution $p_{\hat{\theta}}$ of $\hat{\theta}$ can be approximated by an empirical bootstrap distribution $p_{\hat{\theta}}^{(*)}$ of the samples $\hat{\theta}^{(1)}, \ldots, \hat{\theta}^{(M)}$. We need to assume the validity of the bootstrap principle, i.e. that the distribution p_{S_θ} of S_θ is well approximated by the distribution $p_{S_\theta}^{(b)}$ of the bootstrap samples $S_\theta^{(b)}$, at least for θ in the vicinity of the optimum. The bootstrap principle is valid if the pixel values of f and $g \circ T_\theta$ are independent and identically distributed (i.i.d) in Ω. It is also valid if Ω can be partitioned into several sufficiently big classes such that in each of the classes the pixel values are i.i.d.

Since we want to make the number of bootstrap data sets M reasonably small to reduce the computational overhead, it is advisable to calculate only some simple statistics on $p_{\hat{\theta}}^{(*)}$ such as the bootstrap mean [9]

$$\mu_{\hat{\theta}}^{(*)} = \frac{1}{M} \sum_{b=1}^{M} \hat{\theta}^{(b)}$$

and covariance matrix

$$\Sigma_{\hat{\theta}}^{(*)} = \frac{1}{M-1} \sum_{b=1}^{M} \left(\hat{\theta}^{(b)} - \mu_{\hat{\theta}}^{(*)} \right) \left(\hat{\theta}^{(b)} - \mu_{\hat{\theta}}^{(*)} \right)^T \tag{2}$$

or alternatively the perhaps the more relevant expected square error

$$\mathbf{C}_{\hat{\theta}}^{(*)} = \frac{1}{M} \sum_{b=1}^{M} \left(\hat{\theta}^{(b)} - \hat{\theta} \right) \left(\hat{\theta}^{(b)} - \hat{\theta} \right)^T$$

Note that the convergence of the above estimates in particular requires smoothness of $\hat{\theta}$ with respect to the input data, see [7] for details. The estimators can also be biased.

2.3   Geometrical Error Estimation

A mean squared geometrical error can be defined as

$$\varepsilon^2 = \operatorname*{mean}_{\mathbf{x} \in \Omega} \| T_{\hat{\theta}}(\mathbf{x}) - T_{\text{true}}(\mathbf{x}) \|^2$$

where T_{true} is the true transformation. Assuming that $T_{\mu_{\hat{\theta}}^{(*)}}$ approximates T_{true} well, we can construct the bootstrap estimate for the expected value of ε^2

$$\mathrm{E}\left[\varepsilon^2\right] \approx e^2 = \frac{1}{M-1} \sum_{b=1}^{M} \frac{1}{\|\Omega\|} \sum_{\mathbf{x} \in \Omega} \| T_{\hat{\theta}^{(b)}}(\mathbf{x}) - T_{\mu_{\hat{\theta}}^{(*)}}(\mathbf{x}) \|^2 \tag{3}$$

An estimate of the expected geometrical error of $\hat{\theta}$ is obtained by using $\hat{\theta}$ instead of $\mu_{\hat{\theta}}^{(*)}$. A geometrical error in a particular direction can be also easily constructed.

3   Block Matching

To illustrate the ideas from the preceding section, we shall apply them on the well-known 2D block matching algorithm [18,39,40] in the context of motion estimation from an ultrasound sequence for elastography [13,14]. The algorithm itself is not our main interest here; we have deliberately chosen to make it very simple, in order not to confuse the description and also to make the bootstrap calculations reasonably fast.

We divide the scalar 2D image ($n = 1$, $m = 2$) into a set of possibly over-lapping blocks Ω_i. Here, for simplicity, we shall use rectangular blocks of size $w_x \times w_y$. The block centers $\mathbf{z}_i$ will be placed on a uniform Cartesian grid. For each Ω_i, we independently estimate the motion parameters θ_i by minimizing a standard sum of squared differences (SSD) criterion:

$$\hat{\theta}_i = \arg\min_{\theta \in \Theta} J(S_{i,\theta})$$

with
$$S_{i,\theta} = \left\{ \left(f(\mathbf{x}), g(T_{i,\theta}(\mathbf{x})) \right) ; \; \mathbf{x} \in \Omega_i \right\}$$

and
$$J(S_{i,\theta}) = \sum_{(f',g')} \left(f' - g' \right)^2 \quad \text{for} \quad (f', g') \in S_{i,\theta}$$

In each block, we shall search for a translation ($d = 2$)

$$T_\theta(\mathbf{x}) = \mathbf{x} + \theta \tag{4}$$

This way, we shall have in each block Ω_i information about the local translation.

3.1   Interpolation

The image g is interpolated using uniform cubic B-spline interpolation [41,42,43] which provides continuous derivatives and good approximation properties. The B-spline coefficients are calculated beforehand.

3.2   Minimization

We use a quasi-Newton type optimizer [44] — second–order information (Hessian matrix H) is used to obtain quadratic convergence. We iteratively update the estimate of H^{-1} using the BFGS strategy [44,45]. The minimum is only sought within an a priori chosen interval of 'reasonable' values of θ.

In our application we know that the displacement at the top edge should be zero, since the ultrasound probe is in contact with the tissue there. We go through the image from top to bottom and from center to the left and to the right [46], using the value of θ found in the block immediately above or next to the current one as a starting guess.

3.3   Bootstrap Accuracy Estimation

For each block we evaluate the expected geometrical error e^2 (3) which in the translation case (4) simplifies to $e^2 = \text{tr}\, \Sigma_{\hat{\theta}}^{(*)}$ with the correlation estimator $\Sigma_{\hat{\theta}}^{(*)}$ defined by (2).

4   Experiments

Experiments were performed on a sequence of ultrasound images acquired by a standard Philips Envisor scanner for the elastography experiments. We have used the Gammex 429 Ultrasound Biopsy Phantom[1] that mimics normal tissue and contains eleven test objects filled with low or high density gel, simulating lesions. The movement between images of the sequence is caused by varying the pressure applied on the ultrasound probe.

A key parameter for our bootstrap uncertainty estimation is the number of bootstrap resampling M. According to the literature [7], to estimate simple statistics such as correlation, $M = 50$ is often enough. Hence, we ran the following experiments with $M = 10$ and $M = 100$. Surprisingly, there was a little difference between the results. All results presented here were calculated with $M = 10$ which appears to be enough for the present application.

The algorithm was implemented in the Ocaml language[2]. Our experience suggests that a reimplementation in an optimized C code might bring another $30 \sim 50\,\%$ speed-up. The times reported are on a computer with a Pentium M 1400 MHz processor.

4.1   Synthetic Displacement Field

To have the ground truth information available, we have generated an artificial displacement field (Figure 1) that attempts to be simple yet similar to displacement fields encountered in real data. The right half of the images is undeformed, to create an abrupt transition. In the left half the vertical displacement increases linearly from top to bottom. The horizontal displacement increases linearly from top to bottom and from right to left; in addition there is a low amplitude harmonic component.

The block matching algorithm (Section 3) with bootstrap uncertainty estimation was run on the original grayscale images (Figure 1, top) of size 541×426 pixels. We used overlapping blocks of 29×29 pixels whose centers lie on a uniform grid with spacing of 5×5 pixels. In Figure 2 we show the recovered displacements (to be compared with Figure 1, top), the estimated and the true geometrical error.

Note that even though the amplitude of the error has not been estimated exactly, the results are in the right order of magnitude. Perhaps more importantly, the algorithm has correctly identified the areas where errors are likely — around the vertical edge where the motion is discontinuous and around the 'lesion' area where texture is missing. The registration took about 3 hours.

4.2   Window Size

The bootstrap accuracy estimate permits us to optimize the parameters of the registration itself, for example the window size. Figure 3 shows the de-

---

[1] www.gamex.com

[2] http://caml.inria.fr

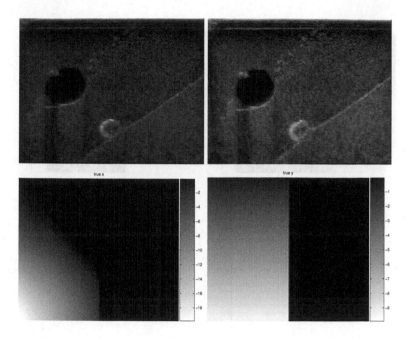

Fig. 1. The original image (top left) and its deformed version (top right). The horizontal and vertical components of the artificial deformation (bottom left and bottom right, respectively).

pendency of the real and estimated geometric error on the window size. Even though the error estimation is not exact, it is nevertheless quite close to the reality and it permits us to correctly identify the trade-off between a window too small which provides a noisy estimate, and a window too big in which the movement is not sufficiently homogeneous and cannot be explained by a translation. One reason for the disparity is that the estimator incorrectly assumes that the true transformation is a translation. The whole experiment took 8 min.

4.3   Real Images

Finally, we have taken two images from the ultrasound sequence a few frames apart and applied the registration algorithm on them (Figure 4) with the same parameters as in Section 4.1. The recovered displacements seem to be realistic and the uncertainty estimation correctly identified the problematic zone of the 'lesion' without texture. The calculation took also about 3 hours.

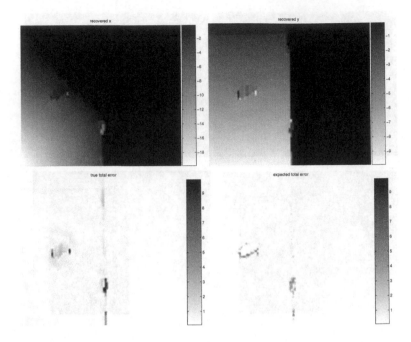

Fig. 2. The estimated horizontal and vertical displacements (top left and top right, respectively). The true geometrical error ε and its bootstrap estimate e (bottom left and bottom right, respectively). All values are in pixels.

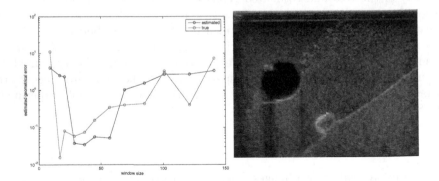

Fig. 3. The dependence of the true end expected geometric error (ε resp. e) on the window size in pixels (left). The location of the window center is marked by the red dot on the deformed image (right).

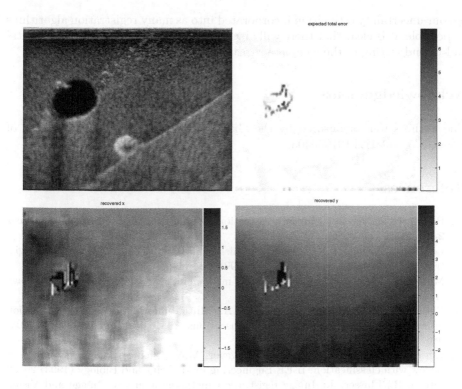

Fig. 4. Two images from the ultrasound sequence (top left, in green and red channels) and the recovered horizontal and vertical displacement (bottom left an right, respectively). The expected geometrical error e (top right).

5 Conclusions

We have described a bootstrap-based uncertainty estimation procedure that can be applied to a wide class of pixel-based image registration algorithms. Unlike any other registration algorithm known to us, it can estimate the registration accuracy using only the input images, yet it does not limit the class of the representable transformations, nor it assumes a specific noise or image intensity distribution. We have shown experimentally that the uncertainty estimates produced by the algorithm are reasonable.

Bootstrap algorithms can take full advantage of the abundant computing power available today. Even though for the simple registration algorithm presented here the computational time was just about acceptable, in more complex cases parallel processing might be advisable.

The algorithm presented here is only a proof of concept, there is a number of ways how to extend it, some of which were already mentioned in the introduction. Finally, note that the algorithm can only estimate the stochastic part of the error inherent to the registration itself. Therefore, even though we would be happy to see our uncertainty estimation incorporated into as many registration algorithms as possible, it is clear that there will always be a need for a careful experimental end-to-end testing of the complete registration chain.

Acknowledgements

The authors were sponsored by the Grant Agency of the Czech Academy of Sciences, grant 1ET101050403.

References

1. Brown, L.: A survey of image registration techniques. ACM Computing Surveys **24**(4) (1992) 326–376
2. Lester, H., Arridge, S.R.: A survey of hierarchical non-linear medical image registration. Pattern Recognition **32**(1) (1999) 129–149
3. Maintz, J., Viergever, M.A.: A survey of medical image registration. Medical Image Analysis **2**(1) (1998) 1–36
4. Pluim, J., Maintz, J.B.A., Viergever, M.A.: Mutual-information-based registration of medical images: A survey. IEEE Transactions on Medical Imaging **22**(8) (2003) 986–1004
5. van den Elsen, P.A., Pol, E.J.D., Viergever, M.A.: Medical image matching—A review with classification. IEEE Engineering in Medicine and Biology (1993) 26–39
6. Zitová, B., Flusser, J.: Image registration methods: a survey. Image and Vision Computing (21) (2003) 977–1000
7. Efron, B., Tibshirani, R.: An Introduction to the Bootstrap. Number 57 in Monographs on Statistics and Applied Probability. Chapman & Hall, CRC (1993)
8. Zoubir, A.M., Boashash, B.: The bootstrap and its applications in signal processing. IEEE Signal Processing Magazine (1998) 56–76
9. Duda, R.O., Hart, P.E., Stork, D.G.: Pattern classification. 2nd edn. Wiley Interscience Publication. John Wiley, New York (2001)
10. Ophir, J., Kallel, F., Varghese, T., Konofagou, E., Alam, S.K., Garra, B., Krouskop, T., Righetti, R.: Elastography: Optical and acoustic imaging of acoustic media. C. R. Acad. Sci. Paris **2**(8) (2001) 1193–1212 serie IV.
11. Ophir, J., Alam, S., Garra, B., Kallel, F., Konofagou, E., Krouskop, T., Varghese, T.: Elastography: ultrasonic estimation and imaging of the elastic properties of tissues. Proc. Instn Mech Engrs **213** (1999) 203–233
12. Washington, C.W., Miga, M.I.: Modality independent elastography (MIE): A new approach to elasticity imaging. IEEE Transactions on Medical Imaging (2004) 1117–1126
13. Kybic, J., Smutek, D.: Estimating elastic properties of tissues from standard 2d ultrasound images. In Walker, W.F., Emelianov, S.Y., eds.: Medical Imaging 2005: Ultrasonic Imaging and Signal Processing. Volume 6 of Progress in Biomedical Optics and Imaging., Bellingham, Washington, USA, SPIE (2005) 184–195
14. Kybic, J., Smutek, D.: Computational elastography from standard ultrasound image sequences by global trust region optimization. In Šonka, M., Christensen, G., eds.: Proceedings of IPMI, Lecture Notes in Computer Science. Number 3565, Heidelberg, Germany, Springer Verlag (2005) 299–310

15. Fang, J., Huang, T.S.: Some experiments on estimating the 3-D motion parameters of a rigid body from two consecutive image frames. IEEE Trans. Pattern Anal. Mach. Intell. **3**(65) (1984)
16. Snyder, M.A.: The precision of 3-D parameters in correspondence based techniques: the case of uniform translational motion in rigid environment. IEEE Trans. Pattern Anal. Mach. Intell. **5**(11) (1998) 523–528
17. Haralick, R.M., Joo, H., Lee, C.N., Zhuang, X., Vaidya, V.G., Kim, M.B.: Pose estimation from corresponding point data. IEEE Trans. Systems, Man and Cybernetics **6**(19) (1989) 1426–1446
18. Davis, C.Q., Freeman, D.M.: Statistics of subpixel registration algorithms based on spatiotemporal gradients or block matching. Optical Engineering **4**(37) (1998) 1290–1298
19. Maurer, C.J., Fitzpatrick, J., Wang, M., Galloway, R.J., Maciunas, R., Allen, G.: Registration of head volume images using implantable fiducial markers. IEEE Transactions on Medical Imaging **16**(4) (1997)
20. West, J., Fitzpatrick, J.M., Wang, M.Y., Dawant, B.M., Maurer, C.R.J., Kessler, R.M., Maciunas, R.J., Barillot, C., Lemoine, D., Collignon, A., Maes, F., Suetens, P., Vandermeulen, D., van den Elsen, P.A., Napel, S., Sumanaweera, T.S., Harkness, B., Hemler, P.F., Hill, D.L.G., Hawkes, D.J., Studholme, C., Maintz, J.B.A., Viergever, M.A., Malandain, G., Pennec, X., Noz, M.E., Maguire, G.Q.J., Pollack, M., Pelizzari, C.A., Robb, R.A., Hanson, D., Woods, R.P.: Comparison and evaluation of retrospective intermodality brain image registration techniques. Journal of Computer Assisted Tomography **21**(4) (1997) 554–568
21. Jannin, P., Fitzpatrick, J., Hawkes, D., Pennec, X., Shahidi, R., Vannier, M.: Validation of medical image processing in image-guided therapy. IEEE Trans. on Medical Imaging **21**(12) (2002) 1445–1449
22. Nicolau, S., Pennec, X., Soler, L., Ayache, N.: Evaluation of a new 3D/2D registration criterion for liver radio-frequencies guided by augmented reality. In: Intl. Symp. on Surgery Sim. and Soft Tissue Model. (2003) 270–283
23. Kanatani, K.: Geometric computation for machine vision. Oxford University Press, Inc., New York, NY, USA (1993)
24. Kanatani, K.: Analysis of 3-d rotation fitting. IEEE Trans. Pattern Anal. Mach. Intell. **16**(5) (1994) 543–549
25. Anandan, P.: A computational framework and an algorithm for the measurement of visual motion. International Journal of Computer Vision **2**(3) (1989) 283–310
26. Heeger, D.J.: "optical flow using spatiotemporal filters". International Journal of Computer Vision **1**(4) (1988) 279–302
27. Simoncelli, E.P., Adelson, E.H., Heeger, D.J.: Probability distributions of optical flow. In: Proc Conf on Computer Vision and Pattern Recognition, Mauii, Hawaii, IEEE Computer Society (1991) 310–315
28. Pennec, X., Thirion, J.P.: A framework for uncertainty and validation of 3d registration methods based on points and frames. International Journal of Computer Vision **25**(3) (1997) 203–229
29. Kybic, J., Unser, M.: Fast parametric elastic image registration. IEEE Transactions on Image Processing **12**(11) (2003) 1427–1442
30. Thévenaz, P., Ruttimann, U.E., Unser, M.: A pyramid approach to subpixel registration based on intensity. IEEE Transactions on Image Processing **7**(1) (1998) 1–15
31. Thévenaz, P., Unser, M.: Optimization of mutual information for multiresolution image registration. IEEE Transactions on Image Processing **9**(12) (2000) 2083–2099

32. Szeliski, R., Coughlan, J.: Spline-based image registration. International Journal of Computer Vision **22** (1997) 199–218
33. Maes, F., Collignong, A., Vandermeulen, D., Marchal, G., Suetens, P.: Multimodality image registration by maximization of mutual information. IEEE Transactions on Medical Imaging **16**(2) (1997) 187–198
34. Rösch, P., Weese, J., Netsch, T., Quist, M., Penney, G., Hill, D.: Robust 3D deformation field estimation by template propagation. In: Proceedings of MICCAI. (2000) 521–530
35. Rueckert, D., Clarkson, M.J., Hill, D.L.G., Hawkes, D.J.: Non-rigid registration using higher-order mutual information. In: Proceedings of SPIE Medical Imaging 2000: Image Processing. (2000) 438–447
36. Pluim, J.P.W., Maintz, J.B.A., Viergever, M.A.: Image registration by maximization of combined mutual information and gradient information. IEEE Transactions Med. Imag. **19**(8) (2000)
37. Horn, B., Schunck, B.: Determining optical flow. Artificial Inteligence **17** (1981) 185–203
38. Bro-Nielsen, M., Gramkow, C.: Fast fluid registration of medical images. In Höhne, K.H., Kikinis, R., eds.: Visualization in Biomedical Computing. Springer-Verlag (1996) 267–276
39. Morsy, A., Ramm, O.: 3D ultrasound tissue motion tracking using correlation search. IEEE Trans. Ultr. Ferro. & Freq. Cont. **20** (1998) 151–159
40. Ourselin, S., Roche, A., Prima, S., Ayache, N.: Block matching: A general framework to improve robustness of rigid registration of medical images. In: Third International Conference on Medical Robotics, Imaging And Computer Assisted Surgery (MICCAI 2000). Number 1935 in Lectures Notes in Computer Science, Springer (2000) 557–566
41. Unser, M., Aldroubi, A., Eden, M.: B-Spline signal processing: Part I—Theory. IEEE Transactions on Signal Processing **41**(2) (1993) 821–833 IEEE Signal Processing Society's 1995 best paper award.
42. Unser, M., Aldroubi, A., Eden, M.: B-Spline signal processing: Part II—Efficient design and applications. IEEE Transactions on Signal Processing **41**(2) (1993) 834–848
43. Unser, M.: Splines: A perfect fit for signal and image processing. IEEE Signal Processing Magazine **16**(6) (1999) 22–38
44. Press, W.H., Teukolsky, S.A., Vetterling, W.T., Flannery, B.P.: Numerical Recipes in C. Second edn. Cambridge University Press (1992)
45. Liu, D.C., Nocedal, J.: On the limited memory BFGS method for large scale minimization. Mathematical Programming (45) (1989) 503–528
46. Brusseau, E., Fromageau, J., Rognin, N., Delacharte, P., Vray, D.: Local estimation of RF ultrasound signal compression for axial strain imaging: theoretical developments and experimental design. IEEE Engineering in Medicine and Biology Magazine **21**(4) (2002) 86–94

SIFT and Shape Context for Feature-Based Nonlinear Registration of Thoracic CT Images*

Martin Urschler[1], Joachim Bauer[2], Hendrik Ditt[3], and Horst Bischof[1]

[1] Institute for Computer Graphics & Vision, Graz University of Technology, Austria
{urschler, bischof}@icg.tu-graz.ac.at
[2] VRVis Research Centre, Graz, Austria
bauer@vrvis.at
[3] Siemens Medical Solutions, CTE PA, Forchheim, Germany
hendrik.ditt@siemens.com

Abstract. Nonlinear image registration is a prerequisite for various medical image analysis applications. Many data acquisition protocols suffer from problems due to breathing motion which has to be taken into account for further analysis. Intensity based nonlinear registration is often used to align differing images, however this requires a large computational effort, is sensitive to intensity variations and has problems with matching small structures. In this work a feature-based image registration method is proposed that combines runtime efficiency with good registration accuracy by making use of a fully automatic feature matching and registration approach. The algorithm stages are 3D corner detection, calculation of local (*SIFT*) and global (*Shape Context*) 3D descriptors, robust feature matching and calculation of a dense displacement field. An evaluation of the algorithm on seven synthetic and four clinical data sets is presented. The quantitative and qualitative evaluations show lower runtime and superior results when compared to the Demons algorithm.

1 Introduction

Many medical image analysis applications require a nonlinear (deformable) registration of data sets acquired at different points in time. Especially when dealing with soft tissue organs, like lung or liver during breathing, there are almost always motion differences that have to be compensated for further analysis. The contributions in this paper focus on thoracic CT images coming from CT angiography (CTA) studies for clinical diagnosis of pulmonary embolism [1]. Nonlinear registration is necessary to guarantee that the same anatomical regions are subtracted from each other since patients in bad condition often have problems holding their breath. Despite the focus on thoracic CTA studies the developed algorithm is in principle suitable for other applications as well.

The registration literature distinguishes intensity- and feature-based nonlinear registration methods. Surveys on nonlinear registration methods in medical imaging can be found in Maintz and Viergever [2] or Zitova and Flusser [3]. Often

---

* This work was funded by Siemens MED CT, Forchheim and Siemens PSE AS, Graz.

R.R. Beichel and M. Sonka (Eds.): CVAMIA 2006, LNCS 4241, pp. 73–84, 2006.

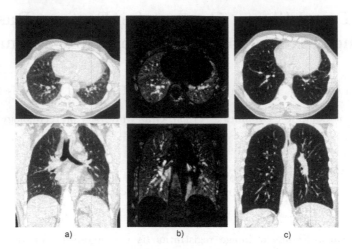

Fig. 1. Evaluation data set F with axial slices in top and sagittal slices in bottom row. a) and c) show the differences in inspiration and exspiration. b) gives the difference image after Demons registration. Note the misregistered vessel structures.

feature-based methods are more accurate than intensity-based methods as long as the feature extraction or segmentation steps are reliable and accurate. Due to the reduction of the problem space, feature-based methods are also significantly faster to compute. On the other hand, segmentation of the organs of interest is not always an easy task and inaccuracies in the segmentation or feature extraction process have severe effects on a subsequent registration step, making the intensity based methods perform better in many practical applications.

This paper presents a novel nonlinear registration approach based on automatically extracted and matched feature points. Although intensity-based approaches are getting more attention by the research community, they face two kinds of practical problems when applied to large thoracic data sets. First, due to their mathematical complexity they require large computational effort. Second, those approaches that are computationally feasible often tend to misregister small structures in the lung like vessels and airways. Further, intensity variations that occur when comparing inhaled and exhaled lungs are not modeled due to implicit brightness constancy assumptions. Fig. 1 shows a nonlinear registration example on lung CT data where the widely-used Demons algorithm [4] leads to misregistrations of vessel structures. Starting from this problem, an automatic feature matching and registration pipeline was established using state of the art techniques from the computer vision community. This pipeline contains Foerstner corner detection [5], forward-backward matching using a 3D scale invariant feature transform (SIFT) descriptor [6] and a global descriptor similar to shape context [7] and dense displacement field estimation in the thin-plate spline (TPS) framework [8]. Especially SIFT and shape context have proved to be very powerful approaches in traditional computer vision applications like wide-baseline matching or object recognition. The main contributions of this work are the 3D extension and the runtime optimization of these stages and their application to medical images. Related work on feature-based registration was presented in Rohr [9] showing an approximating thin-plate spline registration using manually defined landmarks. In Johnson and Christensen [10] a combined landmark and intensity based approach that establishes a consistent deformation field was proposed. Chui et al. [11] have shown a unified nonlinear feature registration approach using a joint clustering and matching framework. Note that none of these works addresses the problem of fully automatic feature extraction, matching and registration.

2   Methods

Breathing motion mainly stems from two sources, the diaphragm and the rib cage muscles. Expected tissue deformations are not extremely large even in the case of matching full exhalation to full inhalation and they change smoothly over the image domain. These considerations imply that a robust and reproducible feature extraction step producing large numbers of feature candidates followed by the automatic matching of feature descriptors is a valid approach to find corresponding structures in the images (see Fig. 2 for the matching and registration pipeline). Due to the large similarity of local neighborhoods in lung images it is important to not only look at local feature descriptors but also add a notion of global correspondence. Mortensen et al. [12] have recently proposed a combined local and global descriptor for the matching of repetitive patterns. Their ideas were adapted to solve the ambiguities with locally similar structures. After establishing sparse corresponding features a dense displacement field has to be calculated. Bookstein [8] motivated the thin-plate spline (TPS) framework as the appropriate way of displacement field interpolation. However, the interpolating behavior of TPS is not desirable since it may lead to foldings. To overcome this problem the decision to use TPS approximation [9] was made.

The large size of current routinely acquired CT volume data poses runtime and memory restrictions on practically useful algorithms. Acquired CT data

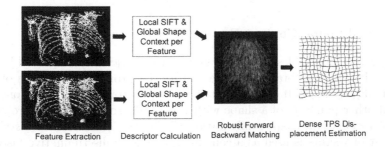

Fig. 2. Nonlinear matching and registration pipeline. The feature extraction stage only shows extracted bone corners, while the method also extracts lung and tissue features.

sets easily require hundreds of MB in memory, so it is necessary to consider computational and memory effort when designing algorithms. In the presented pipeline two performance bottlenecks were identified due to the large number of detected feature points. First, the calculation of the shape context descriptor is critical due to its internally used log-polar histogram bin structure. Therefore an approximation using axis-aligned histogram bins was developed. Second, the calculation of the final dense displacement field is very expensive when confronted with a large number of matched points. Consequently, the global TPS transform was replaced with a k-d tree based locally restricted TPS (LRTPS). The following subsections describe the different pipeline stages in more detail.

2.1   Feature Extraction

The first step in the nonlinear registration pipeline is fast and reproducible feature extraction. This was already extensively investigated by Rohr [9]. His evaluations of several different 3D anatomical feature detection operators resulted in the recommendation of the structure tensor based 3D Foerstner operator [5].

2.2   Local SIFT Feature Descriptor

For each detected feature a distinctive local SIFT feature descriptor [6] is built. SIFT descriptors are robust to local deformations and to errors in feature detection. Performance evaluations show its excellent matching behavior on various kinds of transformations [13]. In this work only the SIFT descriptor representation is used, since keypoint localization is performed using Foerstner corners. To apply the SIFT descriptor representation on volume data an extension to 3D is necessary. The 3D SIFT descriptor quantizes gradient locations in a 2x2x2 grid while gradient orientations are quantized into two 8-bin orientation histograms. Each 512-dimensional descriptor is normalized by its L_2-norm. In contrast to the 2D SIFT formulation, the proposed 3D SIFT descriptor is not rotation-invariant, since this saves computation time and breathing motion is assumed not to lead to strong rotation-like local deformations.

2.3   Global Shape Context Feature Descriptor

The 3D shape context descriptor [7] assumes that objects are captured by point sets $P = \{p_1, ..., p_n\}$ obtained from a feature detector or as locations of edges from an edge detector. If one looks at the set of vectors emitted from one point p_k to all other points p_i of a shape with $i \neq k$, this set can be interpreted as a rich description of the shape configuration relative to p_i. The *relative distribution* of this set of vectors is used as a compact, yet highly discriminative histogram descriptor. This histogram uses bins that are uniform in a 3D spherical coordinate system (θ, ϕ, r). The r coordinate axis is logarithmically scaled, so positions of nearby sample points have stronger influence on the descriptor. The log-polar histogram binning of this method was identified as a performance problem when

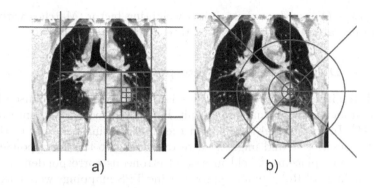

Fig. 3. Approximated global context (a) vs shape context (b) histogram bin structure

applied to a large number of extracted feature points. Therefore an approximation of the shape context descriptor was used, which offers good matching results compared to the classical approach. Here the log-polar histogram bin structure is replaced with a bin structure based on rectangular, axis-aligned image patches. Fig. 3 compares the equivalent 2D histogram bin structures of the classical and the approximated descriptors. The patch size increases exponentially with growing distance from the feature point. This strategy preserves local information close to the feature point and generalizes at larger distance to a coarser quantization. If one uses a 3D integral image representation to store feature point locations, this descriptor is extremely efficient to compute due to its axis-aligned bin structure. The integral image allows to count feature points per rectangular patch in constant time, so for each feature point the histogram is calculated in logarithmic instead of linear time.

2.4 Robust Feature Matching

To find corresponding feature points a matching algorithm has to be used. The previous stages have established a local and a global descriptor for each feature point, the task of the matching stage now is to find those point pairs from two volumes that minimize a cost function derived from the descriptors. Forward-backward matching, a simple but robust approach in terms of consistency, occlusions and erroneous feature extraction, was presented by Fua [14] on stereo matching problems. The basic idea is to perform the matching step twice by reversing the roles of the two volumes V_1, V_2 and considering only those matches as valid for which the corresponding points $P_{i,1}$ and $P_{i,2}$ are identical when matching from V_1 to V_2 and from V_2 to V_1. The cost function used in the two matching steps is a weighted linear combination of distance metrics. The distance metric d_{SIFT} for the SIFT feature descriptor is the Euclidean distance in the 512-dimensional feature space. Shape context descriptors SC_i and SC_j are compared using a χ^2 statistic $d_{SC} = \chi^2 = \frac{1}{2} \sum_k \frac{(SC_{i,k} - SC_{j,k})^2}{SC_{i,k} + SC_{j,k}}$. Both distance metrics are normalized between 0 and 1. The total cost function is given by

$d = \omega d_{SIFT} + (1 - \omega)d_{SC}$ where ω is a weighting factor. Matches with a cost function value above some user-defined threshold T_d are discarded.

2.5   Dense Displacement Field Interpolation

The final step in the registration pipeline is the estimation of a dense displacement field from the sparse matching result. For this purpose a TPS interpolation is used [8,9]. In its original formulation the interpolating behavior of the TPS often is too restrictive and might lead to overfitting to the correspondences or folding of the displacement field in case of erroneous correspondences. In this work the findings of Rohr [9] for approximating TPS mappings were considered. A regularization term is added to the formulation, which is steered by a parameter λ, weighting the tradeoff between interpolation and smoothness of the solution. Further, a landmark error term is introduced to give each pair of corresponding features an uncertainty measure, which is directly derived from the matching costs of the feature matching stage.

It is desirable that the matching stage produces a large number of feature correspondences n_{match}. On typical volume data sets thousands of correspondences might be achieved. In this case the warping of large volume data sets is very costly, since for each voxel a multiplication with $O(n_{match})$ weighted landmarks including the calculation of $O(n_{match})$ vector norms is involved. Therefore a locally restricted version (LRTPS) of the normally global TPS transform is used. The source points of the feature correspondences are put into a k-d tree structure to give efficient access to its neighbor features. For each feature point a TPS transform restricted to a pre-defined number of neighbors is calculated. So only a subset of the total set of correspondences in the volume is taken for locally estimating the transform. The dense displacement field approximation step always looks for the nearest feature correspondence in the k-d tree and takes the stored local TPS transform to compute a displacement.

3   Experiments and Results

To assess the validity of the feature-based registration approach qualitative and quantitative evaluations were performed on synthetically transformed and clinical thorax CT data sets. For the synthetic deformation experiments two different kinds of deformations were used. The first deformation model is a *Simulated Breathing Transformation* simulating rib-cage and diaphragm muscle behavior. The second synthetic transformation makes use of evenly distributed landmarks that are moved in random directions. The synthetic experiments give numbers on the RMS of the intensity differences before and after registration, compares the registered and the synthetic displacement fields and compares the method with the Demons algorithm. Real data experiments show the decrease in the RMS of the intensity differences, compare the RMS with the Demons algorithm and give qualitative difference images. All experiments were performed on a dual 2GHz AMD Opteron system with 8GB RAM running Linux.

3.1   Synthetic Deformation Experiments

Synthetic experiments were performed on seven test data sets (A,B,C,D,E,F,G) taken at inspiration, each of them having a volume size of 512 by 512 by 256 voxels. The first synthetic transformation intends to model breathing behavior. The nonlinear transformation $d(x, y, z) : \mathcal{R}^3 \rightarrow \mathcal{R}^3$ simulates diaphragm and rib cage movement. Diaphragm movement is applied as a translational force in the data sets negative z direction. Nonlinearity is introduced by weighting the constant vertical translation $t_{vertical}$ with a two-dimensional Gaussian distribution that depends on the x and y coordinates of the data set. Mathematically a displacement vector $d_1 = (0, 0, z')^T$ is applied to each point $(x, y, z)^T$ that maps it to $(x, y, z')^T$ with

$$z' = z - t_{vertical} e^{-\frac{(x-\mu_x)^2+(y-\mu_y)^2}{2\sigma^2}}$$

where (μ_x, μ_y) is the center of gravity of the diaphragm points and σ is chosen such that points lying at the exterior of the diaphragm surface nearly remain fixed. In a similar fashion, simulation of rib cage behavior during breathing leads to a radial, center-directed translation $t_{inplane}$. It is used to form a second displacement $d_2 = (x', y', 0)^T$ that maps points $(x, y, z)^T$ to $(x', y', z)^T$ with

$$\begin{pmatrix} x' \\ y' \end{pmatrix} = \begin{pmatrix} \mu_x \\ \mu_y \end{pmatrix} + \left(\left| \begin{pmatrix} x-\mu_x \\ y-\mu_y \end{pmatrix} \right| - t_{inplane} * \left(1 - e^{-\frac{(x-\mu_x)^2+(y-\mu_y)^2}{2\sigma^2}} \right) \right) * \frac{\begin{pmatrix} x-\mu_x \\ y-\mu_y \end{pmatrix}}{\left| \begin{pmatrix} x-\mu_x \\ y-\mu_y \end{pmatrix} \right|}$$

Combining displacements d_1 and d_2 results in transformation d. Finally, to simulate a change in lung gray-values due to inhalation, all gray values smaller than -800 Hounsfield Units (HU) are increased by a random number drawn from a normal distribution centered at 25 HU with a standard deviation of 3 HU.

The seven test data sets were synthetically transformed with a small and a large deformation. The small deformation is defined by the translations $t_{vertical} = 25mm$ and $t_{inplane} = 10mm$ while the large deformation is defined by $t_{vertical} = 55mm$ and $t_{inplane} = 25mm$. Fig. 4 a)-c) shows the effects of these deformations on data set A. First, the feature matching produces corresponding points which can be compared to the ground truth simulated breathing transformation in terms of the RMS of the displacement difference vectors (RMS_{disp}) and the maximum of the lengths of the displacement difference vectors (MAX_{disp}) over all correspondences. Evaluations showed that the RMS_{disp} varies between 0.265mm and 0.314mm for the small and between 0.558mm and 2.479mm for the large deformation over the data sets. Accordingly MAX_{DISP} varies between 2.62mm and 8.59mm for small and between 14.95mm and 28.37mm for large deformations respectively.

Table 1 gives the results of the synthetic registration experiments. All comparisons are always performed only on those regions which are present in both registered data sets. The RMS of the intensity differences before ($RMSD_{initial}$) and after ($RMSD_{feature}$) registration are calculated, as well as the difference of

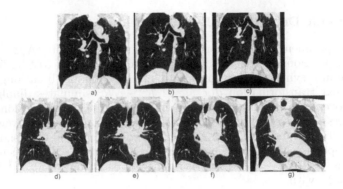

Fig. 4. Synthetic transformations. a) original data set A, b) the small and c) the large simulated breathing deformation. d) original data set B, e) randomly displaced landmark transformation -8...+8, f) displacement -24...+24, g) displacement -48...+48.

Table 1. Simulated breathing transformation. Registration results in terms of RMS intensity differences and displacement difference vectors.

	Measure		A	B	C	D	E	F	G	Mean
SimBreath 25-10	$RMSD_{initial}$	[HU]	385.99	327.25	303.92	359.49	318.73	316.58	316.45	332.63
	$RMSD_{demons}$	[HU]	114.44	115.56	92.05	100.06	96.33	90.21	105.95	102.08
	$RMSD_{feature}$	[HU]	45.18	45.71	43.43	50.78	46.09	41.64	47.91	45.82
	$RMS_{disp,demons}$	[mm]	4.564	5.961	5.412	4.842	4.756	4.931	5.741	5.172
	$RMS_{disp,feature}$	[mm]	0.662	0.769	0.59	0.66	0.601	1.338	1.025	0.806
	$MAX_{disp,demons}$	[mm]	34.55	38.56	38.06	29.95	28.45	35.26	37.59	34.63
	$MAX_{disp,feature}$	[mm]	8.59	9.56	8.02	8.52	8.87	12.64	11.79	9.71
	# matches		2678	2121	2330	2022	1805	5204	3714	2825.9
SimBreath 55-25	$RMSD_{initial}$	[HU]	549.02	477.81	446.84	521.65	477.07	472.65	442.95	484
	$RMSD_{demons}$	[HU]	134.46	135.69	128.57	181.32	145.77	153.67	153.11	147.51
	$RMSD_{feature}$	[HU]	69.35	82.24	71.09	96.98	70.11	74.78	78.93	77.64
	$RMS_{disp,demons}$	[mm]	6.844	7.384	6.912	5.822	5.113	7.012	6.992	6.583
	$RMS_{disp,feature}$	[mm]	1.059	1.382	1.327	1.331	1.252	2.256	2.03	1.519
	$MAX_{disp,demons}$	[mm]	39.45	38.12	39.99	41.72	38.09	43.01	42.95	40.48
	$MAX_{disp,feature}$	[mm]	15.22	21.44	19.84	23.49	18.24	24.14	21.66	20.58
	# matches		1940	1424	1709	1287	1277	2778	2856	1895.9

Table 2. Synthetic TPS transformation results. Registration results in terms of RMS intensity differences and displacement difference vectors.

Measure		-8...+8	-16...+16	-24...+24	-32...+32	-48...+48
$RMSD_{initial}$	[HU]	164.89	233.48	289.76	333.94	397.89
$RMSD_{demons}$	[HU]	161.13	188.67	193.75	184.12	253.81
$RMSD_{feature}$	[HU]	90.58	169.89	236.83	271.113	360.72
$RMS_{disp,demons}$	[mm]	5.834	9.374	13.874	17.099	19.933
$RMS_{disp,feature}$	[mm]	4.802	8.355	11.172	15.792	18.562
# matches		1729	1101	426	312	87

the resulting and the synthetic displacement fields in terms of the RMS of the displacement vector field RMS_{disp} and the maximum of the lengths of the displacement difference vectors MAX_{disp}. The algorithms performance is compared to the widely used Demons [4] algorithm. Its implementation was taken from the Insight Segmentation and Registration Toolkit [1]. The Demons algorithm uses a five level multi-resolution framework to calculate a smooth displacement field with a fixed number of iterations per multi-resolution level (between 100 and 15 from coarse to fine) in a gradient-descent scheme. Fig. 5 a)-c) shows difference images of data set D which had the worst behavior in terms of decreasing the RMS of the intensity differences using the large simulated breathing deformation.

The second synthetic transformation is calculated using a number of evenly distributed landmark points and randomly assigning displacements to these landmarks. The amount of the displacement is increased up to the sampling size of the landmark distribution. These displacements are not physically motivated and the larger the assigned displacements are the harder it is to correct them. The dense synthetic displacement field is calculated using a TPS interpolation. Note that we use TPS interpolation here not TPS approximation. For data sets size 512x512x256 every 64 voxels a landmark is placed in the original image. This leads to a grid of 7x7x3 landmarks. Now a random displacement is calculated for each landmark coordinate in the range from -8 to +8 voxels. This is repeated five times while always doubling the displacement range. Evaluations are solely performed on data set B, Fig. 4 d)-g) shows the effect of these synthetic displacements. The main motivation of these experiments is to determine the degree of deformation where the algorithms are not capable to register the data anymore. Table 2 gives the results of these experiments.

3.2 Clinical Data

The algorithm was also evaluated on four clinical thoracic data sets consisting of two scans at different breathing states. The data sets show different problem characteristics. Data sets B and G differ by a small breathing deformation and intensity variations due to contrast agent application. Data set G additionally shows a lung disease in the upper lobe region. Data sets E and F differ by large breathing deformations and the images have intensity differences due to a lung disease making them very hard to register. For the clinical data no gold standard displacement was available for comparison, therefore solely the decrease in the RMS of the intensity differences before and after registration are calculated. Again the novel feature-based algorithm is compared with the Demons algorithm. The RMS of data set B was decreased from 201.57HU to 129HU (Demons) and to 104.83HU (feature-based). Data set E decreased from 403.49HU to 235.88HU and to 197.45HU, data set F from 413.62HU to 288.31HU and to 294.98HU and finally data set G from 367.66HU to 274.14HU and to 241.43HU. The numbers of found correspondences lies between 685 and 1632. For qualitative results difference images are shown in Fig. 5 d)-f) for data set B and g)-i) for data set E.

---

[1] http://www.itk.org

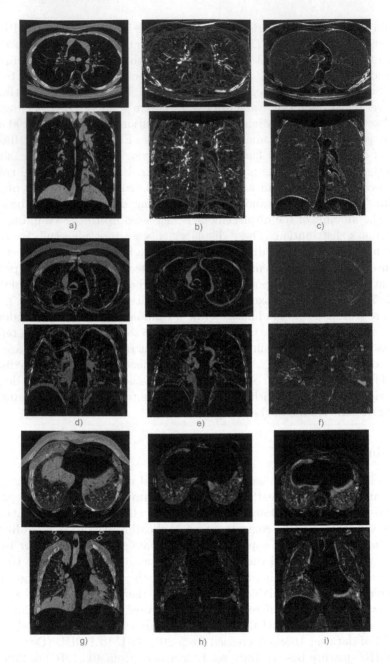

Fig. 5. Selected Results. Top row always axial, bottom row always sagittal slices. Left image shows difference image before, middle image after Demons and right image after feature-based registration. a)-c) shows synthetic results of data set D with a simulated breathing transformation of $t_{vertical} = 55$mm and $t_{inplane} = 25$mm. d)-f) shows results on real data set B, g)-i) on real data set E.

4   Discussion and Outlook

The different stages of the proposed feature-based algorithm require some parameters to be chosen. In the matching stage normalized local and global descriptors are used to form the matching cost function. A meaningful threshold T_d has to be found to exclude bad matches which was empirically chosen between 0.25 and 0.35. The matching stage also produces some outliers. The MAX_{disp} measures reflect this fact, especially in the matching evaluation. However, the registration stage with the approximating TPS framework takes the magnitude of the matching cost into account, such that outlier matches have a low influence on the final dense displacement field. Parameter λ of the TPS displacement field approximation was selected as $\lambda = 0.005$ after experimenting with several data sets. The LRTPS implementation needs a choice on the number of neighboring points that defines a local TPS, this parameter was set to 150.

The two goals of the proposed algorithm, to be faster and at least as accurate as a state-of-the-art nonlinear intensity-based registration algorithm, were both met. Computation time of the feature-based algorithm on the 512x512x256 data sets ranges between 1632s and 2282s, depending on the number of identified correspondences. The largest part (more than 50%) of the algorithm runtime still goes into the calculation of the dense displacement field. The Demons algorithm takes on average around 2540s for registration of two 512x512x256 data sets. If one further increases data sets size a feature-based algorithm will be even more efficient due to its inherent reduction of matching complexity.

Registration accuracy of the feature-based algorithm exceeds the Demons algorithm in most of the synthetic examples. Demons only performs better on the evenly distributed landmark TPS experiments with a high degree of random deformation where the feature-based approach is not able to find enough correspondences. However, these deformations are physically implausible and not representative. Especially the simulated breathing transformation was very accurately registered using the feature-based approach. This is reflected in the substantial decrease of the RMS of the intensity difference and the RMS of the displacement difference vector fields (in the order of 0.5mm to 2.0mm). The difference images of the simulated breathing experiment (Fig. 5) illustrate the problems of the Demons approach with the vascular structures. The real data experiments show that the performance of the feature-based algorithm is comparable to Demons. Performance on data sets B and G was better, while the performance on the very difficult data sets E and F is similar. Although Demons shows lower RMS values, the difference images of the feature-based approach have the same quality. However, the feature-based approach also has some problems with registration of vessel structures on the difficult data sets. The largest disadvantage of the feature-based approach is to get a large number of robust, evenly distributed feature matches. This can not be guaranteed in the current implementation, which explains the registration problems and can also lead to artifacts at the edges of the local TPS regions.

Future work will investigate methods to further speed-up the algorithm in its time-consuming stages. Another important point is to find a way to guarantee a good distribution of matching features. For evaluation a comparison with a more elaborate intensity-based registration approach will be performed. The fusion of this algorithm with a suitable intensity-based method seems to be a very promising direction, since the fast feature-based matching should provide a very good initial condition.

References

1. Wildberger, J.E., Klotz, E., Ditt, H., Mahnken, A.H., Spüntrup, E., Günther, R.W.: Multi-slice CT for Visualization of Acute Pulmonary Embolism: Single Breath-hold Subtraction Technique. Fortschritte auf dem Gebiet der Roentgenstrahlen und der bildgebenden Verfahren **177** (2005) 17–23
2. Maintz, J., Viergever, M.: A Survey of Medical Image Registration. Medical Image Analysis **2**(1) (1998) 1–36
3. Zitova, B., Flusser, J.: Image registration methods: A survey. Image and Vision Computing **21**(11) (2003) 977–1000
4. Thirion, J.P.: Image matching as a diffusion process: An analogy with Maxwell's demons. Medical Image Analysis **2**(3) (1998) 243–260
5. Förstner, W.: A Feature Based Correspondence Algorithm for Image Matching. Int. Arch. of Photogrammetry and Remote Sensing **26**(3) (1986) 150–166
6. Lowe, D.G.: Distinctive Image Features from Scale-Invariant Keypoints. International Journal on Computer Vision **60**(2) (2004) 91–110
7. Belongie, S., Malik, J., Puzicha, J.: Shape matching and object recognition using shape contexts. IEEE PAMI **24**(4) (2002) 509–522
8. Bookstein, F.: Principal Warps: Thin-Plate Splines and the Decomposition of Deformations. IEEE PAMI **11**(6) (1989) 567–585
9. Rohr, K.: Landmark-Based Image Analysis Using Geometric and Intensity Models. Computational Imaging and Vision. Kluwer Academic Publishers (2001)
10. Johnson, H.J., Christensen, G.E.: Consistent Landmark and Intensity-Based Image Registration. IEEE Transactions on Medical Imaging **21**(5) (2002) 450–461
11. Chui, H., Win, L., Schultz, R., Duncan, J., Rangarajan, A.: A unified non-rigid feature registration method for brain mapping. Medical Image Analysis **7** (2003) 113–130
12. Mortensen, E.N., Deng, H., Shapiro, L.: A SIFT Descriptor with Global Context. In: IEEE CVPR 2005. (2005) 184–190
13. Mikolajczyk, K., Schmid, C.: Performance Evaluation of Local Descriptors. IEEE PAMI **27**(10) (2005) 1615–1630
14. Fua, P.: A Parallel Stereo Algorithm that Produces Dense Depth Maps and Preserves Image Features. Machine Vision and Applications **6** (1993) 35–49

Consistent and Elastic Registration of Histological Sections Using Vector-Spline Regularization

Ignacio Arganda-Carreras[1,3], Carlos O.S. Sorzano[1,5], Roberto Marabini[1,3], José María Carazo[1], Carlos Ortiz-de-Solorzano[2], and Jan Kybic[4]

[1] Biocomputing Unit, National Centre of Biotechnology,
Universidad Autónoma de Madrid, 28049 Cantoblanco, Madrid, Spain
{iarganda, coss, roberto, carazo}@cnb.uam.es
http://biocomp.cnb.uam.es/
[2] Cancer Imaging Laboratory, Centre for Applied Medical Research (CIMA),
31008 Pamplona, Spain
codesolorzano@unav.es
http://www.cima.es/index_english.html
[3] Escuela Politécnica Superior, Universidad Autónoma de Madrid,
28049 Madrid, Spain
{Ignacio.Arganda, Roberto.Marabini}@uam.es
http://www.ii.uam.es/esp/welcomii.php?idioma=eng
[4] Center for Machine Perception, Czech Technical University,
121 35 Prague 2, Czech Republic
kybic@fel.cvut.cz
http://cmp.felk.cvut.cz/
[5] Escuela Politécnica Superior, Univ. San Pablo CEU, 28003 Madrid, Spain
coss.eps@ceu.es
http://www.uspceu.com/

Abstract. Here we present a new image registration algorithm for the alignment of histological sections that combines the ideas of B-spline based elastic registration and consistent image registration, to allow simultaneous registration of images in two directions (direct and inverse). In principle, deformations based on B-splines are not invertible. The consistency term overcomes this limitation and allows registration of two images in a completely symmetric way. This extension of the elastic registration method simplifies the search for the optimum deformation and allows registering with no information about landmarks or deformation regularization. This approach can also be used as the first step to solve the problem of group-wise registration. . . .

1 Introduction

Studying the three-dimensional organization of complex histological structures requires imaging, analyzing and registering large sets of images taken from serially sectioned tissue blocks. We have developed an integrated microscopy system that automates or greatly reduces the amount of interaction required for these tasks [1,2] and provides volumetric renderings of the structures in the tissue.

R.R. Beichel and M. Sonka (Eds.): CVAMIA 2006, LNCS 4241, pp. 85–95, 2006.

Proper section alignment is the first step towards an accurate 3D tissue reconstruction, as it is in other imaging modalities [3,4]. In our case we perform a coarse alignment of the sections using an automatic rigid-body registration method [5]. This method can not correct some non-linear distorting effects (e.g. tissue folding, stretching, tearing, etc.) caused by the manual sectioning process. Moreover, the distance between sections causes significant differences between the same structures of interest in consecutive sections, which could be misinterpreted by a complete linear registration process. Therefore, a non-linear or local method is strongly needed in order to refine the first registration step.

In this paper we present a new method for elastic and consistent registration of histological sections. All the examples described in the paper used mammary gland tissue samples; however, the same algorithm could be equally applied to other tissue sources and image modalities.

2   Methodology

The properties of B-splines have been largely proved to be very useful when modeling deformations in many biomedical imaging problems; such as tracking the movement of the left ventricle from MRI images [6], reconstructing the 3-D motion of the cardiac cycle [7] or modeling the motion of the breast by dynamic MR imaging [8].

The registration of a source image with a target image can be defined as the problem of finding a deformation field that transforms coordinates of the target image into coordinates of the source image. The main problem of using B-spline deformation fields is that the estimated field might not be invertible (which is not a problem since depending on the specific case, the true deformation field may not be invertible neither). However, in case it were invertible, the inverse deformation field can be computationally expensive. Either it is invertible or not, it is convenient to have also a way of transforming coordinates in the source image into coordinates of the target. This would define a second deformation field that is close to the inverse of the original field and it has proven to be useful as a way of regularizing the registration problem [9,10]. This two-way registration is known as consistent registration. [10] achieves the consistency by forcing the deformation field to be a diffeomorphism (continuous, differentiable, and invertible, its inverse must also be continuous and differentiable). This is a too strong constraint for our images, although it has the advantage of not having to compute two separate fields since the diffeomorphism condition automatically guarantees the existence of the deformation inverse. [9] computes two independent deformations whose composition should be as close as possible to the identity transformation. Thus, one is not the inverse of the other. This closeness to identity is explicitly introduced into the objective function.

In this work we combine the idea of elastic registration using vector-spline regularization [11] with that of a consistent registration [9]. We combine both ideas and extend them in order to overcome their limitations. The standard registration method presented in [11] propose the calculation of the elastic deformation field trough the minimization of an energy functional composed by three terms: the energy of the similarity error between both images (represented by the pixelwise mean-square distance), the error of the mapping of soft landmarks, and a regularization term based on the divergence and the curl of the deformation to ensure its smoothness. This minimization is optimized by a variant of the robust Levenberg-Marquardt method.

We transform the energy functional presented in [11] into a new functional that incorporates a factor of the deformation field consistency. Unlike in [11], we are now looking for two transformations at the same time (direct and inverse). Therefore, the vectors passed to the Levenberg-Marquardt optimizer are now twice as long. Besides the measurement of dissimilarity between the source and target images (now in both directions) E_{img}, the optional landmark constraint E_μ and the regularization term $(E_{\text{div}} + E_{\text{rot}})$, we add a new energy term E_{cons} that expresses the geometrical consistency between the elastic deformation in one direction (from source to target) and the other direction (from target to source). Therefore, the energy function is now given by

$$E = w_i E_{\text{img}} + w_\mu E_\mu + (w_d E_{\text{div}} + w_r E_{\text{rot}}) + w_c E_{\text{cons}} . \tag{1}$$

Where w_x are the specific weights given to the different energy terms.

2.1   Consistency Term

The consistency energy represents the geometrical distances between the pixel coordinates after applying both transformations (direct-inverse or inverse-direct), i.e. the amount by which the composed transformation differs from identity. The standard approach [11] for this type of registration is to find a deformation function

$$g^+(x) : \mathbb{R}^2 \to \mathbb{R}^2 . \tag{2}$$

This function transforms the source image I_s into an image as similar as possible to the target image I_s. This transformation g^+ maps coordinates in I_s into coordinates in I_t. Here, following [9], we will also simultaneously look for its corresponding inverse function

$$g^-(x) : \mathbb{R}^2 \to \mathbb{R}^2 . \tag{3}$$

This function maps the coordinates in I_t into coordinates in I_s.

Following this notation, our consistency energy term is given by

$$E_{\text{cons}} = E_{\text{cons}}^+ + E_{\text{cons}}^-$$
$$= \int_{\mathbf{x} \in \mathbb{R}^2} \|\mathbf{x} - g^-(g^+(\mathbf{x}))\|^2 \, d\mathbf{x} + \int_{\mathbf{x} \in \mathbb{R}^2} \|\mathbf{x} - g^+(g^-(\mathbf{x}))\|^2 d\mathbf{x} . \tag{4}$$

If we approximate the integrals by discrete sums and restrict the integration domain, we obtain

$$E_{\text{cons}}^+ = \frac{1}{\#\Omega^+} \sum_{\mathbf{x} \in \Omega^+} \|\mathbf{x} - g^-(g^+(\mathbf{x}))\|^2 . \tag{5}$$

$$E_{cons}^{-} = \frac{1}{\#\Omega^{-}} \sum_{\mathbf{x} \in \Omega^{-}} \|\mathbf{x} - g^{+}(g^{-}(\mathbf{x}))\|^2 \ . \tag{6}$$

Where , Ω^+, Ω^- define sets of relevant pixels common to the target and source images:

$$\Omega^+ = \left\{ \mathbf{x} \in \Omega_s \cap \mathbb{Z}^2 : g^+(\mathbf{x}) \in \Omega_t \cap \mathbb{Z}^2 \right\} \ . \tag{7}$$

$$\Omega^- = \left\{ \mathbf{x} \in \Omega_t \cap \mathbb{Z}^2 : g^-(\mathbf{x}) \in \Omega_s \cap \mathbb{Z}^2 \right\} \ . \tag{8}$$

And where $\#\Omega^+$ and $\#\Omega^-$ are the number of pixels in the masks.

2.2 Deformation Representation

Following [11] we represent the deformation fields as a linear combination of B-splines. For instance, g^+:

$$
\begin{aligned}
g^+(\mathbf{x}) &= g^+(x, y) \\
&= \left(g_1^+(x, y), g_2^+(x, y) \right) \\
&= \sum_{k,l \in \mathbb{Z}^2} \begin{pmatrix} c_{1,k,l}^+ \\ c_{2,k,l}^+ \end{pmatrix} \beta^3 \left(\frac{x}{s_x} - k \right) \beta^3 \left(\frac{y}{s_y} - l \right) \ .
\end{aligned} \tag{9}
$$

Where β^3 is the B-spline of degree 3, $c_{k,l}$ are the B-spline coefficients, and s_x and s_y are scalars (sampling steps) controlling the degree of detail of the representation of the deformation field.

2.3 Explicit Derivatives

The chosen optimizer uses gradient information. We will now calculate the derivatives of the energy function with respect to all the parameters, starting with E_{cons}. It can be easily shown that the derivative of E_{cons}^+ with respect to any of the deformation coefficients defining the first component (x in our case) of the direct deformation field g^+, is given by

$$\frac{\partial E_{cons}^+}{\partial c_{1,k,l}^+} = -2 \sum_{\mathbf{x} \in \Omega^+} \left(\mathbf{x} - g^-(g^+(\mathbf{x})) \right) \cdot \left(\frac{\partial}{\partial c_{1,k,l}^+} \left(g^-(g^+(\mathbf{x})) \right) \right) \ . \tag{10}$$

Where

$$\frac{\partial}{\partial c_{1,k,l}^+} \left(g^-(g^+(\mathbf{x})) \right) = \left(\left. \frac{\partial g_1^-}{\partial x} \right|_{x',y'}, \left. \frac{\partial g_2^-}{\partial y} \right|_{x',y'} \right) \left. \frac{\partial g_1^+}{\partial c_{1,k,l}^+} \right|_{x,y} \ . \tag{11}$$

And where

$$\mathbf{x} = (x, y) \ . \tag{12}$$

And

$$(x, y) = g^+(x, y) \ . \tag{13}$$

Again, following the definition of the transformation function we express its derivative with respect to the coefficients of the first component as

$$\frac{\partial g_1^+(x, y)}{\partial c_{1,k,l}^+} = \beta^3 \left(\frac{x}{s_x} - k \right) \beta^3 \left(\frac{y}{s_y} - l \right) \ . \tag{14}$$

This derivative is the same in the case of the second component.

The derivative of E_{cons}^+ with respect to any of the deformation coefficients of the second component of the direct deformation field is calculated in an analogous way.

Let us see now the derivate of E_{cons}^+ with respect to the coefficients of the first component of the inverse transformation:

$$\frac{\partial E_{\text{cons}}^+}{\partial c_{1,k,l}^-} = -2 \sum_{\mathbf{x} \in \Omega^+} \left(\mathbf{x} - g^-(g^+(\mathbf{x})) \right) \cdot \left(\frac{\partial}{\partial c_{1,k,l}^-} \left(g^-(g^+(\mathbf{x})) \right) \right) \ . \tag{15}$$

Where

$$\frac{\partial}{\partial c_{1,k,l}^+} \left(g^-(g^+(\mathbf{x})) \right) = \frac{\partial}{\partial c_{1,k,l}^+} \left(g^-(x', y') \right) = \beta^3 \left(\frac{x'}{s_x} - k \right) \beta^3 \left(\frac{y'}{s_y} - l \right) \ . \tag{16}$$

The derivative of E_{cons}^+ with respect to any of the deformation coefficients of the second component of the inverse deformation field can be calculated in an analogous way. The derivatives of E_{cons}^- are easily inferred in a similar way. We refer to the original article [11] for the derivatives of E_{img}, E_μ and $(E_{\text{div}} + E_{\text{rot}})$.

3   Choice of w_c

All the energy terms of the functional represent different measurements over the images or the deformations, thus presenting different units. Therefore, the terms are not comparable and a weight term is needed. We determined the optimum value experimentally. While value of zero is useful to compare results with the previous algorithm, weight values around 10.0-30.0 often showed the best compromise between the final similarity and the deformation consistency for our images. Higher values make the consistency constraint too rigid and consequently decrease the images similarity. Lower values cause the lack of relevance between g^+ and g^- in the optimization process and thus do not achieve symmetric transformations. Fig. 1 shows the evolution of the similarity and consistency errors with respect to w_c. The consistency error decreases with the weight but causes a significant increase in the similarity error when approaching to values close to 100. The similarity error is defined as the energy of the difference between the target and the warped source image, while the consistency error is the consistency energy explained above.

For the rest of weight terms we refer to [11]. From our own experience we recommend to set w_i to 1.0 and if necessary, w_μ to 1.0 and w_d and w_r to 0.1.

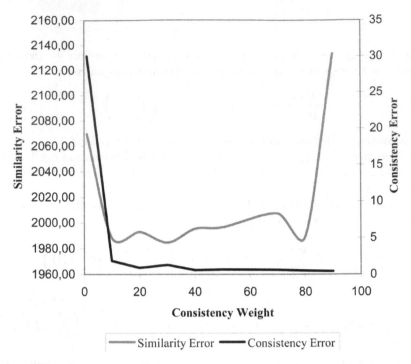

Fig. 1. Evolution of the similarity and consistency error with increasing values of the consistency weight

4   Results

To evaluate our algorithm we tested its performance using synthetic images. We applied some known deformations to the images and then checked whether our method could correct the deformation. That also allowed us to compare our algorithm with the standard one [11]. For instance, in Fig. 2 we have registered a Lena picture with a deformed version of the same image. In this case, the standard method properly registers the deformed image with the original one, but is unable to find the inverse deformation field without using soft landmarks, regularization values and a specific image mask. In the same example, our algorithm finds simultaneously both deformation fields (direct and inverse) using only the similarity term and the consistency term of the energy function.

Fig. 3, 4, and 5 contain a relevant example of the results obtained applying our algorithm compared to the results obtained with the original method (lacking the consistency term) using two consecutive histological sections from breast cancer tissue.

Fig. 4 shows the deformation fields calculated with both methods. It is easy to see how our method guarantees the consistency between the direct and the inverse transformation while the traditional method does not.

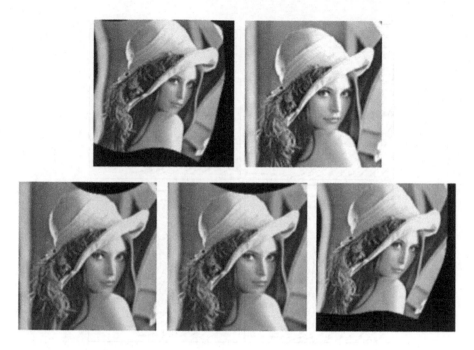

Fig. 2. From top to down, left to right: source image, target image, registered source image (by the standard method), registered source image (by our new method), registered target image (by our new method)

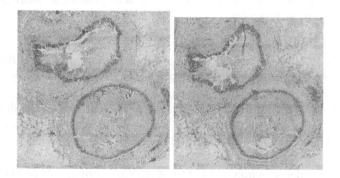

Fig. 3. Two consecutive histological sections from a human biopsy presenting two big tumors

In Fig. 5 we show the result of subtracting the deformed source and target images. We can appreciate how for the inverse transformation our method achieves a much better result than the standard method, as we expected by observing the deformation fields on Fig. 4. These results were also evaluated numerically obtaining an average of similarity error 31.63 of and 32.68 for the deformations calculated with the original method (direct-inverse and inverse-direct) and an average

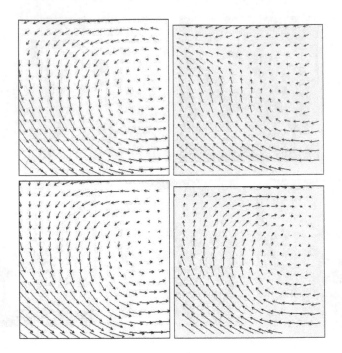

Fig. 4. Comparison of the deformation fields obtained with the original method described in [11] and our new algorithm over the images in Figure 2. The first row shows the deformation when registering image 1 to 2 (left) and image 2 to 1 (right), applying the traditional energy functional. The second row shows the same deformations when using the proposed improvement.

of 31.48 and 31.66 for the deformations of our new method. The differences between the inverse-direct averages provoke visible changes on the registration as shown in the deformation fields representations on Fig. 4.

The gray-scale sample images in Fig. 3 have respectively 325x325 pixels and 300x312 pixels and it took 18 seconds to properly register them in an Intel Pentium M, 1.60 GHz, 589 MHz, 512MB of RAM memory, under a SuSE Linux system.

Fig. 6 is another example with breast tissue sample where the standard method is unable to approach any proper deformation between the source and target images based in the images similarity but where our new method achieves easily the right deformation thanks to the consistency term.

As inferred from the experimental results using our bidirectional method, in most cases only the similarity and the consistency term are needed to achieve a proper registration. This involves a simplification of the energy functional to be minimized and therefore, a reduction in the computational time and complexity. At the same time, forgetting about placing soft landmarks in the images allows us reducing the human interaction in the registration process, which is another advantage of our algorithm over the previous method.

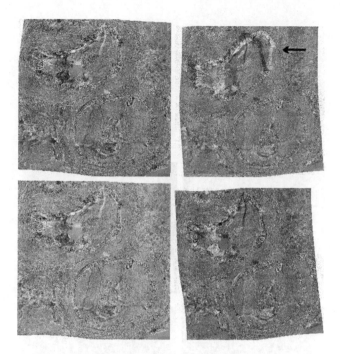

Fig. 5. The top row shows the subtractions of the deformed images and the target ones in both senses, using the traditional method. The bottom row shows the result when applying our method. The black arrow points the most relevant error committed by the standard method.

5   Conclusion and Future Work

A new algorithm for consistent elastic registration has been presented. It combines the ideas of elastic image registration based on B-splines models and consistent image registration. The method improves the results obtained without the consistency factor in the energy function, as it has been qualitative and numerically shown in the results section, and accelerates the search for the optimum. We are aware that a more detailed quantitative evaluation of the algorithm is necessary. This evaluation is currently in progress.

This method can be extended increasing the number of images involved in the registration to do group-wise registration. For this case, the explicit derivatives must be recalculated and a method for composing the deformation fields needs to be proposed.

Acknowledgments

Ignacio Arganda-Carreras is being supported by a predoctoral FPI-CAM fellowship since October 2003. Carlos Ortiz-de-Solorzano is supported by a Ramon y Cajal (Spanish Ministry of Education and Science ryc-2004-002353)

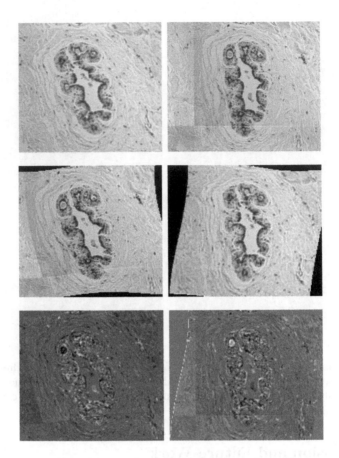

Fig. 6. Example with two transversals cuts of a mammary duct. From top to down, left to right: source image, target image, registered target image, registered source image, difference source image, difference target image.

and a Marie Curie International Reintegration Grant (FP6-518688). Jan Kybic was sponsored by the Czech Ministery of Education under project number MSM210000012. Partial support is acknowledged to Comunidad de Madrid through grant GR/SAL/0234, to Instituto de Salud Carlos III-Fondo de Investigaciones Sanitarias (FIS) through the IM3 Network and grant 040683 and to the Plan Nacional de Investigación Científica, Desarrollo e Innovación Tecnológica (I+D+I).

References

1. Fernandez-Gonzalez, R., Jones, A., Garcia-Rodriguez, E., Chen, P.Y., Idica, A., Barcellos-Hoff, M.H. and Ortiz-de-Solorzano, C.: "A System for Combined Three-Dimensional Morphological and Molecular Analysis of Thick Tissue Speciments", Microscope Research and Technique 59(6): 522-530, 2002.

2. Fernandez-Gonzalez, R., Deschamps, T., Idica, A., Malladi, R. and Ortiz-de-Solorzano, C.: "Automatic segmentation of histological structures in mammary gland tissue sections", Journal of Biomedical Optics, vol. 9, pp. 444-453, 2004.
3. Hajnal, J. V., Hill, D. L. G., and Hawkes, D. J.: Eds., Medical image registration, CRC Press, 2001.
4. Maintz, J. B. A. and Viergever, M. A.: "A survey of medical image registration", Medical Image Analysis, vol. 2, no. 1, pp. 1-36, 1998.
5. Arganda-Carreras, I., Fernandez-Gonzalez, R. and Ortiz-de-Solorzano, C.: "Automatic Registration of Serial Mammary Gland Sections", The 26th International Conference of the IEEE Engineering in Medicine and Biology Society (EMBS), 1-5th September, 2004, San Francisco, California.
6. Radeva, P., Amini, A. A., Huang, J.: "Deformable B-Solids and Implicit Snakes for 3D Localization and Tracking of SPAMM MIR Data", Computer Vision and Image Understanding, vol. 66, no. 2, May, pp. 163-178, 1997.
7. Huang, J., Abendschein D., Dávila-Román V. G., Amini, A. A.: "Spatio-Temporal Tracking of Myocardial Deformations with a 4-D B-Spline Model from Tagged MRI", IEEE Transactions on Medical Imaging, vol. 18, no. 10, October 1999.
8. Rueckert, D., Sonoda L. I., Hayes, C., Hill, D. L. G., Leach, M. O., Hawkes D. J.: "Nonrigid Registration Using Free-Form Deformations: Application to Breast MR Images", IEEE Transactions on Medical Imaging, vol. 18, no. 8, August 1999.
9. Christensen, G.E. and He, J.: "Consistent nonlinear elastic image registration", Mathematical Methods in Biomedical Image Analysis, MMBIA 2001, IEEE.
10. Avants, B. B., Schoenemann, P. T., Gee, J. C.: "Lagrangian frame diffeomorphic image registration: Morphometric comparison of human and chimpanzee cortex", Medical Image Analysis (in press).
11. Sorzano, C.O.S., Thévenaz, P. and Unser, M.: "Elastic Registration of Biological Images Using Vector-Spline Regularization", IEEE Transactions on Biomedical Engineering, vol. 52, no. 4, pp. 652-663, April 2005.

Comparative Analysis of Kernel Methods
for Statistical Shape Learning

Yogesh Rathi, Samuel Dambreville, and Allen Tannenbaum*

Georgia Institute of Technology, Atlanta, GA, 30332, USA
{yogesh.rathi, samuel.dambreville, tannenba}@bme.gatech.edu

Abstract. Prior knowledge about shape may be quite important for image segmentation. In particular, a number of different methods have been proposed to compute the statistics on a set of training shapes, which are then used for a given image segmentation task to provide the shape prior. In this work, we perform a comparative analysis of shape learning techniques such as linear PCA, kernel PCA, locally linear embedding and propose a new method, kernelized locally linear embedding for doing shape analysis. The surfaces are represented as the zero level set of a signed distance function and shape learning is performed on the embeddings of these shapes. We carry out some experiments to see how well each of these methods can represent a shape, given the training set.

1 Introduction

Image Segmentation has been a topic of extensive research in the computer vision community [1,2,3,4].One of the challenges in the field of image segmentation is the incorporation of prior shape knowledge in the segmentation process [5]. Many different methods (using both parameterized or implicit representation of shapes) have been proposed [6,7,8,9,10] to perform statistical shape analysis on a given set of training shapes. In this work, we perform a comparative analysis of several key techniques such as linear PCA (LPCA), kernel PCA (KPCA), locally linear embedding (LLE), and then propose a new method, kernelized locally linear embedding (KLLE) which will be compared with the aforementioned techniques.

There is a large body of literature available for representing a curve or surface using parameterized as well as implicit methods; see [3,11,12] and the references therein. A number of methods have been proposed, using these representations, to study the statistical variations in a given set of training shapes. Cootes *et al.* [6] developed a parametric point distribution model for describing the segmenting curve by using linear combinations of eigenvectors that reflect variations from the mean

* This research was supported by grants from NSF, NIH (NAC P41 RR-13218 through Brigham and Women's Hospital), AFOSR, ARO, MURI, and MRI-HEL, and the Technion, Israel Insitute of Technology. This work was done under the auspices of the National Alliance for Medical Image Computing (NAMIC), funded by the National Institutes of Health through the NIH Roadmap for Medical Research, Grant U54 EB005149.

R.R. Beichel and M. Sonka (Eds.): CVAMIA 2006, LNCS 4241, pp. 96–107, 2006.
© Springer-Verlag Berlin Heidelberg 2006

shape. In [13], Wang and Staib developed a statistical point model by applying linear PCA to the covariance matrices that capture the statistical variations of the landmark points. Recently, Leventon [9] proposed a more general model wherein PCA was performed on a set of signed distance functions. Kernel PCA has been successfully used by the machine learning community for pattern recognition and image denoising [14]. A Gaussian kernel was used by Cremers et al. [8] for learning shape statistics in the kernel space to provide shape prior for segmentation tasks. Finding the pre-image of the projection in the kernel space is one of the challenging tasks in visualizing and computing the performance of these kernel based techniques. In this work, we use the method proposed by [15] to find the pre-image of the projection in the KPCA space and compare it with LPCA.

Locally linear embedding has been widely used for dimensionality reduction and extracting out the nonlinearities in the training data set. In this work, we use LLE to represent a given shape using a linear combination of its nearest neighbors. We further develop this algorithm and propose a new method to perform LLE in the kernel space, called KLLE, and show that it is better than LLE, LPCA and is comparable to KPCA in terms of performance but with fewer computations. Of course, the literature reviewed above is by no means exhaustive. We merely want to point out a new technique that has some attractive features which may act as an alternative to some already existing methodologies.

The rest of the paper is organized as follows: In the next section we briefly describe LPCA, KPCA, LLE and provide details about KLLE. In section 3, we show with examples how well each of these methods perform on a given data set. Section 4 gives conclusion and future research directions.

2 Statistical Models

This section briefly describes each of the shape learning techniques used later in the sequel. Let τ be the training set $\tau = \{\phi_1, \phi_2, \ldots, \phi_n\}$ consisting of n signed distance functions (SDF) with the shapes represented by the corresponding zero level sets. It is assumed that all the ϕ_i's are aligned using a suitable method of registration [6].

2.1 Linear PCA

Linear PCA is widely used to learn the statistical variations of a given set of data (shapes, in our case). LPCA assumes that the set of permissible shapes form a Gaussian distribution, i.e., all possible shapes can be written as a linear combination of a set of eigenshapes obtained by doing principal component analysis on the training data set [10,9]. The eigenshapes can be obtained as follows: Let ϕ_i represent the signed distance function corresponding to the surface S_i. The mean surface, μ, is computed by taking the mean of the signed distance functions, $\mu = \frac{1}{n} \sum \phi_i$. The variance in shape is computed using PCA, i.e., the mean shape μ is subtracted from each ϕ_i to create a mean-offset map $\bar{\phi}_i$. Each such map, $\bar{\phi}_i$, is placed as a column vector in an $N^d \times n$-dimensional matrix M, where $\phi_i \in \mathbf{R}^{N^d}$. Using Singular Value Decomposition (SVD), the covariance matrix $\frac{1}{n}MM^T$ is decomposed as:

$$U\Sigma U^T = \frac{1}{n}MM^T \qquad (1)$$

where U is a matrix whose column vectors represent the set of orthogonal modes of shape variation (eigenshapes) and Σ is a diagonal matrix of corresponding eigenvalues. An estimate of a novel shape Φ of the same class of object can be obtained from m principal components using an m-dimensional vector of coefficients,

$$\alpha = U_m^T(\Phi - \mu), \qquad (2)$$

where U_m is a matrix consisting of the first m columns of U. Given the coefficients α, an estimate of the shape Φ, namely $\tilde{\Phi}$, can be obtained as [9,10]:

$$\tilde{\Phi} = U_m\alpha + \mu. \qquad (3)$$

2.2   Kernel PCA

Kernel methods, in particular, kernel PCA has been the focus of research in the pattern recognition community[16,17]. The basic idea behind these methods is to map the data in the input space $\phi \in \chi$ to a feature space F via some nonlinear map Ψ, and then apply a linear method in F to do further analysis. Kernel PCA [14] is a nonlinear feature extractor, where PCA is performed in the feature space F which is equivalent to doing nonlinear PCA in the input space χ. Since the nonlinear map Ψ is not known, a challenging problem is to find the pre-image of the projection obtained by doing PCA in the feature space F. As demonstrated by Mika [16], the exact pre-image typically may not exist and one can only settle for an approximate solution. But even this may be non-trivial as the dimensionality of the feature space can be infinite. For certain invertible kernels, this nonlinear problem can be solved using a fixed-point iteration method as proposed by Scholkopf and Mika [14,16]. However, this method is dependent on the initial starting point and is highly susceptible to local minima. To circumvent this problem, [17] and more recently [15] proposed an algorithm to reconstruct an approximate pre-image of the projection as described briefly in the remainder of this section.

Kernel PCA performs the traditional linear PCA in the feature space corresponding to the kernel $k(.,.)$. The kernel defines the inner product between two points in the feature space, i.e., $k(\phi_1, \phi_2) = <\Psi(\phi_1), \Psi(\phi_2)>$. This fact can be used to obtain the eigenvectors in the feature space F even though the non-linear map Ψ is unknown. Analogous to linear PCA, it involves the following eigen-decomposition

$$HKH = U\Sigma U^T,$$

where, K is the kernel matrix with entries $K_{ij} = k(\phi_i, \phi_j)$, H is the centering matrix given by

$$H = I - \frac{1}{n}\mathbf{1}\mathbf{1}^T,$$

I is the $n \times n$ identity matrix, $\mathbf{1} = [11...1]^T$ is an $n \times 1$ vector, $U = [\mathbf{a}_1, ..., \mathbf{a}_n]$ with $\mathbf{a}_i = [a_{i1}, ..., a_{in}]^T$ is the matrix containing the eigenvectors and $\Sigma = diag(\lambda_1, ..., \lambda_n)$ contains the corresponding eigenvalues. Denote the mean of the Ψ-mapped data by $\bar{\Psi} = \frac{1}{n} \sum_{i=1}^{n} \Psi(\phi_i)$ and define the "centered" map $\tilde{\Psi}$ as :

$$\tilde{\Psi}(\phi) = \Psi(\phi) - \bar{\Psi}.$$

The k-th orthonormal eigenvector of the covariance matrix in the feature space can then be shown to be [14]

$$V_k = \sum_{i=1}^{n} \frac{a_{ki}}{\sqrt{\lambda_k}} \tilde{\Psi}(\phi_i).$$

Denote the projection of the Ψ-image of a test point Φ onto the k-th component by β_k. Then,

$$\beta_k = \frac{1}{\sqrt{\lambda_k}} \sum_{i=1}^{n} a_{ki} \tilde{k}(\Phi, \phi_i), \tag{4}$$

where,

$$\tilde{k}(x, y) = <\tilde{\Psi}(x), \tilde{\Psi}(y)> = k(x, y) - \frac{1}{n} \mathbf{1}^T k_x - \frac{1}{n} \mathbf{1}^T k_y + \frac{1}{n^2} \mathbf{1}^T K \mathbf{1}$$

$$\text{with} \quad k_x = [k(x, \phi_1), ..., k(x, \phi_n)]^T \tag{5}$$

The projection of $\Psi(\Phi)$ onto the subspace spanned by the first m eigenvectors is given by :

$$P\Psi(\Phi) = \sum_{k=1}^{m} \beta_k V_k + \bar{\Psi}$$

To obtain an approximate pre-image of $P\Psi(\Phi)$ in the input space, we minimize the error $\rho(\hat{\Phi}) = \| \Psi(\hat{\Phi}) - P\Psi(\Phi) \|^2$. Following the exposition in [15], for a Gaussian kernel (also known as radial basis function) given by :

$$k(\phi_i, \phi_j) = e^{-\frac{d^2(\phi_i, \phi_j)}{2\sigma^2}} \tag{6}$$

where $d^2(\phi_i, \phi_j)$ is a distance measure in the input space, one can obtain an approximate pre-image by setting $\nabla_{\hat{\Phi}} \rho = 0$ and using the approximation $\Psi(\hat{\Phi}) \approx P\Psi(\Phi)$. Here, we directly state the result for finding the pre-image $\hat{\Phi}$ (in the input space χ) of the projection $P\Psi(\Phi)$ [15]:

$$\hat{\Phi} = \frac{\sum_{i=1}^{n} \tilde{\gamma}_i \left(\frac{1}{2}(2 - \tilde{d}^2(P\Psi(\Phi), \Psi(\phi_i))) \right) \phi_i}{\sum_{i=1}^{n} \tilde{\gamma}_i \left(\frac{1}{2}(2 - \tilde{d}^2(P\Psi(\Phi), \Psi(\phi_i))) \right)} \tag{7}$$

where $\gamma_i = \sum_{k=1}^{n} \beta_k a_{ki}$ and $\tilde{\gamma}_i = \gamma_i + \frac{1}{n}(1 - \sum_{j=1}^{n} \gamma_j)$ and $\tilde{d}^2$ can be computed only in terms of the kernel using the following expression [15,17]:

$$
\tilde{d}^2(\Psi(\phi_i), P\Psi(\Phi)) = \left(k_\Phi + \frac{1}{n}K\mathbf{1} - 2k_{\phi_i} \right)^T H^T M H \left(k_\Phi - \frac{1}{n}K\mathbf{1} \right)
$$
$$
+ \frac{1}{n^2}\mathbf{1}^T K\mathbf{1} + K_{ii} - \frac{2}{n}\mathbf{1}^T k_{\phi_i} \tag{8}
$$

where $M = \sum_{k=1}^{n} \frac{1}{\lambda_k} \mathbf{a}_k \mathbf{a}_k^T$ and $K_{ii} = k(\phi_i, \phi_i)$.

In this work, we have used the following shape similarity measure given by [18]:

$$
d^2(\phi_i, \phi_j) = \int_{p \in Z(\phi_i)} EDT_{\phi_j}(p)dp + \int_{p \in Z(\phi_j)} EDT_{\phi_i}(p)dp, \tag{9}
$$

where EDT_{ϕ_i} is the Euclidean distance function of the zero level set of ϕ_i (one can think of it as the absolute value of ϕ_i), and $Z(\phi_i)$ is the zero level set of ϕ_i. This distance measure allows for partial shape matching and was shown [15] to perform better (empirically) than the Euclidean L_2 norm. Note that, $\hat{\Phi}$ is only an approximate pre-image of the projection, since an exact pre-image may not exist.

If we use the kernel $k(\phi_i, \phi_j) = <\phi_i, \phi_j>$, then KPCA is equivalent to doing LPCA. Thus, linear PCA is a particular case of kernel PCA. Choosing the right kernel for a given data set is a topic of active research. In this work we have used the Gaussian kernel (6), which is the most commonly used kernel in the machine learning community.

2.3   Locally Linear Embedding

The LLE algorithm [19] is based on certain simple geometric principles. Suppose the data consists of n vectors ϕ_i sampled from some smooth underlying manifold. Provided there is sufficient data, we expect each data point and its neighbors to lie on or close to a locally linear patch of the manifold. We can characterize the local geometry of these patches by a set of coefficients that reconstruct each data point from its neighbors. In the simplest formulation of LLE, one identifies k nearest neighbors for a data point. Reconstruction error is then measured by the cost function: $E(W) = \left(\Phi - \sum_j w_j \phi_j \right)^2$. We seek to minimize the reconstruction error $E(W)$, subject to the constraint that the weights w_j that lie outside the neighborhood are zero and $\sum_j w_j = 1$. With these constraints, the weights for points in the neighborhood of Φ can be obtained as [20]:

$$
E(W) = \left(\Phi - \sum_{j=1}^{k} w_j \phi_j \right)^2 = \sum_{j=1}^{k} \sum_{m=1}^{k} w_j w_m Q_{jm} \Rightarrow w_j = \frac{\sum_{m=1}^{k} R_{jm}}{\sum_{p=1}^{k} \sum_{q=1}^{k} R_{pq}},
$$

$$
\text{where } Q_{jm} = (\Phi - \phi_j)^T (\Phi - \phi_m) \quad \text{and} \quad R = Q^{-1}. \tag{10}
$$

In applications where dimensionality reduction is the major objective, one proceeds further and computes a low dimensional vector corresponding to each ϕ_i, preserving the neighborhood structure by keeping the weights w_j constant [20]. This work uses LLE only for obtaining the neighborhood structure in the training set and not for dimensionality reduction. Thus, we assume that a closed surface S can be represented by a linear combination of its k nearest neighbors. Stacking all the columns of ϕ_i one below the other, one can obtain a vector of dimension D^2, if ϕ_i is of dimension $D \times D$. Thus, given a test point Φ, one can obtain the weights using equation (10) that minimize the reconstruction error $E(W)$. The nearest neighbors are obtained from the training set by finding the squared distance d^2 (equation 9) between Φ and each of the shapes ϕ_i in the training set.

2.4   Kernel LLE

Mercer kernels have been used quite successfully for learning in Support Vector Machines (SVM) and in KPCA as mentioned before. The above LLE algorithm can be generalized for nonlinear manifolds by employing the kernel trick [14]. In [21], the author compares the discriminative power of LLE, KLLE and LPCA by projecting the training data to a lower dimensional space and thereby comparing the recognition rate of a given test sample. The methods presented in this work are quite different than those proposed in [21], since we do not compute a low dimensional data for LLE or KLLE, but compare their performances in the input space itself. This is quite essential for shape analysis in which one needs to compute how accurately a given data point can be reproduced in the input space using these techniques. Thus, the method proposed in [21] uses LLE, KLLE only for classification purposes, while we utilize it to see its performance in the input space. A major contribution of this work is the formulation of a method to find the pre-image of the projection in the kernel space, given the fact that we do not know the mapping Ψ.

The basic idea behind KLLE is to minimize the error (given a test point Φ) $E(W) = \left(\Psi(\Phi) - \sum_j w_j \Psi(\phi_j) \right)^2$. Proceeding as shown in LLE before, we get the following expression for the weights:

$$w_j = \frac{\sum_{m=1}^k R_{jm}}{\sum_{p=1}^k \sum_{q=1}^k R_{pq}} \quad \text{where,}$$

$$Q_{jm} = (\Psi(\Phi) - \Psi(\phi_j))^T (\Psi(\Phi) - \Psi(\phi_m)) = k(\Phi, \Phi) - k(\Phi, \phi_m)$$
$$- k(\Phi, \phi_j) + k(\phi_j, \phi_m) \quad \text{and} \quad R = Q^{-1}. \tag{11}$$

The weights w_j so obtained minimize the error $E(W)$ in the feature space F, i.e., $\Psi(\Phi) = \sum_{j=1}^k w_j \Psi(\phi_j) + \sqrt{E} = \Psi(\hat{\Phi}) + \sqrt{E}$. Assuming E to be small, we have $\Psi(\Phi) \approx \Psi(\hat{\Phi})$. Our goal now is to find the pre-image of $\Psi(\Phi)$. However, an exact pre-image of $\Psi(\Phi)$ may not exist [16], hence we find an approximate pre-image of $\Psi(\Phi)$ in the input space χ. Thus, we want to find the point $\Psi(z)$ which is closest to $\Psi(\Phi)$ and for which the pre-image can be computed. This can be achieved by minimizing the following:

$$\rho(z) = \| \Psi(z) - \Psi(\Phi) \|^2 \approx k(z, z) - 2 \sum_j w_j k(z, \phi_j) + k(\Phi, \Phi),$$

where we have substituted the approximation for $\Psi(\Phi)$. Setting $\nabla_z \rho(z) = 0$ and using the kernel $k(z, \Phi) = \exp(-\frac{\|z-\Phi\|^2}{2\sigma^2})$, one gets the following expression for finding z:

$$z = \frac{\sum_{j=1}^{k} w_j k(z, \phi_j) \, \phi_j}{\sum_{j=1}^{k} w_j k(z, \phi_j)} \tag{12}$$

This equation contains z on both sides of the equation and hence can be solved by fixed-point iteration technique. However, the solution will depend on the starting point and will be very susceptible to local minima. A unique (but approximate) solution to z can be found by noting that

$$k(z, \phi_j) = \; < \Psi(z), \Psi(\phi_j) > \; \approx \; < \Psi(\Phi), \Psi(\phi_j) > \; = \; k(\Phi, \phi_j)$$

where we assume $\Psi(\Phi) \approx \Psi(z)$. Note that this assumption is valid since we are trying to find the point $\Psi(z)$ that is closest to $\Psi(\Phi)$. The error in the computed pre-image will be proportional to the error in approximating $\Psi(z) = \Psi(\Phi)$, which in general can be assumed to be small. As shown in [15], better results can be obtained if the distance measure (9) (for d^2) is used in the Gaussian kernel instead of the Euclidean L_2 norm and hence we use it in all our experiments as described in the next section.

A pre-image can be computed not only for a Gaussian kernel, but for any invertible kernel. If we assume a polynomial kernel $k(\phi_i, \phi_j) = \left(c + \phi_i^T \phi_j\right)^d$, where d is the degree of the polynomial and c is any constant, then the pre-image z of a point $\Psi(\Phi)$ is given by

$$z = \frac{\sum_{j=1}^{k} w_j k(\Phi, \phi_j)^{\frac{d-1}{d}} \, \phi_j}{k(\Phi, \Phi)^{\frac{d-1}{d}}} \tag{13}$$

Thus, LLE is a particular case of KLLE with a polynomial kernel of degree $d = 1$ and $c = 0$. Once again, the k nearest neighbors can be computed using the distance relation (9) or any other metric on the space of shapes [22,11,7,23,24,25].

3   Experiments

In this section, we describe two experiments to test how well each method performs given a training set of shapes. The first set of 3D shapes consists of the left caudate nucleus and the second set consists of the left hippocampus. These are structures in the brain for which a shape prior is often used in segmentation algorithms. A typical measure to test the performance of these methods is to see how well an unknown shape gets projected by each of these methods. In this work, a quantitative measure was calculated by finding the number of voxels that got mislabelled, i.e., by finding the set symmetric difference between the projection and the original test shape.

The training set for the caudate nuclei consisted of 26 elements, each of them embedded in a signed distance function. Figure 1 shows a few shapes in the training set. In Figure 2, an "unseen shape" (i.e., a shape not in the training set) is shown and also the pre-image of the projection using each of the methods. Table 1 shows the number of mislabeled voxels for each of the methods. For LPCA and KPCA, 20 coefficients were used in finding the projection while for LLE and KLLE 20 nearest neighbors were used so that we do not obtain biased results in favor of a particular method. Clearly, the kernel methods perform better than their linear counterparts. More specifically, KLLE performs almost as well or better than KPCA, but with a smaller computational burden.

Table 1. Mislabelled voxels for left caudate nucleus

Volume	Volume Size	LPCA	LLE	KPCA	KLLE
1	2750	119	50	**37**	42
2	3774	134	105	92	**81**
3	2489	108	66	57	**52**

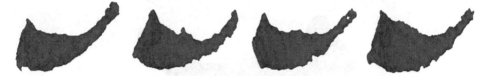

Fig. 1. Sample shapes of left Caudate nucleus from the training set

The second training set of the hippocampii data contained 22 elements. Figure 3 shows a few shapes from the training set and figure 4 shows the original and pre-images of projection for each of the methods. For this experiment, we used 15 coefficients for LPCA and KPCA and 15 nearest neighbors for LLE and KLLE. Table 2 gives the number of mislabelled voxels for each of the methods. Figure 5 shows the weights assigned to each of the neighbors (for all the three test shapes) using LLE and KLLE. Clearly, KLLE assigns larger weights to points closer to the test shape than to points farther away. Thus, only points in the locally linear patch of the feature space are assigned significant weights, whereas other points are assigned weights close to zero. This nonlinear distribution is expected since we used a Gaussian kernel. Once again, it is clear that KLLE performs better than all the other methods. It should be noted that, LLE and KLLE can perform even better with the proper choice of the number of nearest neighbors as given in [20]. To make a fair assessment of each method, we kept k (nearest neighbors) fixed and did not optimize the algorithm as given in [20].

Table 2. Mislabelled voxels for left hippocampus

Volume	Volume Size	LPCA	LLE	KPCA	KLLE
1	1117	440	378	322	**296**
2	1108	306	258	212	**205**
3	1568	804	574	494	**371**

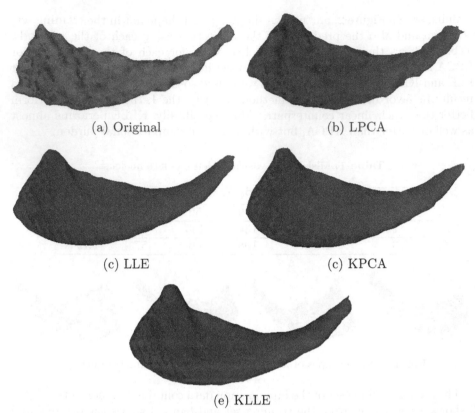

(a) Original   (b) LPCA

(c) LLE   (c) KPCA

(e) KLLE

Fig. 2. Projection of left Caudate nucleus (Volume 1) using each of the methods

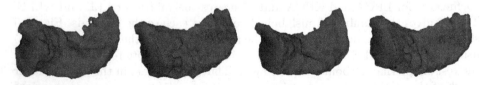

Fig. 3. Sample shapes of left hippocampus from the training set

In all of the experiments above, the parameter σ used in the Gaussian kernel was fixed to be some function of the average minimum distance between shapes in the training set [8], i.e., $\sigma^2 = c \frac{1}{n} \sum_{i=1}^{n} \min_{j \neq i} d^2(\phi_i, \phi_j)$., where c is a user defined real number. The training data (hand segmented shapes) was obtained from the NAMIC data repository of the Brigham and Women's Hospital, Boston, MA. The entire code was written in C++ using the ITK and VTK libraries.

4   Remarks

In this paper, we have proposed a new algorithm for finding an approximate pre-image of a point in the kernel space in the context of Kernel LLE which

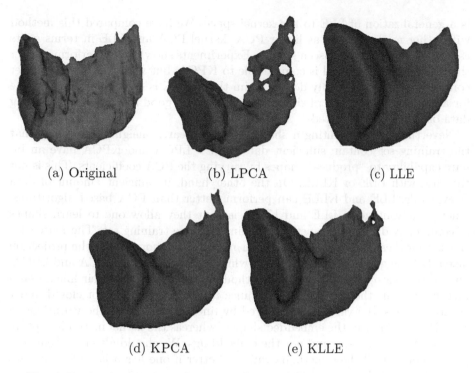

(a) Original   (b) LPCA   (c) LLE

(d) KPCA   (e) KLLE

Fig. 4. Projection of left Hippocampus (Volume 3) using each of the methods

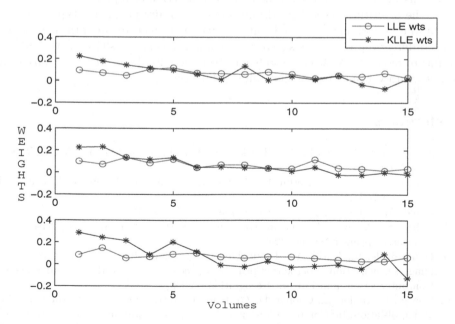

Fig. 5. Weights assigned to the 15 nearest neighbors by LLE and KLLE for each of the test shapes of hippocampus. On the x-axis, 1 is the closest neighbor, 15 is the farthest.

is a generalization of LLE to the kernel space. We have compared this method with other methods such as linear PCA, kernel PCA and LLE in terms of its capability to represent unseen shapes. Experiments show that it performs better than LPCA and LLE and is comparable to KPCA, but with considerably fewer computations. We certainly do not claim that KLLE is the best method to use for any given training set of shapes, but it did give good results on the training data on which it was tested.

Nevertheless, representing a shape using its nearest neighbors requires that the training set contain sufficient data points. LPCA and KPCA have an innate capability to "produce" shapes by varying the PCA coefficients. This is not the case with LLE or KLLE. On the other hand, if sufficient amount of data is available, LLE and KLLE can perform better than PCA based algorithms. Another advantage of LLE and KLLE is that they allow one to learn shapes of completely different geometries, within the same training set. The reason for this is that these methods use only their nearest neighbors to find the projection instead of using the entire training set which is the case with KPCA and LPCA. One of the reasons why the kernel methods work better than their linear counterparts is that, the set of signed distance functions (SDF) is not closed under addition. Thus, the variations captured by linear methods are the variations in the SDF's and not in the embedded shapes, whereas the kernel methods capture the variations in shapes and not the embeddings. We should also note that, the performance of all these methods will get better if one has a large training set (with shapes of the same object).

In this work, we have used signed distance function to represent shapes. However, the algorithms used here do not depend on any particular type of representation. Performing a detailed comparative analysis using all of these methods with different representations (parametric and implicit) for shapes is the subject of future research. We would also like to test these methods on a wide variety of shapes with varying sizes of the training data set.

References

1. Terzopoulos, D., Szeliski, R.: Tracking with Kalman Snakes. In: Active Vision. MIT Press (1992) 3–20
2. Ayache, N., Cohen, I., Herlin, I.: Medical image tracking. In: Active Vision. MIT Press (1992) 3–20
3. Blake, A., Yuille, A., eds.: Active Vision. MIT Press (1992)
4. Osher, S., Paragios, N.: Geometric Level Set Methods in Imaging, Vision and Graphics. Springer Verlag (2003)
5. Dambreville, S., Rathi, Y., Tannenbaum, A.: Shape-based approach to robust image segmentation using kernel pca. In: Proceedings of the IEEE Conference on Computer Vision and Pattern Recognition. (2006)
6. Cootes, T., Taylor, C., Cooper, D., Graham, J.: Active shape models, their training and application. In: Computer Vision and Image Understanding. Volume 61. (1995) 38–59

7. Faugeras, O., Gomes, J.: Dynamic shapes of arbitrary dimension: the vector distance functions. In Cipolla, R., Martin, R., eds.: Proceedings of the Ninth IMA Conference on Mathematics of Surfaces. The Mathematics of Surfaces IX, Springer (2000)
8. Cremers, D., Kohlberger, T., Schnorr, C.: Nonlinear shape statistics in mumford-shah based segmentation. In: 7th ECCV '02. Volume 2351. (2002) 93–108
9. Leventon, M., Grimson, E., Faugeras, O.: Statistical shape influence in geodesic active contours. In: Proc. CVPR, IEEE (2000) 1316–1324
10. Tsai, A., Yezzi, A., Wells, W., Tempany, C., Tucker, D., Fan, A., Grimson, E., Willsky, A.: A shape-based approach to the sementation of medical imagery using level sets. IEEE Trans. on Medical Imaging **22** (2003) 137–153
11. Gomes, J., Faugeras, O.: Shape representation as the intersection of $n - k$ hyper-surfaces. Technical Report 4011, INRIA (2000)
12. Osher, S.J., Sethian, J.A.: Fronts propagation with curvature dependent speed: Algorithms based on hamilton-jacobi formulations. Journal of Computational Physics **79** (1988) 12–49
13. Wang, Y., Staib, L.: Boundary finding with correspondence using statistical shape models. In: Proc. CVPR. (1998) 338–345
14. Scholkopf, B., Smola, A., Muller, K.R.: Nonlinear component analysis as a kernel eigenvalue problem. Technical report, Max-Planck-Institute fur biologische Kybernetik (1996)
15. Rathi, Y., Dambreville, S., Tannenbaum, A.: Statistical shape analysis using kernel pca. In: SPIE, Electronic Imaging. (2006)
16. Mika, S., Scholkopf, B., Smola, A., K.R.Muller, M.Scholz, G.Ratsch: Kernel pca and de-noising in feature spaces. (Advances in Neural Information Processing Systems 11)
17. Kwok, J., Tsang, I.: The pre-image problem in kernel methods. In: 20th Intl. Conference on Machine Learning. (2003)
18. Funkhouser, T., Kazhdan, M., Shilane, P., Min, P., Kiefer, W., Tal, A., Rusinkiewicz, S., Dobkin, D.: Modeling by example. In: ACM Transactions on Graphics (SIGGRAPH 2004). (2004)
19. Saul, L.K., Roweis, S.: An introduction to locally linear embedding. (http://www.cs.toronto.edu/ roweis/lle/papers/lleintro.pdf)
20. D.Ridder, Duin, R.: Locally linear embedding for classification. Technical Report PH-2002-01, Pattern Recognition Group, Delft University of Technology (2002)
21. DeCoste, D.: Visualizing mercer kernel feature spaces via kernelized locally-linear embeddings. In: 8th Intl. Conf. on Neural Information Processing. (2001)
22. Chan, T., Zhu, W.: Level set based shape prior segmentation. Technical report, Computational Applied Mathematics, UCLA (2003)
23. Srivastava, A., Joshi, S., Mio, W., Liu, X.: Statistical shape analysis: Clustering, learning and testing. Trans. PAMI (2005)
24. Yezzi, A., Mennucci, A.: Metrics in the space of curves. http://arxiv.org/abs/ math.DG/ 0412454 (2004)
25. Michor, P., Mumford, D.: Riemannian geomtries of space of plane curves. (http:// front.math.ucdavis.edu/math.DG/0312384.)

Segmentation of Dynamic Emission Tomography Data in Projection Space

Evgeny Krestyannikov, Jussi Tohka, and Ulla Ruotsalainen

Institute of Signal Processing,
Tampere University of Technology,
P.O. Box 553, FI-33101 Tampere, Finland
{evgeny.krestyannikov, jussi.tohka, ulla.ruotsalainen}@tut.fi

Abstract. Dynamic emission tomography is a technique used for quantifying the biochemical and physiological processes within the body. For certain neuroimaging applications, like kinetic modelling in positron emission tomography (PET), segmenting the measured data into a fewer number of regions-of-interest (ROI) is an important procedure needed for calculation of regional time-activity curves (TACs). Conventional estimation of regional activities in image domain suffers from substantial errors due to the reconstruction artifacts and segmentation inaccuracies. In this study, we present an approach for separating the dynamic tomographic data directly in the projection space using the least-squares method. Sinogram ROIs are the fractional parts of different tissue types measured at each voxel. Regional TACs can be estimated from the segmented sinogram ROIs, thereby avoiding the image reconstruction step. The introduced technique was validated with the two dynamic synthetic phantoms simulated based on ^{11}C- and ^{18}F-labelled tracer distributions. From the quantitative point of view, TAC estimation from the segmented sinograms yielded more accurate results compared to the image-based segmentation.

1 Introduction

Dynamic emission tomography is a quantitative technique able to provide important information about physiological parameters indicating the functional state of the inspected tissue. The physiology relates to dynamic or temporal processes and, therefore, collecting also temporal information is necessary for the quantitative analysis of these processes unlike in structural imaging. In emission tomography, for example positron emission tomography (PET), the spatial distribution of a specific chemical compound containing radioactive nuclei across the time instances is assessed. At each time interval the measurements are recorded as a number of coincident positron and electron annihilations occurred along the path, or the line of response (LOR). The collection of such events (counts) detected at each LOR is conventionally called a *sinogram*. A sequence of acquisitions at contiguous time intervals ranging from a few seconds to tens of minutes yields the dynamic sinogram data (usually 4-D volumes). Dynamic images are further independently reconstructed from the raw data using various image reconstruction algorithms.

R.R. Beichel and M. Sonka (Eds.): CVAMIA 2006, LNCS 4241, pp. 108–119, 2006.

In the field of dynamic PET imaging, considerable attention has been focused on image quantification and estimation of kinetic physiological parameters [1]. Such parametric images provide quantitative information and are extensively used in clinical and research environments to assess and describe the tracer's behavior in homogeneous regions [2]. Reliable identification of regions-of-interest (ROIs) matching the anatomical structures is an important step, followed by the spatial averaging of the PET activity over the regions at each time frame. A set of kinetic parameters are further estimated by fitting a kinetic model to the time sequence of averaged regional activities.

The typical approach for ROI extraction involves manual grouping (segmenting) the time-averaged image voxels into spatial regions, and further, projecting those ROIs framewise to the dynamic data. Apparently, manual segmentation is often expensive, time-consuming, and operator-dependent task. Automatic methods for dynamic PET classification have gained particular interest during last decade. Most of them utilize the distinctive characteristics of tissue-dependent time activity curves (TACs) to partition the dynamic images into a smaller number of classes. This process is often called an image-based segmentation. Previous studies addressing the automatic segmentation to cluster analysis [3]-[7], principal component analysis [8], and independent component analysis [9] can be emphasized.

An approach based on analyzing the dynamic behavior of voxel intensities in the image space suffers from two serious drawbacks. First, it involves the time-consuming reconstruction of the whole volume of sinogram data prior to segmentation (e.g. 840 2-D sinograms for the dataset consisting of 24 time frames and 35 spatial planes). Moreover, reconstruction process tends to introduce various kinds of artifacts to the obtained images due to noise and finite amount of measured data. Hence, the segmented image may often become an inaccurate estimate for the required ROIs, while the estimated regional tissue-TACs may suffer from the reconstruction and segmentation errors.

In this work, we present a method for segmenting the dynamic projection data directly in the sinogram space. This strategy allows skipping the image reconstruction routine and, as a consequence, alleviating the additional noise effects. The algebraic formulation of the discrete Radon transform forms the basis of the sinogram segmentation approach. The main advantage is that the direct least-squares solution to the problem via pseudo-inverse exists, and no iterative approximation is needed. Thus, the segmentation is fast, simple, and flexible as it can be applied to high resolution 4-D scans. The work relates to the earlier direct methods for ROI evaluation in a projection space by Formiconi [11] and Reutter [12].

The noiseless segmentation model can be directly transformed into more realistic one, when measurement errors and statistical variations are present in the observations. The probabilistic model describing the true TAC as a realization of random variable with known distribution is described in section 2.2.

A new segmentation approach is beneficial for quantification. With numerical simulations we show that the mean tissue TACs extracted from the noisy measurement data does not depend upon the errors coming from erroneous segmentation and image reconstruction. This is a significant advance which improves the quantification accuracy and speeds up the acquisition of physiological parameters.

2   Sinogram Segmentation

2.1   Deterministic Approach to the Sinogram Segmentation

Let the dynamic image $x = [x_1(t), x_2(t), \dots, x_N(t)]^T$ be a sequence of N deterministic variables, where $[\cdot]^T$ denotes vector or matrix transpose. We view x as a vector consisting of N voxels, where each voxel $x_i(t) = [x_i(1), \dots, x_i(M)]$ is itself represented as an M-dimensional vector and describes the concentration of the tracer at time frame $t = 1, \dots, M$. The vector $x_i(t)$ is conventionally called the *time activity curve* (TAC). We assume that x consists of a known number of tissue components K, while each voxel contains the structure of only one dominant type.

The projection of the image x to the discrete Radon transform space as a set of simultaneous linear equations is defined as [10]

$$g = \mathbf{H}x, \tag{1}$$

where $g = [g_1(t), g_2(t), \dots, g_D(t)]^T$ is the resulting sinogram sequence. Each bin $g_d(t) = [g_d(1), \dots, g_d(M)]$ is again viewed as an M-dimensional sinogram time-intensity vector. The length of g is equal to D that gives the total number of lines of response (LORs) for all detection pairs. $\mathbf{H}$ is the matrix of weighting factors with entries $h_{di} : d = 1, \dots, D; \ i = 1, \dots, N$ that represent the contribution of the i-th pixel to the d-th detector. In more informative way, the factor h_{di} is equal to the fractional area of the i-th voxel intercepted with the d-th LOR. In a matrix-vector form (1) can be rewritten as

$$
\begin{bmatrix} g_1(t) \\ g_2(t) \\ \vdots \\ g_D(t) \end{bmatrix}
=
\begin{bmatrix} h_{11} & h_{12} & \dots & h_{1N} \\ h_{21} & h_{22} & \dots & h_{2N} \\ \vdots & \vdots & \ddots & \vdots \\ h_{D1} & h_{D2} & \dots & h_{DN} \end{bmatrix}
\begin{bmatrix} x_1(t) \\ x_2(t) \\ \vdots \\ x_N(t) \end{bmatrix}.
$$

The set of linear simultaneous equations (1) is often referred to as algebraic formulation for the discrete Radon transform. Due to the large size of $\mathbf{H}$, direct matrix inversion (for square $\mathbf{H}$) or the least-squares methods via pseudo-inverse (when $N \neq D$) are often impractical for estimating x from g. A subset of iterative reconstruction algorithms, historically called algebraic reconstruction (AR) techniques, have been proposed in literature to solve a set of D linear equations (see e.g. [10]).

Assume that the N-dimensional vector x is partitioned with a set of K homogeneous regions. The TAC at each region is assumed to be space invariant, hence x consists of a multiple copies of K tissue-TACs. Let $\mathcal{Z} = \{z_k(t), k = 1, \dots, K\}$

be a set comprising of K true time activity vectors such that $x_i(t) \in \mathcal{Z}$. Then $z = [z_1(t), z_2(t), \ldots, z_K(t)]^T$ be the sequence corresponding to the set $\mathcal{Z}$, where each element $z_k(t)$ is again viewed as an M-dimensional vector.

The discrete Radon transform of the image x can be written in terms of a few TACs z describing the structures of interest as

$$g = \mathbf{B}z, \tag{2}$$

or in matrix-vector form as

$$
\begin{bmatrix} g_1(t) \\ g_2(t) \\ \vdots \\ g_D(t) \end{bmatrix} = \begin{bmatrix} b_{11} & b_{12} & \ldots & b_{1K} \\ b_{21} & b_{22} & \ldots & b_{2K} \\ \vdots & \vdots & \ddots & \vdots \\ b_{D1} & b_{D2} & \ldots & b_{DK} \end{bmatrix} \begin{bmatrix} z_1(t) \\ z_2(t) \\ \vdots \\ z_K(t) \end{bmatrix}.
$$

Matrix $\mathbf{B}$ is the mixing matrix defining the constant multiplicative factors for the vector z. The element b_{dk} of the matrix $\mathbf{B}$ relates to the elements h_{di} of the matrix $\mathbf{H}$ through the following equation

$$b_{dk} = \sum_{i \in \Omega_k} h_{di}, \tag{3}$$

where Ω_k denotes the set of image voxels belonging to a homogeneous region k. In other words, we explain each sinogram voxel $g_d(t)$ in terms of K latent variables $z_k(t)$ mixed linearly with the respective coefficients b_{dk}. The equation (2) is a direct generalization of the model for ROIs evaluation derived by Formiconi [11] for static projections. In [12] Reutter has used a similar parameterization for estimating the spatiotemporal distribution in dynamic SPECT.

We suppose that the knowledge about the TAC for each structure (i.e. the matrix z) is known *a priori*. So, the task of sinogram segmentation is recasted to estimating the unknown matrix $\mathbf{B}$.

2.2 Probabilistic Formulation of the Sinogram Segmentation Approach

The real-world emission tomography images are the product of a radioactive decay that is a random process. The detected number of counts per each voxel $x_i(t)$ taken from the particular structure k can be modelled as a realization of a random variable distributed with the multivariate Poisson density[1]

$$p(x_i(t); \lambda_k(t)) = p(z_k(t); \lambda_k(t)) = \frac{\lambda_k(t)^{z_k(t)} e^{-\lambda_k(t)}}{z_k(t)!}, \tag{4}$$

---

[1] We take into account only noise coming from a statistical nature of the decay process, while leaving the additional sources of errors due to e.g. attenuation correction, accidental coincidences, detector normalization and biological variations aside. This is done solely for the sake of simplicity.

which is fully characterized by the M-dimensional mean vector $\lambda_k(t)$. The detected sinogram counts $g_d(t)$ at voxel location d are the sum of realized outcomes $x_i(t)$ along the ray path. Since the sum of independent Poisson random variables is also a Poisson random variable, $g_p(t)$ has the following density function

$$p(g_d(t); \mu_d(t)) = \frac{\mu_d(t)^{g_d(t)} e^{-\mu_d(t)}}{g_d(t)!} \tag{5}$$

with mean $\mu_d(t) = \sum_{k=1}^{K} b_{dk} \lambda_k(t)$.

2.3   Estimation of Matrix B

The d-th sinogram voxel intensity from (2) can be written as

$$g_d(t) = b_d z, \tag{6}$$

where b_d is the d-th row of matrix $\mathbf{B}$. For each sinogram TAC $g_d(t)$ we have to solve M equations with K unknowns. Since the number of observations M is usually larger than the number of distinct components K, matrix system (6) is overdetermined, and the least-squares solution to this problem can be found by minimizing

$$\min_{b_d} \| g_d(t) - b_d z \|_2. \tag{7}$$

At each $g_d(t)$, K pure tissue types from the image x are mixed with the respective multiplicative coefficients $b_{d1}, \ldots, b_{dk}$. Equation (7) can be solved, for example, via the pseudo-inverse of z. If the matrix z is ill-conditioned, regularized solution to the system of overdetermined equations can be found (e.g. with the truncated singular value decomposition (TSVD) [13]).

2.4   Extraction of Average Tissue TACs in Image and Sinogram Domains

In parametric imaging the primary goal is to produce images which specify the kinetic parameters related to the tracer specific block-model. These parameters are typically estimated based on the mean TACs calculated within each homogeneous ROI [2].

In the image domain the task of calculating the k-th mean tissue TACs is realized by averaging the PET activity frame-wise over the respective region-of-interest

$$\tilde{z}_k(t) = \frac{1}{N_k} \sum_{i \in \Omega_k} x_i(t), \tag{8}$$

where Ω_k is the set of image voxels belonging to the k-th ROI, and N_k is the total number of voxels in Ω_k.

In the sinogram domain, once the segmented sinogram matrix $\mathbf{B}$ has been estimated, the average TACs can be extracted by minimizing the criterion function with respect to z

$$\min_{z} \| g - \mathbf{B} z \|_2. \tag{9}$$

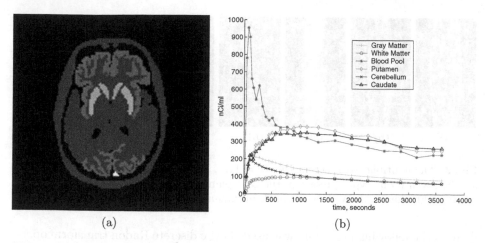

(a)   (b)

Fig. 1. (a) Time-averaged 28th plane of the Raclopride phantom. (b) TACs from six tissue types.

3 Numerical Experiments

3.1 Sinogram Segmentation from Noiseless Simulations

In this study, we examined the performance of the sinogram segmentation using an anatomical Zubal phantom [14] for the ^{11}C Raclopride tracer. The ^{11}C-labelled Raclopride is used to assess the local density of D_2 dopamine receptors in the brain. The phantom consisted of eight distinct structures: caudate nuclei (right and left), putamen (right and left), white matter (WM), gray matter (GM), cerebellum, blood pool, skin and fat/muscle structures. Realistic TACs' characteristics of Raclopride were determined from human studies and assigned to appropriate structures [15]. The simulated imaging protocol lasted for 1 hour: 1 frame of 15 s, 5 frames of 30 s, 1 frame of 45 s, 6 frames of 60 s, 1 frame of 90 s, 4 frames of 120 s, 1 frame of 210 s, 6 frames of 300 s, and 1 frame of 150 s. In total, phantom consisted of 27 time frames of data volumes with $128 \times 128 \times 63$ voxels per each frame. Synthesized images were re-projected to a noiseless sequence of dynamic 2-D sinograms each comprised of 336 angular projections and 275 bins per each projection. Figure 1(a) shows the time-averaged plane 28 of the phantom which includes seven different structures. The TACs from six representative tissue types are displayed in figure 1(b).

For each sinogram bin $g_d(t)$, system (6) contained 28 equations and 3 unknowns. By finding the minimum norm solution to the equation (7), the multiplicative factors b_k for every tissue type were found. They are depicted in figure 2 as separate sinograms.

3.2 Extraction of Average TACs from Noisy Simulations

The average TAC extraction from noisy simulations was performed in the image and sinogram domains, and results were quantitatively compared. In the image

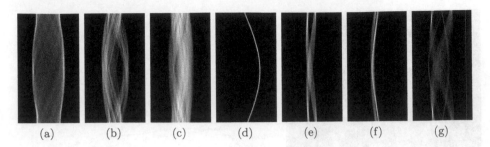

Fig. 2. The multiplicative factors $\{b_k : k = 1, \ldots, K\}$ depicted as separate sinograms for the seven tissue types present in the 28th plane of the Raclopride phantom. From left to right: skin, GM, WM, blood pool, putamen, caudate, fat/muscle.

domain the following procedure was used: 1) the discrete Radon transform operator was applied for projecting the dynamic Raclopride phantom to the sinogram space, 2) the Poisson noise was generated for the every sinogram bin $g_d(t)$ using pseudo-random number generator, 3) the constructed sequence of noisy sinograms was reconstructed back to the image space using filtered-backprojection (FBP) reconstruction algorithm, 4) given the vector $\lambda_k(t)$, the Bayes classifier was applied for each tissue type

$$\omega_i = \arg \max_{i=1,\ldots,K} \pi_k p(x_i(t); \lambda_k(t)), \tag{10}$$

where ω_i is the label of the voxel i, and π_k is the prior probability for the class k. The mean tissue TACs $\{\tilde{z}_k(t) : k = 1, \ldots, K\}$ were obtained by averaging the voxels belonging to the same structure, as given by (8).

In the sinogram domain the TACs were retrieved from the sequence of noisy sinograms projected from the phantom data. Knowing the mean vector of the Poisson activity $\lambda_k(t)$, the segmented sinogram matrix **B** was found using the least-squares method. The averaged TACs were directly evaluated using equation (9).

For both methods 3-D ROIs were delineated, and averaging was applied for all the voxel intensities belonging to a particular ROI. For each structure the root mean-square error (RMSE) between the true and estimated TAC was evaluated by the following equation

$$\text{RMSE} = \sqrt{\frac{1}{M} \sum_{t=1}^{M} (z_k(t) - \tilde{z}_k(t))^2}. \tag{11}$$

The errors for different structures and different evaluation methods are summarized in Table 1.

For the image-based segmentation (reconstruction + ROI estimation) the results varied significantly for different tissues. Skin TAC was underestimated due to the certain amount of background pixels incorrectly labelled as belonging to skin structure. Sizeable portion of caudate and cerebellum voxels were classified

Table 1. The root mean-square error (measured in nCi/ml) between the true TACs and average TACs estimated in the image and sinogram domains

Structure	Image-based segmentation			Sinogram-based segmentation
	Reconstruction + ROI estimation	Reconstruction + true labelling	No reconstruction + ROI estimation	
Skin	2.061	1.106	0.005	0.009
GM	1.075	2.682	0.011	0.017
WM	0.133	0.398	0.060	0.086
Blood pool	10.661	12.237	0.101	0.101
Putamen	3.898	4.404	0.105	0.151
Caudate	5.386	5.474	0.067	0.103
Cerebellum	1.093	0.803	0.016	0.017
Fat/Muscle	0.232	0.946	0.007	0.008

as putamen and gray matter, respectively, that yielded to a large deviation from the true activity values.

The total error in the image-based approach sums up from the following two reasons: the errors coming from the image reconstruction and the errors coming from the erroneous segmentation. We carried out two additional experiments to separate the reconstruction errors and to evaluate their significance on TACs' estimation. First, we excluded the segmentation errors by averaging the tissue-TACs for each structure within the true ROIs. In the second experiment, we generated the Poisson noise directly to the phantom data and estimated the TACs within the delineated ROIs. No re-projection to the sinogram domain and reconstruction were done, hence, the reconstruction errors were left out.

The results showed that the segmentation inaccuracies produce no significant effect on the total RMSE. For certain structures the regional curves estimated by averaging within the true ROI were even more biased than the ones averaged within the erroneous ROI. For image-based method the reconstruction justified to be the primary source of errors degrading accurate quantification of average radioactivity within the ROI. Sinogram-based approach operating directly in the projection space demonstrated very accurate extraction of TACs comparable to the image-based estimation from the non-reconstructed phantom.

3.3 Effect of the Structure's Size on TACs Estimation

The accuracy of TAC estimation depends largely upon the size of the ROI. To quantify how does the image reconstruction affect the estimation error for ROIs of different size we carried out the following experiment. A simple dynamic cylindrical phantom with a single ROI was simulated from a fluorine ^{18}F-labelled tracer distribution. It consisted of 24 time frames of the size 64×64 voxels each. The TAC for the cylinder ROI is depicted in figure 3. Further, we duplicated the phantom six times decreasing the radius of the cylinder by a factor of two each time in such a way that the ROI in the last cylinder shrank to a point source. The noiseless phantoms were re-projected to the sinogram domain, and the Poisson

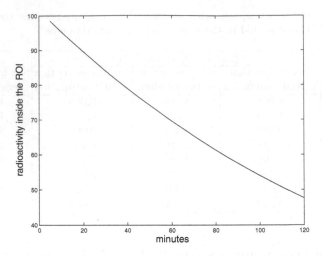

Fig. 3. The TAC inside the cylindrical phantom

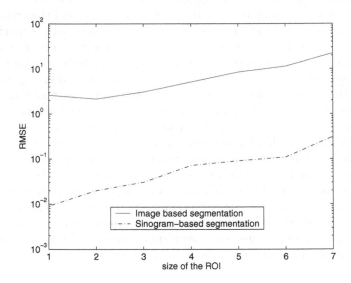

Fig. 4. The impact of ROI's size on the accuracy of TAC estimation for the sinogram and image-based methods. Label 1 along the x-axis refers to the initial ROI size, label 7 to the point source.

noise was generated to the projection data. Given the true region-TAC and the ROI segmentation for each cylinder, the activity curves were estimated from the noisy sinogram data using (7). Image-based TAC extraction was accomplished according to the procedure described in section 3.2.

The logarithmic dependence between the RMSE and the size of the ROI is demonstrated in figure 4. The results showed that the estimation error increases for the ROIs of smaller size. For the image-based approach the accuracy of calculated regional values was significantly worsened by the reconstruction procedure.

4 Discussion

In kinetic modelling the goal of segmentation is to define ROIs for calculating the mean radioactivity within them. These average TACs are further used to estimate the kinetic rate constants of the compartmental model. We introduced an algebraic deterministic model for segmenting the dynamic projection data. Its main difference from the AR techniques used in image reconstruction is the small size of system matrix. Hence, direct numerical approaches can be applied to solve the set of simultaneous equations. For overdetermined noise-free system, the least-squares estimates produce exact separation of dynamic sinogram into constituent projected components.

We compared the image-based approach for extracting the average tissue TACs from the noisy Poisson observations to the direct sinogram-based scheme. The image-based method exhibited fairly poor performance even with the known true ROI segmentation. The image reconstruction step was shown to be the main reason for that. The sinogram-based method allowed producing more stable and accurate results owing to the fact that ROIs were estimated from the projection data which are free of reconstruction artifacts. The attractive feature of the sinogram-based segmentation approach is its low computational demand. For a 4-D dataset consisting of $128 \times 128 \times 63 \times 27$ pixels the average time of segmentation was just a few seconds on a computer with 2 GHz Pentium 4 processor.

A crucial issue in the dynamic projection imaging concerns the parameter estimation for the true TACs from the data. In the present study, the segmentation problem was relaxed by assumption that the mean vector for each tissue-TAC $\lambda_k(t)$ is known beforehand. In practice this is not true, and the maximum likelihood approach can be employed to develop an algorithm for learning parameters $\lambda_k(t)$ and b_{dk}. We address this issue to our future work.

Another important fact that deserves a separate discussion is that the segmented sinogram ROIs are not limited for use in the sinogram space only. In general, reconstruction is possible and it yields the segmented ROIs in the image space.

There is an interesting link to sinogram segmentation with independent component analysis (ICA). In e.g. [16] authors modelled the dynamic sinogram as a linear mixture of unknown sources to separate the functional components in PET. In contrast to our approach, they imposed the deterministic nature on the TACs $z_k(t)$ and the stochastic (non-Gaussian) nature on the columns of matrix **B**. The major drawback of ICA separation is that it lacks the ability to find the amplitude (scaling) of the estimated signals. Without knowing the exact quantitative values, segmented ROIs in sinogram domain are useless for quantitation. Therefore, the ICA-based separation can be found practical only in conjunction with reconstructing the segmented sinogram ROIs to an image domain.

5 Conclusion

A novel sinogram-based segmentation approach for dynamic emission tomography data is introduced. It benefits the advantage of estimating the local ROI values directly in sinogram space, thereby skipping the time consuming image reconstruction process which tends to introduce substantial errors and artifacts to the reconstructed volumes. Using two computer-simulated phantoms we demonstrated that the higher accuracy can be achieved for quantitative parameters computed from raw data in comparison to the image-based segmentation.

Acknowledgment

The work was supported by Tampere Graduate School in Information Technology (TISE); the Academy of Finland under the Grants No 108517, 104834, and 213462 (Finnish Centre of Excellence program (2006-2011)).

References

1. Kamasak, M.E., Bouman, C.A., Morris, E.D., Sauer, K.: Direct reconstruction of kinetic parameter images from dynamic PET data. IEEE Tran. Med. Imag. 24(5) (2005) 636-650
2. Passchier, J., Gee, A., Willemsen, A., Vaalburg, W., van Waarde, A.: Measuring drug-related receptor occupancy with positron emission tomography. Methods 27 (2002) 278-286
3. Ashburner, J., Haslam, J., Taylor, C., Cunningham, V.J., Jones, T.: A cluster analysis approach for the characterization of dynamic PET data. In: Myers, R., Cunningham, V., Bailey, D., Jones, T. (eds.): Quantification of Brain Function using PET, San Diego, CA: Academic (1996) 301-306
4. Chen, J.L., Gunn, S.R., Nixon, M.S., Gunn, R.N.: Markov random field models for segmentation of PET images. In: Insana, M.F., Leahy, R.M. (eds.): Proceedings of Information Processing in Medical Imaging (IPMI), LNCS 2082 (2001) 468-474
5. Wong, K-P., Feng, D., Meikle, S., Fulham, M.: Segmentation of dynamic PET images using cluster analysis. IEEE Trans. Nucl. Sci. 49(1) 2002 200-207
6. Brankov, J.G., Galatsanos, N.P., Yang, Y.Y., Wernick, M.N., Segmentation of dynamic PET or fMRI images based on a similarity metric. IEEE Trans. Nucl. Sci. 50(5) (2003) 1410-1414
7. Kim, J., Feng, D.D., Cai, T.W., Eberl, S.: Automatic 3D temporal kinetics segmentation of dynamic emission tomography image using adaptive region growing cluster analysis. In: Nucl. Sci. Symposium Conf. Record 3 (2002) 1580-1583
8. Parker, B., Feng, D.D.: Variational segmentation and PCA applied to dynamic PET analysis. In: Jin, J.S., Eades, P., Feng, D.D., Yan, H. (eds.): Proc. Pan-Sydney Workshop on Visual Information Processing (VIP2002), Adelaide, Australia. Conferences in Research and Practice in Information Technology, 22 (2002) 89-92
9. Koivistoinen, H., Tohka, J., Ruotsalainen, U.: Comparison of pattern classification methods in segmentation of dynamic PET brain images. In: Proc. of Sixth Nordic Signal Processing Symposium, NORSIG 2004 (2004) 73-76
10. Kak, A.C., Slaney, M.: Principles of Computerized Tomographic Imaging. Society of Industrial and Applied Mathematics (2001)

11. Formiconi, A.R.: Least squares algorithm for region-of-interest evaluation in emission tomography. IEEE Tran. Med. Imag. **12** (**1**) (1993) 90-100
12. Reutter B.W., Gullberg G.T., Huesman, R.H.: Direct least-squares estimation of spatiotemporal distributions from dynamic SPECT projections using a spatial segmentation and temporal B-splines. IEEE Tran. Med. Imag. **19**(**5**) (2000) 434-450
13. Trefethen, L.N., Bau III, D.: Numerical linear algebra. Society of Industrial and Applied Mathematics, Philadelphia (1997)
14. Zubal, I., Hurrell, C., Smith, E., Rattner, Z., Gindi, G., Hoffer, P.: Computerized three-dimensional segmented human anatomy. Med. Phys. **21**(**2**) (1994) 299-302
15. Reilhac, A., Lartizien, C., Costes, N., Sans, S., Comtat, C., Gunn., R.N., Evans, A.C.: PET-SORTEO: A Monte Carlo-based simulator with high count rate capabilities . IEEE Trans. Nuc. Sci. **51**(**1**) (2004) 46-52
16. Magadan-Mendez, M., Kivimäki, A., Ruotsalainen, U.: ICA separation of functional components from dynamic cardiac PET data. In: IEEE Nucl. Sci. Symposium Conference Record, **4** (2003) 2618-2622

A Framework for Unsupervised Segmentation of Multi-modal Medical Images

Ayman El-Baz[1], Aly Farag[1], Asem Ali[1], Georgy Gimel'farb[2],
and Manuel Casanova[3]

[1] Computer Vision and Image Processing Laboratory
University of Louisville, Louisville, KY, USA
{elbaz, farag, asem}@cvip.uofl.edu
http://www.cvip.louisville.edu
[2] Department of Computer Science, Tamaki Campus
University of Auckland, Auckland, New Zealand
g.gimelfarb@auckland.ac.nz
[3] Department of Psychiatry, University of Louisville, USA
manuel.casanova@louisville.edu

Abstract. We propose new techniques for unsupervised segmentation of multi-modal grayscale images such that each region-of-interest relates to a single dominant mode of the empirical marginal probability distribution of gray levels. We follow most conventional approaches such that initial images and desired maps of regions are described by a joint Markov–Gibbs random field (MGRF) model of independent image signals and interdependent region labels. But our focus is on more accurate model identification. To better specify region borders, each empirical distribution of image signals is precisely approximated by a linear combination of Gaussians (LCG) with positive and negative components. Initial segmentation based on the LCG-models is then iteratively refined by using the MGRF with analytically estimated potentials. The convergence of the overall segmentation algorithm at each stage is discussed. Experiments with medical images show that the proposed segmentation is more accurate than other known alternatives.

1 Introduction

Applications of vision-guided robotics, automatic navigation, and medical image analysis need only fast and accurate special-purpose segmentations of multi-model images. Therefore, the supervised general-purpose segmentation algorithms based on training samples from previously segmented images [1,2,3,4] are insufficient for these applications in terms of accuracy and computational complexity; necessitating the use of unsupervised algorithms for multi-modal images (see e.g. [5]).

The currently popular deformable model methods for the segmentation of multi-modal images (see e.g. [6,7,8] to cite a few) also have some serious drawbacks in practical applications, namely, the high computational complexity, limited capabilities in detecting boundaries with concavities, and typically manual

R.R. Beichel and M. Sonka (Eds.): CVAMIA 2006, LNCS 4241, pp. 120–131, 2006.

initialization of an initial model within a desired object. Known automatic initialization schemes in [7,9] assume either a given approximate prototype of the average region boundary to match to the image or only a specific uniform spatial arrangement of signals in each region, respectively.

Although sometimes looking reasonably simple, the difficulty of the segmentation of multi-model images arises due to the intermixing object boundaries. In the mixed marginal frequency distribution of multi-modal images, each object is related to individual modes (or dominant peaks) of the distribution. In the case of dull edges, even if the dominant modes of an empirical signal mixture are clearly separated, object boundaries may not be accurately detected because of the intersecting tails of the adjacent objects in the signal mixture. Therefore, for accurate segmentation of such images, not only the main body of each such distribution but also its tails have to be precisely recovered from the mixture of these distributions.

To bypass the aforementioned drawbacks of the current algorithms and to overcome the intersecting tails problem, we revisit in this paper a more conventional scheme of unsupervised segmentation of multi-modal images to show that it is still highly competitive with more recent approaches. The scheme assumes image signals are conditionally independent with different marginal probability distributions for each object, recovers these latter from the mixed empirical signal distribution collected over the image [10,11], and performs the initial segmentation by the low-level pixel-wise classification. A region map obtained is further refined by optimal statistical (Bayesian or maximum likelihood) estimation of a hidden Markov–Gibbs random field (MGRF) model of regions. To specify an iterative estimation process, both the images and region maps are described with a joint two-level MGRF model that combines an unconditional model of interdependent region labels at the higher level and a conditional model of independent image signals in each region at the lower level (see, e.g. [12,13]).

Although this fast scheme is under development for a long time, all its conventional implementations identify the lower-level model only very roughly by assuming a normal density mixture with a single Gaussian per mode. Also, only heuristically chosen Gibbs potentials are typically used to govern the higher-level model. As a result, this scheme encounters difficulties in detecting practically meaningful accurate boundaries between the objects. In contrast to other solutions, we focus on most accurate identification of the low-level and high-level probability models. For this purpose, we propose new efficient techniques for precise approximation of the marginal probability distributions of image signals for each class (object) and precise approximation of Gibbs potentials for the region model [13]. Because empirical signal distributions in each region have quite intricate shapes, we represent in this paper each distribution including its tails with a linear combination of Gaussians (LCG). Each linear combination has both positive and negative components and offers, under the same number of components, much better approximation of empirical data than a conventional normal mixture with only positive components. A mixed probability distribution for the whole image is also an LCG combining the individual LCG models of each class.

2   Joint MGRF Image and Region Model

Let $\mathbf{Q} = \{0,\ldots,Q-1\}$ and $\mathbf{K} = \{1,\ldots,K\}$ denote sets of Q gray levels and K region labels, respectively, K being the number of modes (classes) in the mixed gray level distribution, e.g., $K = 2$ for a bimodal image. We assume each dominant image mode relates to a particular object to be found in the image.

Let $\mathbf{S} = \{(i,j) : 1 \leq i \leq I, 1 \leq j \leq J\}$ be a finite arithmetic grid supporting grayscale images $\mathbf{Y} : \mathbf{S} \to \mathbf{Q}$ and their region maps $\mathbf{X} : \mathbf{S} \to \mathbf{K}$. A two-level probability model of original images and their desired region maps is given by a joint distribution $P(\mathbf{Y},\mathbf{X}) = P(\mathbf{X})P(\mathbf{Y}|\mathbf{X})$ where $P(\mathbf{X})$ is an unconditional probability distribution of maps (the higher level) and $P(\mathbf{Y}|\mathbf{X})$ is a conditional distribution of images, given the map (the lower level of the model).

The Bayesian maximum a posteriori (MAP) estimate $\mathbf{X}^* = \arg\max_{\mathbf{X}\in\mathcal{X}} L(\mathbf{Y},\mathbf{X})$ of the map $\mathbf{X}$, given the image $\mathbf{Y}$, maximizes the log-likelihood function:

$$L(\mathbf{Y},\mathbf{X}) = \frac{1}{|\mathbf{S}|} \log P(\mathbf{Y}|\mathbf{X}) + \frac{1}{|\mathbf{S}|} \log P(\mathbf{X}) \tag{1}$$

Here, $\mathcal{X}$ is the parent population of all K-label maps on $\mathbf{S}$. To find the estimate $\mathbf{X}^*$, we need to identify parameters of the low- and high-level components of the model. In accordance to the chosen conventional scheme, the low-level component is an independent random field of gray levels $\mathbf{Y} = (Y_{i,j} : (i,j) \in \mathbf{S})$ with different distributions $\mathbf{P}_k = \left(p(q|k) : q \in \mathbf{Q}; \sum_{q\in\mathbf{Q}} p(q|k) = 1 \right)$ for each object $k \in K$. The conditional distributions $\mathbf{P}_k$; $k \in \mathbf{K}$, are the model parameters, and the joint conditional distribution $P(Y|X)$ of gray levels is: $P(\mathbf{Y}|\mathbf{X}) = \prod_{(i,j)\in\mathbf{S}} p(Y_{i,j}|X_{i,j})$.

Let $\nu_{\mathbf{X},\mathbf{Y}}(q,k) = |\{(i,j) : (i,j) \in \mathbf{S}; X_{i,j} = k; Y_{i,j} = q\}| \equiv \alpha_{\mathbf{X}}(k) f_{\mathbf{X},\mathbf{Y}}(q|k)|\mathbf{S}|$ be the number of pixels with the gray value q in the class k. Here, $\alpha_{\mathbf{X}}(k)$ and $f_{\mathbf{X},\mathbf{Y}}(q|k)$ are the relative frequencies of the label k in the region map $\mathbf{X}$ and of the gray value q in the image $\mathbf{Y}$ for the pixels of the class k, respectively. Then

$$P(\mathbf{Y}|\mathbf{X}) = \prod_{k\in\mathbf{K}} \prod_{q\in\mathbf{Q}} [p(q|k)]^{\alpha_{\mathbf{X}}(k) f_{\mathbf{X},\mathbf{Y}}(q|k)|\mathbf{S}|}$$

giving the first term of the log-likelihood in Eq. (1) as follows:

$$\sum_{k\in\mathbf{K}} \alpha_{\mathbf{X}}(k) \left(\sum_{q\in\mathbf{Q}} f_{\mathbf{X},\mathbf{Y}}(q|k) \log p(q|k) \right) \tag{2}$$

The high-level unconditional region map model is the simple MGRF with interdependent pairs of region labels in the nearest 8-neighborhood of each pixel. By symmetry considerations, the Gibbs potentials are independent of relative orientations of pixel pairs, which are the same for all objects, and depend only on whether the pairs of labels are equal or not. Under these simplifications, the model is closely similar to the conventional Potts (auto-binomial)

MGRF [14,15,16] except that the Gibbs potentials have no pre-defined heuristic functional form and are analytically estimated.

Let $\mathbf{V} = \{V(k, \kappa) = \gamma$ if $k = \kappa$ and $V(k, \kappa) = -\gamma$ if $k \neq \kappa$: $k, \kappa \in \mathbf{K}\}$ denotes the centered bi-valued Gibbs potential governing probabilities of symmetric pairwise co-occurrences of the region labels. Let the neighborhood $\mathbf{N} = \{(1,0), (0,1), (-1,1), (1,1)\}$ specify the inter-pixel offsets for the 8-neighboring pixel pairs. Let $\mathbf{T_N} = \{((i,j), (i+\xi, j+\eta)) : (i,j) \in \mathbf{S}; (i+\xi, j+\eta) \in \mathbf{S}; (\xi, \eta) \in \mathbf{N}\}$ be a family (with cardinality $|\mathbf{T_N}|$) of the neighboring pixel pairs supporting the Gibbs potentials. Let $f_{eq}(\mathbf{X})$ denote the relative frequency of the equal labels in the pixel pairs of that family in the map $\mathbf{X}$:

$$f_{eq}(\mathbf{X}) = \frac{1}{|\mathbf{T_N}|} \sum_{((i,j),(i+\xi,j+\eta)) \in \mathbf{T_N}} \delta(X_{i,j} - X_{x+\xi,j+\eta})$$

where $\delta()$ is the Kronecker delta function: $\delta(0) = 1$ and 0 otherwise. Then the MGRF model of region maps is specified by the following Gibbs probability distribution (GPD) where $Z_\mathbf{N}$ is the normalizing factor (the partition function):

$$P(\mathbf{X}) = \frac{1}{Z_\mathbf{N}} \exp \left(\sum_{(i,j) \in \mathbf{S}} \sum_{(\xi,\eta) \in \mathbf{N}} V(X_{i,j}, X_{i+\xi,j+\eta}) \right)$$

$$= \frac{1}{Z_\mathbf{N}} \exp \left(\gamma |\mathbf{T_N}| (2 f_{eq}(\mathbf{X}) - 1) \right) \tag{3}$$

To identify this high-level model, we have to estimate only the potential value γ. The close approximation of γ is easily obtained by expanding the second likelihood term, $\frac{1}{|\mathbf{S}|} \log P(\mathbf{X})$, of Eq. (1) in the close vicinity of the zero potential, $\gamma = 0$, into the truncated Taylor's series. This expansion results in the following approximate MLE of γ for a given map $\mathbf{X}$:

$$\gamma = \frac{K^2}{2(K-1)} \left(f_{eq}(\mathbf{X}) - \frac{1}{K} \right) \tag{4}$$

specifying the potentials of the MGRF model for each current region map obtained by Bayesian classification based on the previously identified low-level conditional image model.

To actually compute the second likelihood term for the MAP segmentation, we use the approximate partition function $Z_\mathbf{N}$ given in [14] which is reduced in our case to $Z_\mathbf{N} \approx \exp \left(\gamma |\mathbf{T_N}| (2 - K) \right)$. Then

$$\frac{1}{|\mathbf{S}|} \log P(\mathbf{X}) \approx 4\gamma (2 f_{eq}(\mathbf{X}) + K - 3) \tag{5}$$

3   Segmentation Framework

The log-likelihood of Eq. (1) is a complex multi-modal function of the region map $\mathbf{X}$. To approach the desired MAP estimate $\mathbf{X}^*$, we follow a conventional two-stage framework [12,13] but with far more accurate model identification than in other known algorithms due to the use of the LCG and precise parameter estimates of the LCG and the MGRF.

Initialization: A close initial approximation $\mathbf{X}_{[0]}^*$ of the desired region map by the precise unsupervised estimation of the marginal distributions $\mathbf{P}_k$ for each object $k \in \mathbf{K}$ (Section 4) and the subsequent Bayesian pixel-wise classification. Only the number K of dominant modes is specified by the user and holds during the whole process.

Refinement: An iterative search for a local maximum of the log-likelihood in Eq. (1) which is the closest to the initial approximation refines the initial map. Each iteration involves the following steps:

1. The MGRF region map model, updated by estimating analytically the potential γ in line with Eq. (4), is used together with the image model to refine the current map by stochastic relaxation.
2. The current low-level image model, given the region map, is refined by re-collecting the empirical gray level distributions for the classes and re-approximating the distributions with the LCG in order to update the map using the pixel-wise Bayesian classification.

At each step the approximate log-likelihood of Eq. (1) with the terms of Eqs. (2) and (5) is greater than or at least equal to its previous value, so that the proposed algorithm converges to a local maximum of this criterion.

4 Identification of the Low-Level Model

To most accurately identify the model, we approximate the marginal gray level probability density in each region with a LCG having $C_{p,k}$ positive and $C_{n,k}$ negative components:

$$p(q|k) = \sum_{r=1}^{C_{p,k}} w_{p,k,r}\varphi(q|\theta_{p,k,r}) - \sum_{l=1}^{C_{n,k}} w_{n,k,l}\varphi(q|\theta_{n,k,l}); \qquad (6)$$

such that $\int_{-\infty}^{\infty} p(q|k)dq = 1$. Here, q is the gray level, $\varphi(q|\theta)$ is a Gaussian density having a shorthand notation $\theta = (\mu, \sigma^2)$ for its mean, μ, and variance, σ^2. In contrast to more conventional normal mixture models, the components are now both positive and negative and have only one obvious restriction in line with Eq. (6): $\sum_{r=1}^{C_{p,k}} w_{p,k,r} - \sum_{l=1}^{C_{n,k}} w_{n,k,l} = 1$. These weights are not the prior probabilities, and the LCG of Eq. (6) is considered simply as a functional form of the approximation of a probability density depending on parameters (w, θ) of each component.

In the general case, the actual probability densities belong to a proper subset of the set of all possible LCGs of Eq. (6). In the subset, the weights and parameters of the Gaussians are limited to keeping non-negative values of the combined densities over the whole infinite signal range. The latter restriction is impracticable because it results in strongly interdependent parameters. Nonetheless, in our particular case the interdependence may be ignored. We use the LCG model to better approximate the main bodies as well as the intersecting tails of empirical distributions within a finite and relatively small actual signal range $[0, Q]$. Thus, the model behavior outside the range and the associated restrictions on the model parameters are of no concern. Moreover, the likelihood maximization is also directed towards keeping the probability densities positive at points where they approximate the empirical positive values.

The mixture of K LCGs, $p(q) = \sum_{k=1}^{K} w_k p(q|k)$, has just the same form but with a larger number of the components, e.g., $C_p = \sum_{k=1}^{K} C_{p,k}$ and $C_n = \sum_{k=1}^{K} C_{n,k}$ if all the values $\theta_{p,k,r}$ and $\theta_{n,k,l}$ differ for the individual models:

$$p(q) = \sum_{r=1}^{C_p} w_{p,r} \varphi(q|\theta_{p,r}) - \sum_{l=1}^{C_n} w_{n,l} \varphi(q|\theta_{n,l}) \tag{7}$$

To identify this model in the unsupervised mode, the mixed empirical distribution of gray levels over the image has to be first represented by a joint LCG of Eq. (7) and then partitioned into individual LCG-models for each class $k = 1, \ldots, K$.

Under the fixed number of positive and negative components, C, the model parameters $\mathbf{w} = \{w_c; c = 1, \ldots, C\}$ and $\mathbf{\Theta} = \{\theta_c : c = 1, \ldots, C\}$ maximizing the image likelihood can be found using a modified EM algorithm. It modifies the conventional EM-scheme to take into account the components with alternating signs, for more details see [13].

The modified EM algorithm is sensitive to its initial state specified by the numbers of positive and negative Gaussians and the initial parameters (mean and variance) of each component. To find a close initial LCG-approximation of the empirical distribution, we used the sequential EM algorithm which proposed in [13].

5   Step-Wise Segmentation Framework

Step-by-step implementation of the proposed segmentation algorithm is as follows.

1. Find the empirical probability distribution $\mathbf{F}$ by normalizing the gray level histogram for a given image $\mathbf{Y}$.
2. Use the sequential EM algorithm to initially estimate the numbers and parameters (means, variances, and weights) of the positive and negative Gaussians in the LCG-model.
3. Use the modified EM algorithm to refine the estimated model parameters, and estimate the marginal density for each class.
4. Form the initial region map $\mathbf{X}$ by pixel-wise Bayesian classification using the obtained class models.
5. Estimate the potential (γ) for the Potts model using Eq. (4).
6. Improve the region map $\mathbf{X}$ using pixel-wise stochastic relaxation (Metropolis sampler).

7. Calculate the log-likelihood function of Eq. (1).
8. Repeat Steps 3–8 iteratively until the log-likelihood remains almost the same for two successive iterations.
9. Output the final region map **X**.

6   Experimental Results

We illustrate the performance of the proposed techniques by the example of a medical screening of low dose computer tomographic (LDCT) chest images. The segmentation separates lung tissues from the surrounding anatomical structures such as chest tissues, ribs, and liver so that each LDCT slice has only two dominant objects ($K = 2$): the darker lungs and the brighter background. The lungs have to be accurately separated in such a way that their boundaries closely approach those outlined by a radiologist. Because of grayness some lung tissues (such as arteries, veins, bronchi, and bronchioles) are very close to the chest tissues, the segmentation cannot be based on only image signals but have to also account for spatial relationships between the region labels in order to preserve the details. Figure 1 demonstrates the typical LDCT chest slice, its empirical gray level density, and the initial mixture of two Gaussians approximating the dominant modes. The Levy distance 0.09 between these two distributions indicates a notable mismatch [17]. Figure 2 illustrates the sequential EM-based initialization that estimates ten subordinate Gaussians giving the minimum approximation error and shows the initial estimated LCG-model after the subordinate positive and negative components are added to and subtracted from the dominant mixture, respectively.

Figure 3 represents the final LCG-model and its 12 components obtained by refining the initial model in Fig. 2 by the modified EM-algorithm as well as the successive changes of the log-likelihood at the refining iterations. The first five iterations of the modified EM-algorithm increases the log-likelihood from -5 to -4.2. Then the iterations are terminated since the log-likelihood begins to very slightly decrease (presumably, because of accumulated numerical errors). The resulting Levy distance of 0.02 is much smaller than using the dominant mixture only. The minimum classification error of 0.004 between the lung and background

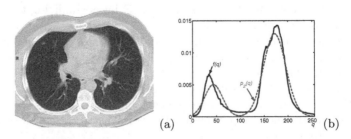

(a)   (b)

Fig. 1. Typical chest slice from a spiral LDCT scan (a) and its empirical signal distribution **F** approximated with the dominant mixture **P**$_2$

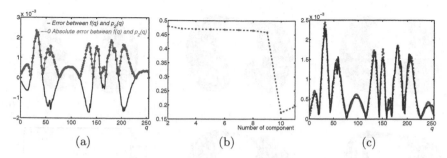

Fig. 2. Deviation and absolute deviation (a) between the empirical $\mathbf{F}$ and dominant $\mathbf{P}_2$ mixtures; the error (b) of approximating the scaled absolute deviation as a function of the number of the subordinate components; the best subordinate mixture (c) estimated for the absolute deviation, and the empirical vs. the estimated distributions for the CT slice in Fig. 1(a) with the 12-component LCG

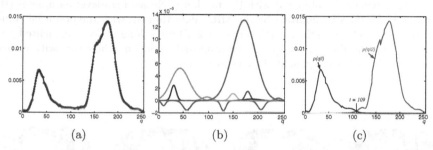

Fig. 3. Final LCG-approximation (a) of the bi-modal distribution; the components of the final LCG (b), and the LCG-models of objects for the best separation threshold $t = 109$ (c)

tissues for the final LCG-model is obtained with the threshold $t = 109$. In this case the LCG-components 1–4 correspond to the the lung tissues and 5–10 to the background ones.

The starting region map obtained by the pixel-wise classification in line with the LCG-models is further refined using the iterative algorithm in Section 3. Changes in the likelihood $L(\mathbf{Y}, \mathbf{X})$ become very small after 12 iterations as shown in Fig. 4. The initial and final potential estimates for the map model are $\gamma = 1.01$ and 1.30, respectively. The final region map produced with the estimated potential and model parameters using stochastic relaxation is shown in Fig. 4. For comparison, we also represent in Fig. 4 the initial region map, and the final map but refined with the randomly (heuristically) selected potential, the segmentation obtained by the MRS algorithm [19], and the "ground truth" outlined by a radiologist. The final refinement involving the whole MGRF model gives only a minor accuracy improvement so that the large errors in the initial region map after using a conventional mixture of positive Gaussians to model the empirical distribution cannot be eliminated.

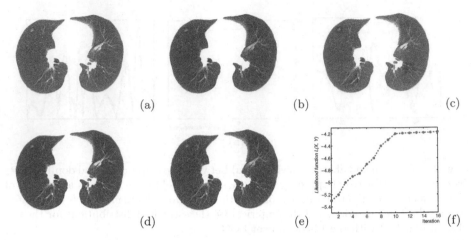

(a)   (b)   (c)

(d)   (e)   (f)

Fig. 4. Initial low-level segmentation (a); the final lung regions with the error of 0.85% (b); the lung regions (c) obtained with the randomly chosen high-level parameter (the error of 1.86%); the segmentation by the MRS algorithm (d) with the potential values 0.3 and three levels of resolution (the error of 2.3%); the lung regions segmented by a radiologist (e), and the convergence of the proposed algorithm (the errors with respect to the ground truth are highlighted by yellow color)

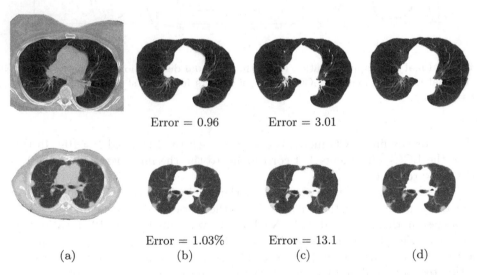

Error = 0.96   Error = 3.01

Error = 1.03%   Error = 13.1

(a)   (b)   (c)   (d)

Fig. 5. Original CT slices (a); our lungs segmentation (b) with errors only around the outer boundary; the segmentation by the IT algorithm in [18] (c), and the ground truth (d) given by a radiologist (the errors are highlighted by yellow color)

Figure 5 compares our segmentation to iterative thresholding (IT) proposed in [18]. In contrast to this method, our segmentation does not lose abnormal lung tissues. In all our experiments, segmentation errors are evaluated by comparing to the "ground truth" map produced by an expert. More segmentation results for lung tissues are shown in Fig. 6.

To show that the proposed approach is not limited to segment lung tissues from LDCT images, we applied the proposed segmentation techniques on two more different types of medical images. These two types are axial human head

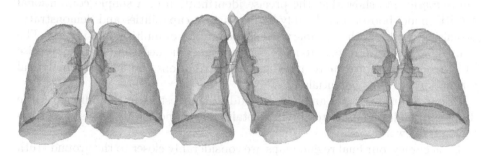

Fig. 6. 3D segmentation results of lung tissues from LDCT images

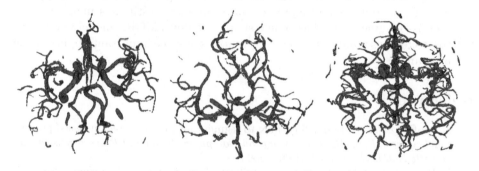

Fig. 7. 3D segmentation results of blood vessels from MRA images

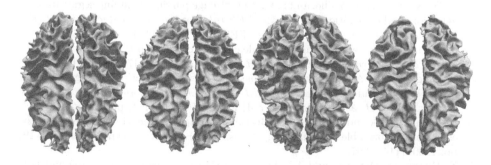

Fig. 8. 3D segmentation results of white matter from MRI images

slices obtained by time-of-flight magnetic resonance angiography (TOF-MRA), and axial human head slices obtained by magnetic resonance imaging (MRI). These images were acquired with the Picker 1.5T Edge MRI scanner. The TOF-MRA 512×512 and MRI 256×256 slices were 1.5 mm thick. The segmentation results for both MRA and MRI images are shown in Fig. 7 and Fig. 8

7   Concluding Remarks

Our experiments show that the precise identification of a simple conventional MGRF-model boosts considerably its descriptive capabilities and demonstrates promising results in the unsupervised segmentation of multi-modal images. The main difference with respect to more conventional schemes is in the use of precise LCG-models to approximate mixed signal distributions and accurate analytical estimation of Gibbs potentials.

In our future work, we are going to additionally estimate the number of the dominant modes, in order to obtain a totally autonomous unsupervised segmentation framework.

By accuracy, our final region maps are considerably closer to the ground truth than the maps produced by other known segmentation algorithms including the deformable model based ones. Therefore, the more precise LCG-based approximation of distributions and more accurate parameter estimates make the fast unsupervised segmentation based on a simple two-level MGRF model quite competitive to today's more elaborative alternatives in some important applied areas of image analysis.

References

1. J. Kaufhold and A. Hoogs, "Learning to segment images using region-based perceptual features," *Proc. IEEE Int. Conf. on Computer Vision and Pattern Recognition (CVPR 2004)*, vol. 1, pp. 954-961, 2004.
2. X. Ren and J. Malik, "Learning a classification model for segmentation," *Proc. 9th IEEE Int. Conf. on Computer Vision (ICCV 2003), 14–17 Oct. 2003, Nice, France*, IEEE CS Press, vol. 1, pp. 10–17, 2003.
3. Z. Tu, X. Chen, A. L. Yuille, and S. C. Zhu, "Image parsing: Unifying segmentation, detection, and recognition," *Proc. 9th IEEE Int. Conf. on Computer Vision (ICCV 2003), 14–17 Oct. 2003, Nice, France*, IEEE CS Press, vol. 1, pp. 18–25, 2003.
4. S. X. Yu, "Segmentation using multiscale cues," *Proc IEEE Int. Conf. on Computer Vision and Pattern Recognition (CVPR 2004)*, vol. 1, pp. 247-254, 2004.
5. M. Singh and N. Ahuja, "Regression based bandwidth selection for segmentation using Parzen windows," *Proc. 9th IEEE Int. Conf. on Computer Vision (ICCV 2003), 14–17 Oct. 2003, Nice, France*, IEEE CS Press, vol. 1, pp. 2–9, 2003.
6. R. P. Grzeszczuk and D. N. Levin, "Brownian strings: Segmenting images with stochastically deformable contours," *Ieee Trans. Pattern Anal. Machine Intell.*, vol. 19, pp. 1100–1114, 1997.
7. X. Huang, D. Metaxas, and T. Chen, "MetaMorphs: Deformable shape and texture models," *Proc. IEEE Int. Conf. on Computer Vision and Pattern Recognition (CVPR 2004)*, vol. 1, pp. 496-503, 2004.

8. C. Xu and J.L. Prince, "Snakes, shapes, and gradient vector flow," *IEEE Trans. Pattern Anal. Machine Intell.*, vol. 7, no. 3, pp. 359-369, 1998.

9. P. C. Yuen, G. C. Feng, and J. P. Zhou, "A contour detection method: Initialization and contour model," *Pattern Recognition Letters*, vol. 20, pp. 141-148, 1999.

10. R. O. Duda, P. E. Hart, and D. G. Stork, *Pattern Classification*, Wiley, New York, 2001.

11. M. I. Schlesinger and V. Hlavac, *Ten Lectures on Statistical and Structural Pattern Recognition*, Kluwer: Dordrecht, 2002.

12. C. A. Bouman and M. Shapiro, "A multiscale random field model for Bayesian image segmentation," *IEEE Trans. Image Processing*, vol. 3, no. 2, pp. 162–177, 1994.

13. A.A. Farag, A. El-Baz, and G. Gimelfarb, "Density Estimation Using Modified Expectation Maximization for a linear combination of Gaussians," *Proc. of IEEE International Conference on Image Processing (ICIP- 2004)*, Singapore, October 24–27, 2004, vol. I, pp. 194–197.

14. R. C. Dubes and A. K. Jain, "Random field models in image analysis," *J. Applied Statistics*, vol. 16, no. 2, pp. 131–164, 1989.

15. R. W. Picard and I. M. Elfadel, "Structure of aura and cooccurrence matrices for the Gibbs texture model," *J. Math. Imaging and Vision*, vol. 2, no. 1, pp.5–25, 1992.

16. L. Dryden, M. R. Scarr, and C. C. Taylor, "Bayesian texture segmentation of weed and crop images using reversible jump Markov chain Monte Carlo methods," *J. Royal Statistical Society*, vol. 52C, pt. 1, pp. 3150, 2003.

17. J. W. Lamperti, *Probability*, J. Wiley & Sons, New York, 1996.

18. S. Hu and E. A. Hoffman, "Automatic lung segmentation for accurate quantization of volumetric X-Ray CT images," *IEEE Trans. Medical Imaging*, vol. 20, no. 6. pp. 490–498, 2001.

19. C. Bouman and B. Liu, "Multiple resolution segmentation of textured images," *IEEE Trans. Pattern Analysis Machine Intell.*, vol. 13, no. 2, pp. 99-113, Feb. 1991.

An Integrated Algorithm for MRI Brain Images Segmentation

Yinghua Lu[1,2], Jianzhong Wang[2,3], Jun Kong[2,3,*],
Baoxue Zhang[3], and Jingdan Zhang[2]

[1] Computer School, Jilin University, Changchun, Jilin Province, China
[2] Computer School, Northeast Normal University, Changchun, Jilin Province, China
[3] Key Laboratory for Applied Statistics of MOE, China
{luyh, wangjz019, kongjun, bxzhang}@nenu.edu.cn

Abstract. This paper presents an integrated algorithm for MRI (Magnetic Resonance Imaging) brain tissues segmentation. The method is composed of four stages. Noise in the MRI images is first reduced by a versatile wavelet-based filter. Then, the watershed algorithm is applied to brain tissues as an initial segmenting method. Because the result of classical watershed algorithm on grey-scale textured images such as tissue images is over-segmentation. The third stage is a merging process for the over-segmentation regions using fuzzy clustering algorithm (Fuzzy C-Means). But there are still some regions which are not divided completely due to the low contrast in them, particularly in the transitional regions of gray matter and white matter, or cerebrospinal fluid and gray matter. We exploited a method base on Minimum Covariance Determinant (MCD) estimator to detect the regions needed segmentation again, and then partition them by a supervised k-Nearest Neighbor (kNN) classifier. This integrated approach yields a robust and precise segmentation. The efficacy of the proposed algorithm is validated using extensive experiments.

1 Introduction

Many issues inherent to medical image make segmentation a difficult task. The objects to be segmented from medical image are true (rather than approximate) anatomical structures, which are often non-rigid and complex in shape, and exhibit considerable variability from person to person. Moreover, there are no explicit shape models yet available for capturing fully the deformations in anatomy. MRI produces high contrast between soft tissues, and is therefore useful for detecting anatomy in the brain. Segmentation of brain tissues in MRI images plays a crucial role in three-dimensional (3-D) volume visualization, quantitative morphmetric analysis and structure-function mapping for both scientific and clinical investigations.

Because of the advantages of MRI over other diagnostic imaging [2], the majority of researches in medical image segmentation pertains to its use for MR images, and

---

* Corresponding author.
This work is supported by science foundation for young teachers of Northeast Normal University, No. 20061002, China.

there are a lot of methods available for MRI image segmentation [1-12]. Niessen et al. roughly grouped these methods into three main categories: classification methods, region-based methods and boundary-based methods. Just as pointed out in [12], the methods in the first two categories are limited by the difficulties due to intensity in-homogeneities, partial volume effects and susceptibility artifacts, while those in the last category suffer from spurious edges.

In this paper we address the segmentation problem in the context of isolating the brain in MRI images. An integrated method using an adaptive segmentation of brain tissues in MRI images is proposed in this paper. Firstly, we de-noise the images using a versatile wavelet-based filter. Subsequently, watershed algorithm is applied to the brain partition as an initial segmenting method. Normally, result of classical water-shed algorithm on grey-scale textured images such as tissue images is over seg-mented. The following procedure is a merging process for the over segmented regions using fuzzy clustering algorithm (here, we take Fuzzy C-Means). But there are still some regions which are not divided completely, particularly in the transitional regions of gray matter and white matter, or cerebrospinal fluid and gray matter. This moti-vated the construction of a re-segmentation processing approach to partition these regions. We exploited a method base on Minimum Covariance Determinant (MCD) estimator to detect the regions needed segmentation again, and then partition them by a supervised k-Nearest Neighbor (kNN) classifier.

The rest of this paper is organized as follows. In Section 2, we present the versatile wavelet-based de-noising algorithm. Watershed algorithm is briefed in Section 3. In Section 4, we describe the merging process using region-based Fuzzy C-Means (RFCM) clustering. Section 5 presents the proposed a re-segmentation processing approach based on the combination of MCD and kNN. Experimental results are pre-sented in Section 6 and we conclude this paper in Section 7.

2 Wavelet-Based De-noising

The noise type in the MRI magnitude images is Rician, having a signal-dependent mean, and the Rician distribution approaches a Gaussian distribution when the SNR is high [15]. In medical images, noise suppression is a particularly delicate and difficult task. A trade off between noise reduction and the preservation of actual image fea-tures has to be made in a way that enhances the diagnostically relevant image content. To achieve a good performance in this respect, a de-noising algorithm has to adapt to image discontinuities. The wavelet representation naturally facilitates the construction of such spatially adaptive algorithms.

A versatile and spatially adaptive wavelet-based de-noising algorithm [15] is applied in this paper. The algorithm exploits generally valid knowledge about the correlation of significant image features across the resolution scales to perform a preliminary coefficient classification. This preliminary coefficient classification is used to empirically estimate the statistical distributions of the coefficients that represent useful image features on the one hand and mainly noise on the other. The adaptation to the spatial context in the image is achieved by using a wavelet domain indicator of the local spatial activity. This robust method adapts itself to various types of image noise as well as to the preference of the medical expert. **Fig. 1**(a) shows an MRI image simulated from a normal brain phantom [16] with 3% noise level, and **Fig. 1**(b) shows the corresponding wavelet-based de-noising result.

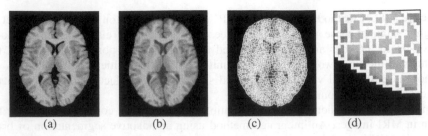

| (a) | (b) | (c) | (d) |

Fig. 1. (a) Original image simulated from MRI brain phantom with 3% noise level, and its processed versions with (b) wavelet-based de-noising. (c) Partition result after using watershed algorithm. (b) Some regions that aren't divided completely.

3 Watershed Algorithm

The input to watershed algorithm is a gray-scale gradient image. Sobel edge detection is applied to get this gradient magnitude image, denoted by I_G. The gradient image is considered as a topographic relief. We apply the Vincent and Soille [13] version of watershed algorithm, which is based on immersion simulation: the topographic surface is immersed from its lowest altitude until water reaches all pixels. The output of watershed algorithm is segmentation of MRI into a set of non-overlapping regions [14]. **Fig. 2**c demonstrates the watershed result of the image shown in **Fig. 1**b.

The watershed transformation constitutes one of the most powerful segmentation tools provided by mathematical morphology. But there are two disadvantages in the watershed algorithm. Firstly, result of classical watershed algorithm on grey images such as tissue images is over-segmentation, as shown in **Fig. 1**c. Secondly, there are some regions which are not divided completely particularly in the transitional regions of gray matter and white matter, or cerebrospinal fluid and gray matter. It is clearly shown in **Fig. 1**d obtained from one part of **Fig. 1**c zoomed in. In Section 4 and Section 5, we will focus our attentions on these questions respectively.

4 Merging the Over-Segmentation Regions

After watershed algorithm being used, there are too many regions because of natural attribute of watershed algorithm -- over segmentation. To overcome this problem, we proposed a region-based FCM (RFCM) clustering method to merge these regions over segmented in this section.

FCM has been applied widely to MRI segmentation [6-9], and regarded as one of the most promising methods [7]. The FCM clustering algorithm assigns a fuzzy membership value to each data point based on its proximity to the cluster centroids in the feature space. In our work, the output of watershed algorithm is the segmentation of I_G into a set of non-overlapping regions denoted by R_i, $i = 1, 2, ..., n$ where n is the number of regions. To implement the merging of similar regions, we use the region based FCM (RFCM) clustering method. The mean value, denoted by $m_i, i = 1, 2, ..., n$ of each region R_i, is needed.

The RFCM clustering algorithm in this paper is formulated as:

$$J_{RFCM}(U,v) = \sum_{i \in \Omega} \sum_{k=1}^{C} u_{ik}^{m} \parallel m_i - v_k \parallel^2 \text{ , subject to } \sum_{k=1}^{C} u_{ik} = 1 \text{ , } \Omega = \{1,2,...,n\}. \quad (1)$$

where the matrix $U = \{u_{ik}\}$ is a fuzzy c-partition of I_G, and u_{ik} gives the membership of region R_i in the kth cluster c_k, c is the total number of clusters and set to 3 in our study, because three brain tissues are of interest: CSF (Cerebrospinal Fluid), GM (Gray Matter), and WM (White Matter), $v = \{v_1, v_2, v_3\}$ is the set of fuzzy cluster centroids, and v_1, v_2, v_3 denote the centroids of CSF, GM and WM respectively, $m \in (1, \infty)$ is the fuzzy index (in our study, $m=2$).

If the difference of intensity mean value of region R_i and v_k is small enough, region R_i will be assigned to a high membership value for the kth cluster c_k. Let the first derivatives of J_{RFCM} with respect to u and v equal to zero yields the two necessary conditions for minimizing J_{RFCM}. The RFCM algorithm is implemented by iterating the two necessary conditions until a solution is reached. After RFCM clustering, each region will be associated with a membership value for each class. By assigning the region to the class with the highest membership value, a segmentation of the region can be obtained.

The result image after merging the over segmentation regions using RFCM on **Fig. 1**c is shown in **Fig. 2**a. We can see the result of some regions which are not partitioned completely obviously in **Fig. 2**b obtained from a part of the image after **Fig. 2**a zoomed in. **Fig. 2**c and d are images after watershed lines removed from **Fig. 2**a and b respectively. From these images (see **Fig. 2**), another disadvantage of the watershed algorithm – segmentation incompletely and inaccurately in some regions is shown clearly.

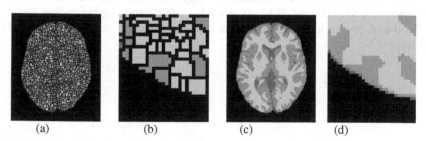

| (a) | (b) | (c) | (d) |

Fig. 2. (a) Image after using RFCM. (b) A partial image of (a) zoomed in. (c) and (d) are images after watershed lines removed from (a), (b) respectively.

5   The Re-segmentation Processing

Though the image is partitioned into too many regions after the operation of watershed algorithm, there are still some regions which have not been separated completely and accurately, particularly in the transitional regions of gray matter and white matter, or cerebrospinal fluid and gray matter. Therefore, this motivate the construction of a re-segmentation processing method to partition these regions in this section, which is based on the combination of MCD and kNN.

5.1 Searching for the Re-segmentation Regions

As we known, the attribute of transitional regions partitioned incompletely after watershed segmentation is different from that of interior regions of the brain tissues. Now, if the variance of the region R_i is small enough, the region R_i is homogeneous. Otherwise, region R_i may be inhomogeneous and would be partitioned again.

Moreover, if the result after watershed segmentation is complete and accurate, the region's mean value would be close to the centroid of the class it belongs to. While region's mean value is far from the centroid of the class it belongs to, this region may be inhomogeneous. Thus, the feature vector is constructed by the mean value and variance of each region. In **Fig. 3**a, the horizontal axis represents the mean of each region, the vertical axis represents the variance of each region, and the samples are obtained by RFCM clustering result. The dots which are far from the centroids of brain tissues they belong to may be the regions needed re-segmentation in **Fig. 3**a.

For detecting the transitional regions which are not divided completely, the Minimum Covariance Determinant (MCD) estimator is exploited in our study. It is defined to be the mean and covariance of an ellipsoid covering at least half of the data with the lowest determinant of covariance. This method is highly robust, with a high breakdown point. The breakdown point is the fraction of the data that must be moved to infinity so that the estimate also moves to infinity. The MCD estimate has a breakdown point of 0.5, more than half of the data needs to be contaminated to make the estimate be unreasonable.

To speed up the MCD detection, a fast MCD algorithm proposed by Rousseeuw and Van Driessen [17] is used in this section. In **Fig. 4**, these outliers are just the transitional regions needed re-segmentation. **Fig. 4**a, b and c are the fast MCD detection results of CSF, GM and WM respectively. After removing the outlier dots from **Fig. 3**a, the inliers are left (**Fig. 3**b) which is the reliable and validity result of RFCM clustering.

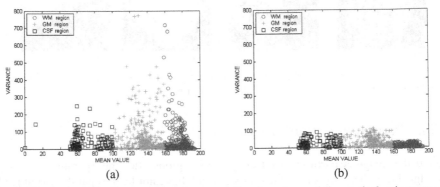

(a)   (b)

Fig. 3. The horizontal axis represents the mean of each region and the vertical axis represents the variance of each region after watershed segmentation. (a) Original samples obtained by RFCM clustering result (b) The samples after removing the outliers.

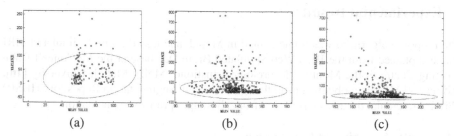

(a)   (b)   (c)

Fig. 4. Fast MCD detection algorithm. (a), (b) and (c) are the detection results of CSF, GM and WM respectively.

The MCD estimator not only can detects the re-segmented regions, but also the inliers of the region class samples can be used as training set for the next k-Nearest Neighbor classification.

5.2 Re-segmentation Using kNN

In this section, we exploited a supervised classifier, the classical k nearest-neighbor (kNN) classifier [18], to partition the regions needed re-segmentation. We choose the means of inlier's regions obtained from fast MCD estimator as the training set. For each data point to be classified in re-segmented regions, kNN compute this point's closest k training samples in feature space. Then the data is classified with the label most represented among these k nearest neighbors. kNN is attractive because it is a non-parametric classifier, and it can learn from the training set.

According to the suggestion which Enas and Choi given in [19], we choose k = 7 in the experiments presented in this paper, and our implementation uses a fast nearest neighbor lookup library [22] which pre-processes using box-decomposition trees to reduce the computation of kNN algorithm.

To illustrate our re-segmentation approach, the re-segmentation result operating on **Fig. 2**a is shown in **Fig. 5**a, and **Fig. 5**b is its result image without watershed lines. **Fig. 5**c is a part of image after **Fig. 5**a zoomed in, and the same part image of **Fig. 5**b zoomed in is shown in **Fig. 5**d. Compared this result (**Fig. 5**c and d) with watershed segmentation result in **Fig. 1**d, the precise and veracity of our method is obviously validated.

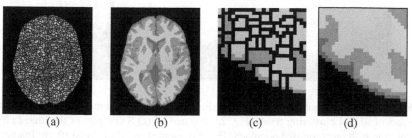

(a)   (b)   (c)   (d)

Fig. 5. (a) Re-segmented result image using our method. (b) Finial result image without watershed lines. (c) and (d) are the same part of (a) and (c) zoomed in respectively.

6 Experimental Results

The proposed algorithm was implemented in Matlab and tested on both simulated MRI images obtained from the BrainWeb Simulated Brain Database at the McConnell Brain Imaging Centre of the Montreal Neurological Institute (MNI), McGill University [16], and on real MRI data obtained from the Internet Brain Segmentation Repository (IBSR) [20]. Extra-cranial tissues are removed from all images prior to segmentation.

6.1 Results Analysis and Comparison

Figure. 6a is a part of the image which is obtained from the partition result after using watershed algorithm (**Fig. 1**c) zoomed in, and it is clearly shown that some regions are partitioned incompletely after the operation of watershed algorithm. This disadvantage of watershed algorithm is obviously shown in **Fig. 6**b obtained from a part of RFCM clustering result (**Fig. 2**a) zoomed in. Using our novel re-segmentation approach, the regions partitioned incompletely are divided again, and the result image is shown in **Fig. 6**c. **Fig. 6**d, e and f are images with watershed lines removed from **Fig. 6**a, b and c respectively. Compared this result (**Fig. 6**c) with watershed segmentation result in **Fig. 6**a, the precise and veracity of our method is obviously validated.

In following, we compare the segmentation results among FCM clustering, segmented result using our proposed approach and the "ground truth" in **Fig. 7**b, c and d. The original image is shown in **Fig. 1**a and **Fig. 7**a is the wavelet-based de-noising image. FCM clustering result (**Fig. 7**b) is partitioned inaccurately, particularly in the transitional regions of gray matter and white matter, or cerebrospinal fluid and gray

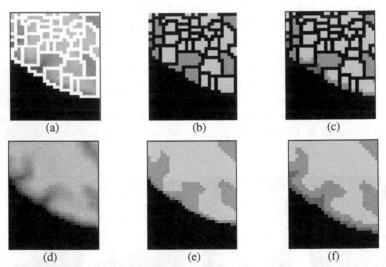

(a)   (b)   (c)

(d)   (e)   (f)

Fig. 6. (a) A part of the partition image after using watershed algorithm (Fig. 1c) zoomed in. (b) Same part of RFCM clustering result (Fig. 2a) zoomed in. (c) Same part of the image after re-segmentation with our proposed approach (Fig. 5a) zoomed in. (d), (e) and (f) are images with watershed lines removed from (a), (b) and (c) respectively.

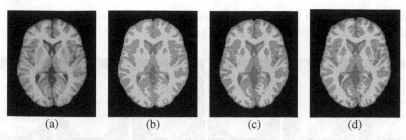

(a)   (b)   (c)   (d)

Fig. 7. (a) Wavelet-based de-noising image. (b) FCM segmentation. (c) Segmented result using our proposed approach. (d) Ground truth.

matter. The segmented result using our approach (**Fig. 7**c) clearly outperforms the result of FCM clustering (**Fig. 7**b).

Three different indices (false positive ratio γ_{fp}, false negative ratio γ_{fn}, and similarity index ρ [21]) are exploited for each of three brain tissues as quantitative measures to compare our method and FCM clustering with the "ground truth". The results are shown in **Table 1**. Our integrated scheme produces a more robust segmentation result than FCM.

Table 1. Comparing our method and FCM clustering with the ground truth

	FCM clustering			Our proposed approach		
	γ_{fp}	γ_{fn}	ρ	γ_{fp}	γ_{fn}	ρ
WM	10.12	7.24	91.44	2.36	6.25	95.01
GM	13.44	12.69	86.98	1.99	8.01	93.25
CSF	6.48	16.10	83.19	5.29	5.18	92.10

6.2 Quantitative Validation

To quantitatively validate our method, test images with known "ground truth" are required. For this purpose, we used the simulated MRI images from a normal brain phantom [16] with T1-weighted sequences, slice thickness of 1 mm, volume size of $217 \times 181 \times 181$ and noise levels of 3%, 5%, 7% and 9% respectively. Background pixels are ignored in our experiment, thus the brain of interest consisting of CSF, GM and WM is extracted and then segmented by our proposed method.

Fig. 8a, d, g and j are simulated MRI images with noise levels of 3%, 5%, 7%, and 9% respectively. The corresponding segmentation results processed by our approach are shown in **Fig. 8**b, e, h and k with their "ground truth" of **Fig. 8**c, f, i and l respectively.

For validating the accuracy and reliability of our method, we also use the three different indices (false positive ratio γ_{fp}, false negative ratio γ_{fn}, and similarity index ρ [21]) for each of three brain tissues as quantitative measures. The validation results are shown in **Table 2**. The similarity index $\rho > 70\%$ indicates an excellent similarity [21]. In our experiments, the similarity indices ρ of all the tissues are larger than 90%

even for a bad condition with 9% noise level, which indicates an excellent agreement between our segmentation results and the "ground truth".

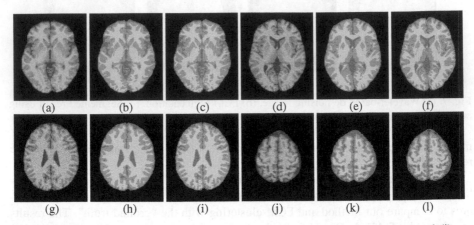

(a)   (b)   (c)   (d)   (e)   (f)

(g)   (h)   (i)   (j)   (k)   (l)

Fig. 8. Segmentation of simulated image from MRI brain phantom. (a), (d), (g) and (j) are images with the noise levels of 3%, 5%, 7% and 9% respectively, with (b), (e), (h) and (k) their corresponding segmentation results using our proposed approach. (c), (f), (i) and (l) are the "ground truth" of (a), (d), (g) and (j) respectively.

Table 2. Validation results for different noise levels

	3% noise			5% noise			7% noise			9% noise		
	γ_{fp}	γ_{fn}	ρ	γ_{fp}	γ_{fn}	ρ	γ_{fp}	γ_{fn}	ρ	γ_{fp}	γ_{fn}	ρ
WM	1.94	6.37	95.44	2.36	7.25	95.01	2.70	7.62	94.13	3.18	9.81	93.27
GM	1.47	8.59	94.27	1.99	9.01	93.25	2.42	10.31	92.95	3.03	12.20	91.32
CSF	6.12	6.10	92.48	6.29	6.18	92.10	7.45	6.98	91.86	10.63	9.15	90.15

6.3 Performance on Actual MRI Data

Fig. 9a shows one slice of real T1-weighted MRI images [17]. **Fig. 9**b is FCM segmentation result. Using our re-segmentation processing, the result image is shown in **Fig. 9**c. Visual inspection shows that our approach produces better segmentation than FCM, especially in the transitional regions of gray matter and white matter, or cerebrospinal fluid and gray matter.

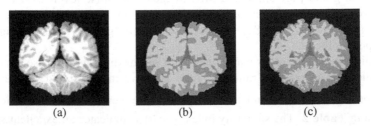

(a)   (b)   (c)

Fig. 9. Segmentation of real MRI image. (a) Original image. (b) FCM segmentation. (c) Re-segmented result using our approach.

7 Conclusions

We propose a novel approach for segmenting brain tissues in MRI images, which is based on the combination of wavelet-based de-noising, watershed algorithm, RFCM and a re-segmentation processing approach. As a result, the quality of the segmentation is improved. The algorithm is composed of four stages. In the first stage, we de-noise the images using a versatile wavelet-based filter. Subsequently, watershed algorithm is applied to brain tissues as an initial segmenting method. Normally, result of classical watershed algorithm on grey-scale textured images such as tissue images is over-segmentation. The following procedure is a merging process for the over segmentation regions using RFCM. But there are still some regions which are not partitioned completely, particularly in the transitional regions of gray matter and white matter, or cerebrospinal fluid and gray matter. This motivated the construction of a re-segmentation processing approach to partition these regions. We exploited a method base on Minimum Covariance Determinant (MCD) estimator to detect the regions needed segmentation again, and then partition them by a supervised k-Nearest Neighbor (kNN) classifier. This integrated scheme yields a robust and precise segmentation.

References

1. Pham DL, Xu CY, Prince JL: A survey of current methods in medical image segmentation. Ann. Rev. Biomed. Eng. 2 (2000) 315—37 [Technical report version, JHU/ECE 99—01, Johns Hopkins University].
2. Wells WM, Grimson WEL, Kikinis R, Arrdrige SR: Adaptive segmentation of MRI data. IEEE Trans Med Imaging, 15 (1996) 429—42.
3. Nowak R.: Wavelet-based Rician noise removal for magnetic resonance imaging. IEEE Trans. Image Process. 8(10), (1999) 1408–1419.
4. LORENZ C, KRAHNSTOEVER N: 3D statistical shape models for medical image segmentation [J]. Proceedings of the Second International Conference on 3-D Digital Imaging and Modeling (3DIM)'99, (1999)394-404.
5. Pham D., Xu C., Prince J.: Current methods in medical image segmentation. Annu. Rev. Biomed. Eng. 2, (2000)315–337.
6. Bezdek J., Hall L., Clarke L.: Review of MR image segmentation techniques using pattern recognition. Med. Phys. 20 (4), (1993)1033–1048.
7. Clark M., Hall L., Goldgof D., Clarke L., Velthuizen R., Silbiger M.: MRI segmentation using fuzzy clustering techniques. IEEE Eng. Med. Biol. Mag. 13 (5), (1994)730–742.
8. Clarke L., Velthuizen R., Camacho M., Heine J., Vaidyanathan M., Hall L., Thatcher R., Silbiger M.: MRI segmentation: methods and application. Magn. Reson. Imaging 13 (3), (1995)343–368.
9. Alan Wee-Chung Liew, Hong Yan: An Adaptive Spatial Fuzzy Clustering Algorithm for 3-D MR Image Segmentation, IEEE Transaction on Medical Imaging, vol 22, No 9 (2003).
10. Niessen W., Vincken K., Weickert J., Haar Romeny B., Viergever M.: Multiscale segmentation of threedimensional MR brain images. Internat. J. Comput. Vision 31 (2/3), (1999)185–202.
11. Kwan R.-S., Evans A., Pike G.: MRI simulation-based evaluation of image-processing and classification methods. IEEE Trans. Med. Imaging 18 (11), (1999)1085–1097.

12. Niessen W., Vincken K., Weickert J., Haar Romeny B., Viergever M.: Multiscale segmentation of threedimensional MR brain images. Internat. J. Comput. Vision 31 (2/3), (1999)185–202.
13. Luc Vincent, Pierre Soille: Watersheds in Digital Spaces: An Efficient Algorithm Based on Immersion Simulations, IEEE Transaction on Pattern Analysis And Machine Intelligence, vol 13, No 6, (1991).
14. Ety Navon, Ofer Miller, Amir Averbuch: Color image segmentation based on adaptive local thresholds, Image and Vision Computing 23 (2005) 69-85.
15. Pizurica A., Philips W., Lemahieu I., Acheroy M.: A versatile wavelet domain noise filtration technique for medical imaging. IEEE Trans. Med. Imaging 22 (3), (2003)323–331.
16. Kwan R.-S., Evans A., Pike G.: MRI simulation-based evaluation of image-processing and classification methods. IEEE Trans. Med. Imaging 18 (11), (1999)1085–1097. Available: http://www.bic.mni.mcgill.ca/brainweb.
17. 17 Rousseeuw, P.J., Driessen, K.: A fast algorithm for the minimum covariance determinant estimator. Technometrics 41 (3), (1999)212-223.
18. Chris A. Cocosco, Alex P. Zijdenbos, Alan C. Evans: A fully automatic and robust brain MRI tissue classification method. IEEE Transaction on Medical Image Analysis, vol.7, (2003) 513-527.
19. Enas, G., Choi, S., 1986. Choice of the smoothing parameter and efficiency of k-nearest neighbour classification. Computers and Mathematics with Applications 12A (2), 235-244.
20. DN Kennedy, PA Filipek, VS Caviness: Anatomic segmentation and volumetric calculations in nuclear magnetic resonance imaging, IEEE Transactions on Medical Imaging, Vol. 8, (1989)1-7. Available: http://www.cma.mgh.harvard.edu/ibsr/.
21. Zijdenbos A., Dawant B.: Brain segmentation and white matter lesion detection in MR images. Crit. Rev. Biomed. Eng. 22 (5–6), (1994)401–465.
22. Mount, D., Arya, S., 1998. ANN: Library for approximate nearest neighbor searching. http://www.cs.umd.edu/_mount/ANN/.

Spatial Intensity Correction of Fluorescent Confocal Laser Scanning Microscope Images

Sang-Chul Lee and Peter Bajcsy

National Center for Supercomputing Applications, University of Illinois at
Urbana-Champaign, 1205 W. Clark St., Urbana, IL 61801, USA
{sclee, pbajcsy}@ncsa.uiuc.edu

Abstract. Fluorescent confocal laser scanning microscope (CLSM) imaging has
become popular in medical domain for the purpose of 3D information extraction. 3D information is extracted either by visual inspection or by automated
techniques. Nonetheless, 3D information extraction from CLSM suffers from
significant lateral intensity heterogeneity. We propose a novel lateral intensity
heterogeneity correction technique to improve accurate image analysis, e.g.,
quantitative analysis, segmentation, or visualization. The proposed technique is
novel in terms of its design (spatially adaptive mean-weight filtering) and application (CLSM), as well as its properties and full automation. The key properties
of the intensity correction techniques include adjustment of intensity heterogeneity, preservation of fine structural details, and enhancement of image contrast.
The full automation is achieved by data-driven parameter optimization and introduction of several evaluation metrics. We evaluated the performance by
comparing with three other techniques, four quality metrics, and two realistic
synthetic images and one real CLSM image.

1 Introduction

Visual inspection of medical specimens is one of the most common techniques in a
medical domain used for diagnosis. Based on the need to investigate specimen characteristics at high spatial resolution, fluorescent Confocal Laser Scanning Microscopy
(CLSM) imaging is frequently used for obtaining images of cross sections. Unfortunately, the intensity information often is distorted due to multiple specimen preparation and image acquisition limitations. Thus, there is a need to investigate techniques
for fluorescent CLSM image intensity adjustment to support visual inspection tasks.
Our work is primarily intended to support visual inspection of 3D volumes in virtual
reality environments [1] to be quantitatively analyzed and correlated with information
from other sensors. Nevertheless, it is well recognized that spatial intensity heterogeneity is a major barrier in acquiring reliable results during the above analyses [2],[3].

There are several known factors that cause spatial intensity heterogeneity, such as
photo-bleaching, fluorescent attenuation along confocal (depth) axis, image acquisition factors [2],[4], variations of illumination exposure rate, spatially uneven distribution of dye and the spatial characteristics of illumination beams [5], and fluorochrome
micro-environment, e.g., pH, temperature, embedding medium, etc [6]. However, it is
infeasible to monitor all exact states of a fluorescent dye in an imaged specimen at a

R.R. Beichel and M. Sonka (Eds.): CVAMIA 2006, LNCS 4241, pp. 143–154, 2006.

pixel resolution. Thus, it is very hard to develop an intensity heterogeneity correction method that would be directly linked to the sources of intensity heterogeneity coming from specimen preparation and image acquisition steps.

In past, intensity correction has been performed based on empirical correction methods for intensity loss [7], constant thresholding [8], iterative correction methods [9], 2D histogram [10], or estimations of intensity decay function [11]. However, most of these methods assume that the rate of photo-bleaching is spatially homogeneous in a lateral plane, can be characterized by an exponential function in depth [4], and mainly contributes to intensity loss along the specimen depth axis (z-axis) [12]. Nonetheless, these assumptions do not hold in a general case.

To solve the intensity correction problem in a lateral (x-y) plane, Histogram Equalization (HE) has been used in early applications [13], which leads to a uniform global intensity distribution in output image. However, it cannot effectively enhance local intensity variation due to its global property. To address this problem, Adaptive Histogram Equalization (AHE) has been used to adjust intensity variation locally by computing local histograms within spatially different windows [14]. A major problem of AHE is high sensitivity to noise, which results in amplification of undesired noise values. An improved approach to adjust local intensity variation is the Contrast Limiting Adaptive Histogram Equalization (CLAHE) [15]. It reduces noise amplification due to AHE by setting clipping limits and so removes boundary artifacts by background subtraction. Nevertheless, the main drawbacks of CLAHE are; (1) the parameters need to be manually selected. (2) There could be loss of fine details caused by intensity saturation. Alternatively, a model based approach is proposed by applying a bias field, e.g., intensity distortion map, to a polynomial function which is defined in prior [16]. However, this method requires prior knowledge about images, e.g., the degree of a polynomial function, and the computational complexity tends to increase exponentially upon the degree of a polynomial function.

In this work, we propose an intensity correction technique with data-driven parameter selection. The technique, we call *mean-weight filtering*, adjusts intensity heterogeneity in x-y plane, preserves fine structural details, and enhances image contrast by performing spatially adaptive filtering, which is understood as highly salient in 3D visualization environment when examined by medical experts [1]. Although the intensity heterogeneity correction problem may be viewed as a restoration problem, we

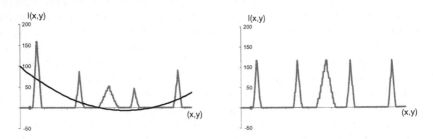

Fig. 1. Intensity Correction Problem: (left) measured intensity profile for CLSM images with intensity bias (solid curve) and (right) corrected intensity profile. Intensity bias has been corrected while preserving local intensity gradients.

formulate the problem as an optimization problem since it is impossible to obtain the true uncorrupted intensity values for comparative purposes. Thus, we formulate the intensity heterogeneity correction problem as a search for an optimal, spatially adaptive, intensity transformation that maximizes intensity contrast with respect to background, minimizes overall spatial intensity variation for large area, e.g., low frequency domain, and minimizes distortion of intensity gradient for local features, e.g., high frequency domain, as shown in Fig. 1. We assume that the input image contains a single band (or a grayscale image) with spatially varying intensities.

2 Mean Weight Filtering

Our approach combines a kernel-based spatial filtering, and incorporates local and global image intensity analysis. The proposed intensity correction process consists of determining the background threshold intensity, optimizing the kernel size, constructing a set of 2D intensity correction maps for the volume, multiplying the intensity correction maps to the frames, and removing outlier pixels (speckle noise) from the corrected images based on statistical value ranges.

2D filter model: An image filtering approach to the presented intensity correction problem can be described as:

$$g_{[a,b]}(x, y) = I(x, y) \cdot w_{[a,b]}(x, y) \tag{1}$$

where $g_{[a,b]}(x, y)$ and $I(x, y)$ are the output and input pixel values at (x, y) and $w_{[a,b]}(x, y)$ is the weighting coefficient computed over a pixel neighborhood $([x-a, x+a], [y-b, y+b])$. The spatial neighborhood $(2a+1) \times (2b+1)$, also denoted as a filtering kernel of size, is introduced to meet the requirement on local intensity gradient. Other requirements on intensity contrast and global spatial intensity variations are incorporated into the filter design by separating background according to a threshold δ, and computing the weighting coefficient $w_{[a,b]}(x, y)$ as Eq. (2).

$$w_{[a,b]}(x, y) = \begin{cases} \dfrac{\mu_G}{\mu_{L[a,b]}(x, y)} & \text{if } I(x, y) > \delta \text{ and } \mu_{L[a,b]}(x, y) \neq 0 \\ 1 & \text{otherwise} \end{cases} \tag{2}$$

where μ_G and $\mu_{L[a,b]}(x, y)$ are the global and local estimated sample means for foreground pixels only, and δ is a background threshold intensity value.

It is apparent that the weighting coefficients could be ill-defined when the local sample mean takes very small values (the spatial kernel belongs to background with some noise, $\mu_{L[a,b]}(x, y) \approx 0$.) To avoid this problem, input image is thresholded first, and then the values of global and local sample means are computed only over foreground pixels. In the filter design, we introduced two parameters, such as a background threshold δ and a kernel size $(2a+1) \times (2b+1)$.

Background separation: In general, the background threshold value could be determined by purely depending on images, such as variogram [17]. However, it is prefer able that the noise model of different imaging techniques should be modeled differently based on known imaging physics such as Exponential, Rayleigh, Gaussian, Gamma, Poisson, or Weibull function [18]. In our background separation, we assume an exponential noise model for the CLSM background noise since it is well known that the noise in laser imaging can be modeled by an exponential function [13].

We derived δ by modeling a frequency function of the pixel intensities, i.e., a histogram, followed by fitting with underlying physical models of CLSM imaging. We model the frequency function of intensity values as a conjunction of background noise $\Lambda(v)$ in a photo-multiplier tube and foreground fluorescent pixel intensity distribution $\Phi(v)$, where v is an intensity value. Assuming that $\Lambda(v)$ and $\Phi(v)$ follow an exponential and unknown exponential family of functional model respectively, we define the frequency functions as $\Lambda(v) = \alpha e^{\beta v}$ and $\Phi(v) = \gamma(v)e^{\kappa(v)}$ where α, β are constants and $\gamma(\cdot), \kappa(\cdot)$ are some functions for foreground intensity values. Since defined components are independent, assuming noise is additive, the frequency function $F(v)$ of output intensity can be modeled as a sum of $\Lambda(v)$ and $\Phi(v)$, which is $F(v) = \Phi(v) + \Lambda(v)$.

In particular, since the background pixels usually appear in low-intensity ranges and we only consider the left tail of the $F(v)$ where foreground intensity starts to contributes to $F(v)$ by fitting our noise model $\Lambda(v)$ to the low intensity range of $F(v)$. To compute the background frequency function, we estimated the parameters α, β using the least-squares methods [19] as following:

$$\begin{bmatrix} \sum_{v=1}^{k} F(v) & \sum_{v=1}^{k} vF(v) \\ \sum_{v=1}^{k} vF(v) & \sum_{v=1}^{k} v^2 F(v) \end{bmatrix} \begin{bmatrix} \alpha \\ \ln(\beta) \end{bmatrix} = \begin{bmatrix} \sum_{v=1}^{k} F(v)\ln(F(v)) \\ \sum_{v=1}^{k} vF(v)\ln(F(v)) \end{bmatrix} \tag{3}$$

where $F(v)$ is the frequency (e.g., pixel count) of the intensity value v in the input image, k is the bin number (intensity value) in $[1, n]$, and n is the number of bins.

In order to find the threshold value which is dominantly determined by the background noise by photo-multiplier tube, we computed the sum of squared error $R(k)$ (Eq. (4)) by increasing k from 3 to n in Eq. (3), where $\Lambda_k(v)$ is an exponential function fit to first k bins.

$$R(k) = \left(\frac{1}{0.1n} \sqrt{\sum_{v=1}^{0.1n} (F(v) - \Lambda_k(v))^2} \right) \tag{4}$$

Since we approximated the foreground pixel intensity distribution for the left tail only, the sum of squared error is calculated for the pixel intensity values in 10% of low intensity value range, i.e., $[1, 25]$ in byte (8-bit) image. It approximates $\Lambda_k(v)$ in the input image well enough since R is not much affected by large intensity values.

Finally, the background threshold value δ is determined by the value k where the estimated function $\Lambda_k(v)$ best fits with the background noise in the input image such as $\delta = \arg\min_{k \in [1,n]} (R(k))$.

Kernel size optimization: In order to compute local sample means $\mu_{L[a,b]}(x,y)$, one has to choose the size and shape of a filtering kernel for an input image. We first constrained the kernel shape to a rectangle. Then we selected a kernel size by maximizing the global contrast while minimizing the gradient distortion, e.g., high frequency distortion. We used a global contrast metric C described in [21] which incorporates one of the requirements of the intensity heterogeneity correction problem as follows.

$$C = \sum_{i=1}^{m} \left\| f_i(I) - E(f(I)) \right\| \times f(I)_i \tag{5}$$

where $f(I)$ is the histogram (estimated probability density function) of all contrast values by using Sobel edge detector in an image I, $f_i(I)$ is the density of i-th bin, $E(f(I))$ is the sample mean of the histogram $f(I)$, and m is the number of distinct contrast values in a discrete case. The equation includes the contrast magnitude term and the term with the likelihood of contrast occurrence. In general, image frames characterized by a large value of C are more suitable for further processing than the frames with a small value of C.

To demonstrate the high frequency image difference between the original image and the processed image, we define a metric D as follows:

$$D = \sum_{v}^{M} \sum_{u}^{N} (I_{hf}^{org}(u,v) - I_{hf}^{adj}(u,v))^2 \tag{6}$$

where I_{hf}^{org} and I_{hf}^{adj} are the high-pass filtered images of the original and the intensity adjusted image respectively. Finally, the filter size is selected by evaluating the maximum value of the ratio C/D denoted as a measure of image saliency.

Speckle noise removal: One of the side products of the mean-weight filtering is an easy detection of speckle noise in the background. Speckle noise is characterized by a pixel with very few or no neighboring pixels and the mean-weight filtering generates very high intensity correction value for the speckle pixels. We have eliminated speckle noise by removing the pixels with abnormally high intensity correction values statistically, and accepted the pixels with values within the range $[0, \mu + 4\sigma]$ (99.99% of pixels are included), where μ and σ are the sample mean and standard deviation of the intensities in the corrected image. Finally, the values within the range $[0, \mu + 4\sigma]$ are normalized to $[0,255]$ to meet the dynamic range of output images (8 bits per pixel).

3 Experimental Results

Simulation Results: Fig. 2 (left) shows a bias-free synthetic image (shown as horizontal and vertical bars with different thickness and spacing, and Fig. 2 (middle) and (right) show intensity distorted images by pre-defined intensity variations (bias fields). Background noise is simulated by adding random exponential synthetic noise with density function $\Lambda(v) = 0.3e^{0.3v}$.

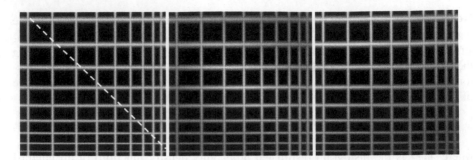

Fig. 2. (left) bias-free image (dotted line is shown to illustrate the intensity profile later in Fig. 7), (middle, right) images with intensity distortion with synthetic noise

Fig. 3. (left) shows the curves of residuals $R(\cdot)$ for the two simulation images in Fig. 2. (middle, right) (see Eq. (4)). The background thresholds are selected based on the minimum value of the curves except the low value range between 1 and 3, which were 20 for both simulation images. Next, to optimize the kernel size for each image, we calculated the image saliency (C/D) for kernel sizes from 3 to 51, shown in Fig. 3. (right). Generally, it is observed that; (1) for small kernels, the contrast C is maximized but the high frequency distortion is large; (2) for large kernels, the high frequency distortion is minimized but the contrast C is compromised. Therefore, the simulation results verified that the optimal kernel size is achieved by maximizing the contrast divided by the high frequency difference (C/D). In our simulation experiments, we calculated C/D using kernel sizes from 3 to 51 pixels wide, and obtained the optimum values equal to 33 and 47 pixel widths respectively (see the peaks in Fig.3 (right)).

Given the background threshold and kernel size in Fig. 3, we show the intensity corrected images by the mean weight filtering in Fig. 4. (left and middle). Fig. 4. (right) shows the intensity correction maps applied to the intensity distorted (uncorrected) images. The intensity correction maps demonstrate higher weight in dark local

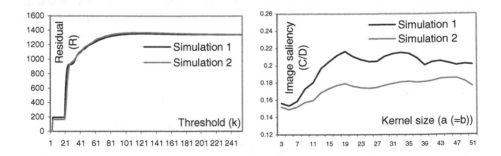

Fig. 3. (left) Residual for background thresholding in Eq, (4), and (right) image saliency as a function of the kernel size (see Eq. (5) and Eq. (6))

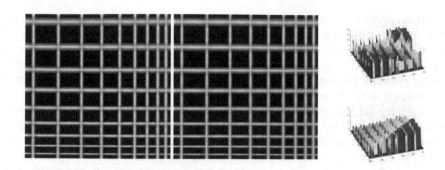

Fig. 4. (left, middle) Intensity corrected images using the mean-weight filtering with the kernel size of 33 (left) and 47 (middle) respectively. (right) Intensity correction maps (pseudo colored) where upper and lower map corresponds to the (left) and (middle) image respectively.

regions than in bright local regions. Regardless of the type of a bias field, all intensity corrected images show noticeable improvement such that the mean weight filtering corrects intensity heterogeneity over spatially large area while preserving the edge gradients (minimum high frequency distortion) over spatially small area.

For visual comparison, we show the intensity correction results for the simulation images using Histogram equalization (HE), Histogram equalization with background

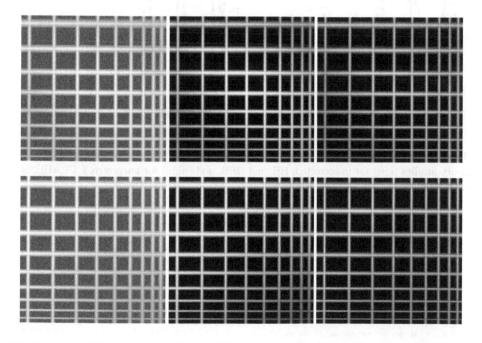

Fig. 5. Result of Histogram Equalization, Histogram Equalization with background thresholding, and CLAHE for simulation 1 (upper three images) and simulation 2 (lower three images)

separation (HEB) (background threshold = 20), and CLAHE (see Fig. 5). One could notice that HE saturated most of pixels, amplified background noise, and removed edge gradient significantly. HEB separated out background noise, but the edge gradient is not preserved well similarly to the HE, and CLAHE relatively well preserved the edge gradient, but the spatial (x-y) intensity heterogeneity has not been corrected in comparison to the Mean weight filtering.

To demonstrate the spatial intensity correction result, Fig. 6. shows the intensity profiles (along the dotted line Fig. 2. (left) for the simulation 2 (see Fig. 2 (right)) of the uncorrected, HE, HEB, CLAHE, and the mean weight filtering. The intensity profile clearly demonstrates that the intensity along x-y plane is best corrected by the mean weight filtering while preserving local intensity gradients, i.e., the peaks of intensity value remains between 190 and 200.

Comparative Results for CLSM Images: We applied the mean weight filtering method to a real CLSM image. The image was acquired with a Leica SP2 laser scanning confocal microscope (Leica, Heidelberg, Germany) using the 40X objective with 605~ 700 nm excitation wavelength range for the test specimens. The image was stored in tagged information file format (TIFF) with 512 by 512 pixel resolution.

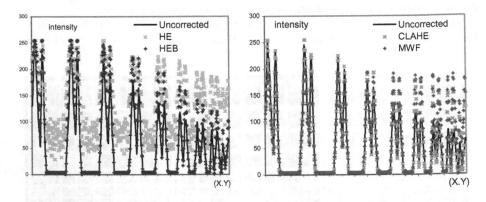

Fig. 6. Intensity profile along the red dotted line in Fig. 3 (left) for the simulation image 2: Intensity profiles (left) for uncorrected, HE, and HEB, and (right) for uncorrected, CLAHE, and mean-weight filtering

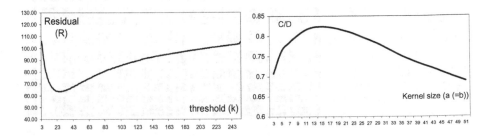

Fig. 7. Residual of the estimated function for the input image in Fig. 8. The intensity threshold minimizing R is 26 (left), and the optimal kernel size (maximizing C/D) is 15 (right).

First, we decided the background threshold and the kernel size by the proposed method in the Section 2, which correspond to $\delta = 26$ and $a = b = 15$ (see Fig. 7.)

In order to quantitatively asses the quality of multiple filtering techniques for real CLSM images, multiple intensity correction results are compared by image contrast C (Eq. (5)), high frequency distortion D (Eq. (6)), the low frequency intensity heterogeneity S (evaluated by the image entropy in low frequency domain [20]), and the number of saturated pixels N as defined in Eq. (7).

$$N = \sum_{v}^{M} \sum_{u}^{N} sat(I^{org}(u,v), I^{adj}(u,v)) \tag{7}$$

where $sat(I^{org}(u,v), I^{adj}(u,v)) = \begin{cases} 1 & \text{if } I^{org}(u,v) \neq l \text{ and } I^{adj}(u,v) = l \\ 0 & \text{otherwise} \end{cases}$, I^{org} and I^{adj} are the original and intensity adjusted images, and l is the maximum intensity value of the original image, e.g. 255 in a byte image. For the best image quality, it is desirable to achieve large C and small S, D, and N.

Fig. 8. shows the input CLSM image with the processed results by existing and the mean-weight filtering method. One could visually notice that the histogram equalization

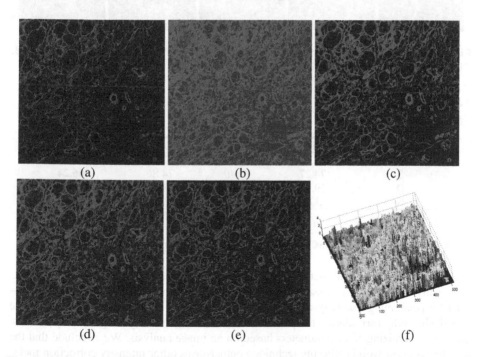

(a)   (b)   (c)

(d)   (e)   (f)

Fig. 8. CLSM test image: (a) Original test image, (b) histogram equalization, (c) histogram equalization with background thresholding, (d) CLAHE ("adapthisteq()" with default setting by Matlab Image Processing Toolbox, Build. R12), (e) mean weight filtering, and (f) intensity correction maps by the mean weight filtering.

method removes best intensity heterogeneity in large spatial regions but maintains low visual saliency and, most importantly, removes edge details (high frequency distortion) (see the second image in Fig. 9.). The histogram equalization with background threshold ($\delta = 26$) and Contrast Limited Adaptive Histogram Equalization demonstrate similar removal of edge gradient and edge details. To demonstrate the effect of edge gradient, we show a sub-region of the intensity corrected images in Fig. 9. They show that most of pixels around the edge were saturated using HE, HEB, or CLAHE while the mean weight filtering well preserves edge gradient.

In addition to visual assessments, we show the quantitative evaluation of the compared techniques with four quality metrics in Table 1. In general, an optimal intensity correction technique has to meet multiple optimization criteria, for example, minimize S, D and N, and maximize C. For both measured test images, Table 1 shows that the mean-weight filtering achieves a normalized metric that is about 1.5 to 1.7 times larger than the second best performing technique.

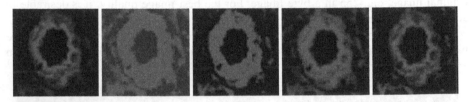

Fig. 9. Sub-region of intensity corrected images in Fig. 8. (from left, original image, HE, HEB, CLAHE, and Mean-weight filtering).

Table 1. Evaluation results in Fig. 8. The first and second best results are shown in bold and italic respectively.

CLSM Image	HE	HEB (26)	CLAHE	MWF (26,15)
C	17.15	**17.34**	*17.20*	16.26
S	74.27	*73.40*	74.86	**66.24**
D	29.88	*23.93*	28.02	**21.98**
N	*330*	*330*	334	**0**

4   Conclusion and Discussion

We introduced an intensity heterogeneity correction technique that adjusts intensity heterogeneity of 2D images, preserves fine structural details, and enhances the image contrast by performing spatially adaptive mean-weight filtering. The proposed technique was designed by formulating the problem requirements, defining image quality metrics, and then optimizing filter parameters based on an image analysis. We conclude that the developed mean-weight filtering technique outperforms other intensity correction methods by at least a factor of 1.5 when applied to fluorescent CLSM images.

Although automatic selection of a kernel size shows optimized the global image saliency, it is worth to consider some images with a mixture of different structures (e.g., edge thickness) that require multiple kernel sizes per image for different regions of interest. If a user chooses to select a kernel size on his own, we would provide the following considerations: (a) A large kernel tends to preserve the detail of rather large area, e.g., thick edge or spatial intensity heterogeneity in a feature region, and extremely large kernels correct minimally intensities in x-y plane. (b) A small kernel generates visually salient images by highlighting sharp intensity changes, e.g., small intensity discontinuities. However, extremely small kernels *correct* high frequency intensity change which is typically considered as edge gradient (and need to be preserved). (c) A kernel size could be selected based on edge thickness: for thin edges, a smaller kernel size is preferred since only high frequency component should be corrected. For thick edges, a larger kernel should be used since a low frequency component should be corrected while preserving a high frequency component. Fig. 10 shows the mean weight filtering results with different kernel sizes.

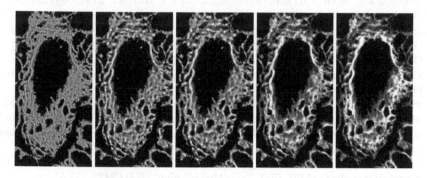

Fig. 10. Mean weight filtering with different kernel sizes: From left, the kernel width is equals to 3,7,9,21,51

References

1. Chen, X., Ai, Z., Rasmussen, M., Bajcsy, P., Auvil, L., Welge, M., Leach, L., Folberg, R.: Three-dimensional reconstruction of extravascular matrix patterns and blood vessels in human uveal melanoma tissue: Preliminary findings. Invest. Ophthal. & Vis. Sci., 44 (2003) 2834-2840
2. Benson, D., Bryan, J., Plant, A., Gotto, A., Smith, L.: Digital Imaging fluorescence microscopy: Spatial heterogeneity of photobleaching rate constants in individual cells. J. Cell Biol. 100 (1985) 1309-1323
3. Jungke, M., Seelen, von W., Bielke, G. , Meindl, S. et al.: A system for the diagnostic use of tissue characterizing parameters in NMR-tomography. Proc. of Info. Proc. in Med. Imaging, IPMI'87, 39 (1987) 471-481
4. Rigaut, J., Vassy, J.: High-resolution 3D images from confocal scanning laser microscopy: quantitative study and mathematical correction of the effects from bleaching and fluorescence attenuation in depth. Anal. Quant. Cytol. 13 (1991) 223-232
5. Oostveldt, P. V., Verhaegen, F., Messen, K.: Heterogenous photobleaching in confocal microscopy caused by differences in refractive index and excitation mode. Cytometry 32 (1998) 137-146
6. Tauer, U., Hils, O.: Confocal Spectrophotometry, in Sci. and Tech. Info., Sp. issue: Confocal Microscopy, CDR 4 (2000) 15-27

7. Rodenacker, K., Aubele, P., Hutzler, M., Adiga, P.: Groping for quantitative digital 3-D image analysis: an approach to quantitative fluorescence in situ hybridization in thick tissue sections of prostate carcinoma. Anal. Cell. Pathol. 15 (1997) 19-29

8. Irinopoulo, T., Vassy, J., Beil, M., Nicolopoulo, P., Encaoua, D., Rigaut, J.: 3-D DNA image cytometry by confocal scanning lasermicroscopy in thick tissue blocks of prostatic lesions. Cytometry, 27 (1997) 99-105

9. Roerdink, J., Bakker, M.: An FFT-based method for attenuation correction in fluorescence confocal microscopy. J. Microsc. 169 (1993) 3-14

10. Liljeborg, A., Czader, M., Porwit, A.: A method to compensate for light attenuation with depth in 3D DNA image cytometry using a confocal scanning laser microscope. J. Microsc. 177 (1995) 108-114

11. Kervrann, C., Legland, D., Pardini, L.: Robust incremental compensation of the light attenuation with depth in 3D fluorescence microscopy. J. Microsc., 214 (2004) 297-314

12. Oostveldt, P., Verhaegen, F., Messens, K.: Heterogeneous photobleaching in confocal microscopy caused by differences in refractive index and excitation mode. Cytometry, 32 (1998) 137-146

13. Gonzalez, R., Woods, E.: Digital Image Processing. 2nd ed., Prentice hall, (2002)

14. Pizer, S. M., Zimmerman, J. B., Stabb, E.: Adaptive grey level assignment in CT scan display. J. Comp. Assist. Tomography, 8 (1984) 300-305

15. Pisano, E., Zong, S., Hemminger, M., De Luca, M., Johnsoton, R., Muller, K., Braeuning, M., Pizer, S.: Contrast Limited Adaptive Histogram Equalization Image Processing to Improve the Detection of Simulated Spiculations in Dense Mammograms. J. Digital Imaging, 11(4) (1998) 193-200

16. Styner M, Brechbuhler C, Szekely G., Gerig G.: Parametric estimate of intensity inhomogeneities applied to MRI. IEEE Trans Med Imaging, 19(3) (2000) 153-65

17. Sanchez-Brea, L.M., Bernabeu, E.: On the standard deviation in CCD cameras: a variogram-based technique for non-uniform images. J. Electronic Imaging 11(2) (2002) 121-126.

18. Hu, J., Razdan, A., Nielson, G., Farin, G., Baluch, D., Capco, D.: Volumetric Segmentation Using Weibull E-SD Fields, IEEE Trans. on Vis. and Comp. Graphics, 9(3) (2003)

19. Weisstein, E. Least Squares Fitting--Exponential. from MathWorld--A Wolfram Web Resource. http://mathworld.wolfram.com/LeastSquaresFittingExponential.html

20. Mangin, J.: Entropy minimization for automatic correction of intensity nonuniformity Math. Method in Biomed. Image Analysis (MMBIA), (2000) 162-169

21. Bajcsy P., Groves, P.: Methodology for Hyperspectral Band Selection, Photo. Eng. and Remote Sensing J., 70 (2004) 793-802

Quasi-conformal Flat Representation of Triangulated Surfaces for Computerized Tomography

Eli Appleboim, Emil Saucan, and Yehoshua Y. Zeevi

Electrical Engineering Department, Technion, Haifa, Israel
{eliap, semil, zeevi}@ee.technion.ac.il

Abstract. In this paper we present a simple method for flattening of triangulated surfaces for mapping and imaging. The method is based on classical results of F. Gehring and Y. Väisälä regarding the existence of quasi-conformal and quasi-isometric mappings between Riemannian manifolds. A random starting triangle version of the algorithm is presented. A curvature based version is also applicable. In addition the algorithm enables the user to compute the maximal distortion and dilatation errors. Moreover, the algorithm makes no use to derivatives, hence it is robust and suitable for analysis of noisy data. The algorithm is tested on data obtained from real CT images of the human brain cortex and colon, as well as on a synthetic model of the human skull.

1 Introduction

In many medical applications of image processing, such as medical imaging for noninvasive diagnosis and image guided surgery, a paramount importance lies in the process of two-dimensional representation by flattening of three-dimensional object scans. For example, it is often advantageous to present three-dimensional MRI or CT scans of the cortex as flat two-dimensional images. Yet in order to do so in a meaningful manner, so that the diagnosis will be accurate, it is essential that the geometric dilatation and distortion, in terms of change of angles and lengths, caused by this representation, will be minimal. However, since most surfaces of medical interest, such as colon, cortex, etc., are not isometric to the plane, a zero-distortion solution is seldom feasible. A reasonable solution to this problem is given by conformal maps ([9], [10]). Mapping the surface conformally to the (complex) plane preserves angles and therefore the local shape.

Naturally, the problem of conformal flattening of surfaces, in particular for medical imaging, has focused the interest of many researchers in the recent years, and there exists a vast literature covering the said problem (see Section 1.1 below). In fact, in all previous works, only approximations of conformal mappings have been achieved, and as such they all suffer from the presence of some amount of distorsion/dilatation. Therefore, one should aim to control the amount of inherent distortion. This can be achieved by quasi-isometric/quasi-conformal maps (i.e. maps that are almost isometries/conformal; precise definition will follow in Section 2). Practically, there is a tradeoff between the cost of an implementation

R.R. Beichel and M. Sonka (Eds.): CVAMIA 2006, LNCS 4241, pp. 155–165, 2006.

on one hand and accuracy on the other. Common to all solutions is the fact, which cannot be avoided because of the inevitable distortion, that the more locally one is willing to focus, the more accurate the results become.

1.1   Related Works

As stated above, the problem of minimal distortion flattening of surfaces attracted, in recent years, a great attention and interest, due to its wide range of applications.

In this section we briefly review some of the methods that were proposed for dealing with this problem.

Variational Methods. Haker et al. ([9], [10]) introduced the use of a variational method for conformal flattening of CT/MRI 3-D scans of the brain/colon for the purpose of medical imaging. The method is essentially based on solving Dirichlet problem for the Laplace-Beltrami operator $\triangle u = 0$ on a given surface Σ, with certain boundary conditions on $\partial \Sigma$. A solution to this problem is a harmonic (thus conformal) map from the surface to the (complex) plane. The solution suggested in [9] and [10] is a PL (piecewise linear) approximation of the smooth solution, achieved by solving a proper system of linear equations.

Circle Packing. Hurdal et al. ([11]) attempt to obtain such a conformal map by using circle packing. This relies on the ability to approximate conformal structure on surfaces by circle packings. The authors use this method for MRI brain images and conformally map them to the three possible models of geometry in dimension 2 (i.e. the 2-sphere, the Euclidian plane and the Hyperbolic plane). Yet, the method is applicable for surfaces which are topologically equivalent to a disk whereas the brain cortex surface is not. This means that there is a point of the brain (actually a neighborhood of a point), which will not map conformally to the plane, and in this neighborhood the dilatation will be infinitely large. Hurdal et al. solve this problem by removing the *corpus callosum*, thus obtaining a surface homeomorphic to a 1-punctured sphere, and thus conformally equivalent to a disk ([11], [12]). An additional problem arises due to the necessary assumption that the surface triangulation is homogeneous in the sense that all triangles are equilateral. Such triangulations are seldom attainable.

Holomorphic 1-forms. Gu et al. ([7], [8], [6]) are using holomorphic 1-forms in order to compute global conformal structure of a smooth surface of arbitrary genus given as a triangulated mesh. holomorphic 1-forms are differential forms (differential operators) on smooth manifolds, which among other things can depict conformal structures. This method indeed yields a global conformal structure hence, a conformal parameterization for the surface however, computing homology basis is extremely time consuming.

Angle Methods. In [13] Sheffer et al. parameterize surfaces via an angle based method in a way that minimizes angle distortion while flattening. However, the surfaces are assumed to be approximated by cone surfaces, i.e. surfaces that are composed from cone-like neighborhoods.

To summarize, all the methods described above compute only approximation to conformal mappings, therefore producing only quasi-conformal mappings, with no precise estimates on the dilatation.

In this paper we propose yet another solution to this problem. The proposed method relies on theoretical results obtained by Gehring and Väisalä in the 1960's ([5]). They were studying the existence of quasi-conformal maps between Riemannian manifolds. The basic advantages of this method resides in its simplicity, in setting, implementation and its speed. Additional advantage is that it is possible guarantee not to have distortion above a predetermined bound, which can be as small as desired, with respect to the amount of localization one is willing to pay (and, in the case of triangulated surfaces, to the quality of the given mesh). In fact, the proposed method is – to the best of our knowledge – the only algorithm capable of computing both length distortion and angle dilatation. The suggested algorithm is best suited to cases where the surface is complex (high and non-constant curvature) such as brain cortex/colon wrapping, or of large genus, such as skeleta, proteins, etc. Moreover, since together with the angular dilatation, both length and area distortions are readily computable, the algorithm is ideally suited for applications in Oncology, where such measurements are highly relevant.

The paper is organized as follows: In the next section we introduce the theoretical background, regarding the fundamental work of Gehring and Väisalä. Afterwards we describe our algorithm for surface flattening, based on their ideas. In Section 4 we present some experimental results of this scheme and in Section 5 we discuss possible extensions of this study.

2 Theoretical Background

2.1 Basic Definitions

Definition 1. *Let* $D \subset \mathbb{R}^3$ *be a domain. A homeomorphism* $f : D \to \mathbb{R}^3$ *is called a* quasi-isometry *(or a* bi-lipschitz mapping*), if there exists* $1 \leq C < \infty$, *such that*

$$\frac{1}{C}|p_1 - p_2| \leq |f(p_1) - f(p_2)| < C|p_1 - p_2|, \text{ for all } p_1, p_2 \in D.$$

$C(f) = \min\{C \mid f \text{ is a quasi} - \text{isometry}\}$ *is called the* minimal distortion *of* f *(in* D).

Remark 1. If f *is a quasi-isometry then* $K_I(f) \leq C(f)^2$ *and* $K_O(f) \leq C(f)^2$ *where* $K_I(f), K_O(f)$ *represent the* inner, *respective* outer dilatation *of* f *(see see* v. *It follows that any quasi-isometry is a quasi-conformal mapping (while – evidently – not every quasi-conformal mapping is a quasi-isometry). Quasi-conformal is the same as quasi-isometry where distances are replaced by angles.*

Definition 2. *Let* $S \subset \mathbb{R}^3$ *be a connected set.* S *is called* admissible *iff for any* $p \in S$, *there exists a quasi-isometry* i_p *such that for any* $\varepsilon > 0$ *there exists a* *neighbourhood $U_p \subset \mathbb{R}^3$ of p, such that $i_p : U_p \to \mathbb{R}^3$ and $i_p(S \cap U_p) = D_p \subset \mathbb{R}^2$, where D_p is a domain and such that $C(i_p)$ satisfies:*

$$(i) \ \sup_{p \in S} C(i_p) < \infty;$$

and

$$(ii) \ \sup_{p \in S} C(i_p) < 1 + \varepsilon.$$

2.2   The Projection Map

Let S be a surface, $\bar{n}$ be a fixed unitary vector, and $p \in S$. Let $V \simeq D^2$, $D^2 = \{x \in \mathbb{R}^2 \mid ||x|| \le 1\}$ be a disk neighbourhood of p. Moreover, suppose that for any $q_1, q_2 \in S$, the acute angle $\angle(q_1 q_2, \bar{n}) \ge \alpha$ (see Figure 2). We refer to the last condition as *the Geometric Condition* or *Gehring Condition*.

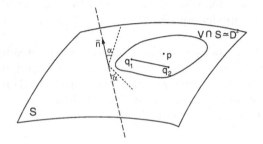

Fig. 1. The Geometric Condition

Then for any $x \in V$ there is a unique representation of the following form:

$$x = q_x + u\bar{n};$$

where q_x lies on the plane through p which is orthogonal to $\bar{n}$ and $u \in \mathbb{R}$.
  Define:

$$Pr(x) = q_x.$$

Note: $\bar{n}$ need not be the normal vector to S at p.

By [5], Section 4.3 and Lemma 5.1, we have that for any $p_1, p_2 \in S$ and any $a \in \mathbb{R}_+$ the following inequalities hold:

$$\frac{a}{A}|p_1 - p_2| \le |Pr(p_1) - Pr(p_2)| \le A|p_1 - p_2|;$$

where

$$A = \frac{1}{2}[(a \csc \alpha)^2 + 2a + 1]^2 + \frac{1}{2}[(a \csc \alpha)^2 - 2a + 1]^2.$$

In particular for $a = 1$ we get that

$$C(f) \leq \cot \alpha + 1 \, ; \tag{1}$$

and

$$K(f) \leq \left(\left(\frac{1}{2} (\cot \alpha)^2 + 4 \right)^{\frac{1}{2}} + \frac{1}{2} \cot \alpha \right)^{\frac{3}{2}} \leq (\cot \alpha + 1)^{\frac{3}{2}} \, ; \tag{2}$$

where

$$K(f) = \max \left(K_O(f), K_I(f) \right)$$

is the *maximal dilatation* of f.

The Geometric Condition. From the discussion above we conclude that $S \subset \mathbb{R}^3$ is an admissible surface if for any $p \in S$ there exists $\bar{n}_p$ such that for any $\varepsilon > 0$, there exists $U_p \simeq D^2$, such that for any $q_1, q_2 \in U_p$ the acute angle $\angle(q_1 q_2, \bar{n}_p) \geq \alpha$, where

$$(i) \ \inf_{p \in S} \alpha_p > 0 \, ;$$

and

$$(ii) \ \inf_{p \in S} \alpha_p < \frac{\pi}{2} - \varepsilon \, .$$

Example 1. Any surface in $S \in \mathbb{R}^3$ that admits a well-defined continuous turning tangent plane at any point $p \in S$ is admissible.

3   The Algorithm

We will present in this section the algorithm that is used for obtaining a quasi-isometric (flat) representation of a given surface. First assume the surface is equipped with some triangulation T. Let N_p stand for the normal vector to the surface at a point p on the surface.

Second, a triangle Δ, of the triangulation must be chosen. We will project a patch of the surface quasi-isometrically onto the plane included in Δ. This patch will be called the patch of Δ, and it will consists of at least one triangle, Δ itself. There are two possibilities to chose Δ, one is in a random manner and the other is based on curvature considerations. We will refer to both ways later. For the moment assume Δ was somehow chosen. After Δ is (trivially) projected onto itself we move to its neighbors. Suppose Δ' is a neighbor of Δ having edges e_1, e_2, e_3, where e_1 is the edge common to both Δ and Δ'.

We will call Δ' *Gehring compatible w.r.t* Δ, if the maximal angle between e_2 or e_3 and N_Δ (the normal vector to Δ), is greater then a predefined measure suited to the desired predefined maximal allowed distortion, i.e. $\max \{\varphi_1, \varphi_2\} \geq \alpha$, where $\varphi_1 = \angle(e_2, N_\Delta)$, $\varphi_2 = \angle(e_3, N_\Delta)$; (cf. (1), (2)).

We will project Δ' *orthogonally* onto the plane included in Δ and insert it to the patch of Δ, iff it is Gehring compatible w.r.t Δ.

We keep adding triangles to the patch of Δ moving from an added triangle to its neighbors (of course) while avoiding repetitions, till no triangles can be

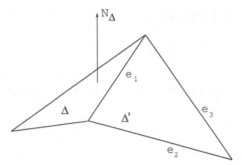

Fig. 2. Gehring Compatible Triangles

added. If by this time all triangles where added to the patch we have completed constructing the mapping. Otherwise, chose a new triangle that has not been projected yet, to be the starting triangle of a new patch. A pseudocode for this procedure can be easily written.

Remark 2. There are two ways for choosing a base triangle for each patch. One is by curvature considerations, i.e. taking a triangle which the sum of the (magnitude of) curvatures of its vertices is minimal, and the other one is by randomly choosing a triangle for each new patch.

Remark 3. One should keep in mind that the above given algorithm, as for any other flattening method, is local. Indeed, in a sense the (proposed) algorithm gives a measure of "globality" of this intrinsically local process.

Remark 4. Our algorithm is best suited for highly folded surfaces, because of its intrinsic locality, on the one hand, and computational simplicity, on the other. However, on "quasi-developable" surfaces (i.e. surfaces that are almost cylindrical or conical) the algorithm behaves similar to other algorithms, with practically identical results.

4   Experimental Results

We now proceed to present some experimental results obtained by applying the proposed algorithm, both on synthetic surfaces and on data obtained from actual CT scans.

In each of the examples both the input surface and a flattened representation of some patch are shown. Details about mesh resolution as well as flattening distortion are also provided. The number of patches needed in order to flatten the surface is also given. In all images, the small rectangle shown on the surface represents a base triangle for the flattened patch. The colored area in each of the images represents the patch being flattened.

The algorithm was implemented in two versions, or more precisely two possible ways of processing, automatic versus user defined.

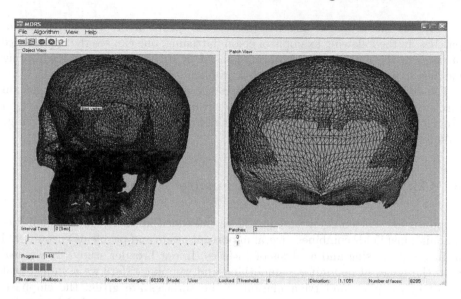

Fig. 3. Skull Flattening: The role of almost flat regions is accentuated. The resolution is of 60,339 triangles. Here α is $10°$ and the dilatation is 1.1763.

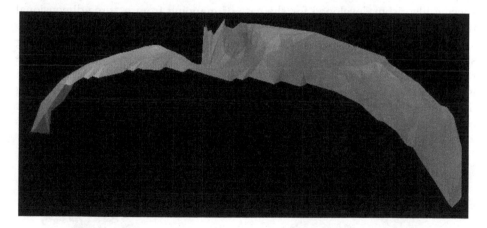

Fig. 4. Colon Section: Observe the highly folded region that a large number of patches while preserving a small dilatation. The image shows the back-side of the colon, whose flattened image is depicted in Fig. 5. (b). CT-data is in curtesy of Dr. Doron Fisher from Rambam Madical Center in Haifa.

- Automatic means that the triangles serving as base points for the patches to be flattened are chosen automatically according to curvature, as stated in Remark 3.2. The discrete curvature measure employed is that of *angular defect*, due to its simplicity and high reliability (see [14]).
- User defined means that at each stage the user chooses a base triangle for some new patch.

Since at this stage we did not address the problem of properly gluing of patches, in the following example of colon flattening, one can see the appearance of holes in the flattened presentation caused by artificially gluing neighboring patches to each other. We refer to this problem in the next section.

Experiments have shown that results of the automatic process are similar, in terms of the dilatation, to those obtained from the user defined process yet, in order to flatten entire surface in the user defined method one needs in average 25% more patches.

5   Concluding Remarks and Future Study

Sampling and flattening of folded surfaces embedded in higher dimensional Riemannian manifolds combines several important facets and problems encountered in image processing and analysis of surfaces. In our broader study [3], we deal with the issues of nonuniform smoothing and sampling. Here we assumed that a proper sampling and triangulation of the surfaces are given. the emphasis was therefore on quasi-conformal and quasi-isometric aspects of the mapping between Riemannian manifolds. While the theory is general and applicable to mapping from any higher to lower dimensional manifolds, here we presented a specific algorithm developed for the case of mapping from a three-dimensional to two-dimensional flat surface.

From the implementation results it is evident that this algorithm while being simple to program as well as efficient, also gives good flattening results and maintains small dilatations even in areas where curvature is large and good flattening is a challenging task. Moreover, since there is a simple way to assess the resulting dilatation/distorsion, the algorithm was implemented in such a way that the user can set in advance an upper bound on the resulting dilatation/distorsion. Let us

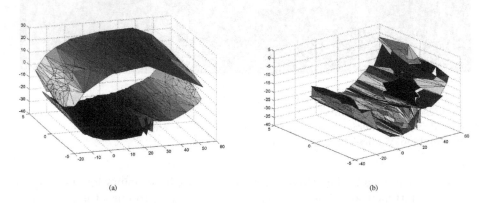

(a)   (b)

Fig. 5. Colon CT-Images: (a) Triangulated colon surface taken from 3 slices of human colon scan and (b) One half of the colon, after flattening. One is able to observe the holes caused by improper gluing of neighbouring patches.

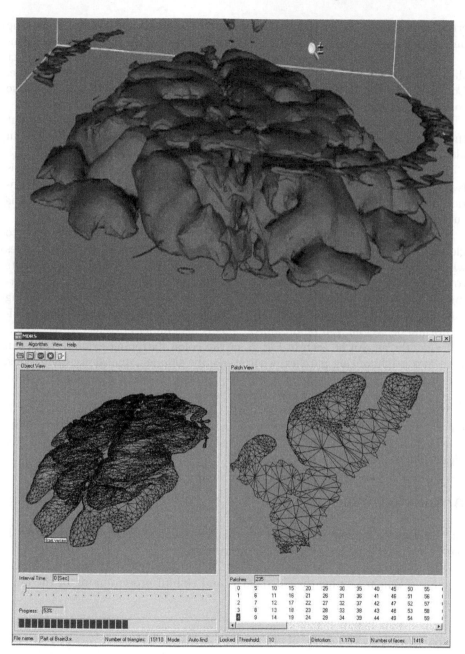

Fig. 6. Cerebral Cortex Flattening: A patch obtained in the flattening of the parietal region. The resolution is 15.110 triangles, the angle chosen is 5°, producing a dilatation of 1.0875.

stress once more that, to the best of our knowledge, our method represents the only algorithm capable of computing both length distortion and angle dilatation.

An additional advantage of the presented algorithm is related to the fact that, contrary to some of the related studies, no use of derivatives is made. Consequently, the algorithm does not suffer from typical drawbacks of derivative computations like lack of robustness, etc.

Moreover, since no derivatives are employed, no smoothness assumption about the surface to be flattened are made, which makes the algorithm presented herein ideal for use in cases where smoothness is questionable (to say the least).

The algorithm may be practical for applications where local yet, good analysis is required such as medical imaging with the emphasis on flattened representation of the brain and the colon (virtual colonoscopy) – see [1]. Further study is currently undertaken.

The main issue for further investigation, remains the transition from local to global in a more precise fashion, i.e. how can one glue two neighbouring patches while keeping fixed bounded dilatation. In more technical terms, this amounts to actually *computing* the *holonomy map* of the surface – see [15]. Computing holonomy tells you exactly how to match-up two areas of a surface having different conformal characteristics so that a bigger patch with controlled quasi-conformal behaviour will be obtained. This is also under current investigation.

Evidently, as can be seen in Fig. 5, of the colon flattening example, one can have two neighbouring patches, with markedly different dilataions/distorsions, which results in different lengths for the common boundary edges. Therefore, "cuts" and "holes" appear when applying a "naive" glueing.

We conclude by remarking that while the the application presented here is for $2D$-images of $3D$-surfaces, the results of Gehring and Väisälä are stated and proven for any dimension (and co-dimension). Therefore, implementations for higher dimensions are also in progress.

Acknowledgment

Emil Saucan is supported by the Viterbi Postdoctoral Fellowship. Research is partly supported by the Ollendorf Minerva Center.

The authors would like to thank Ofir Zeitoun and Efrat Barak and Amiad Segal and Ronen Lev for their dedicated and skillful programming of the algorithms.

References

[1] Appleboim, E., Saucan E., and Zeevi, Y. *Minimal-Distortion Mappings of Surfaces for Medical Imaging*, Proceedings of VISAPP 2006, to appear.
[2] Appleboim, E., Saucan, E., and Zeevi, Y.Y. *On Sampling and Reconstruction of Surfaces*, Technion CCIT Report, 2006.
[3] Appleboim, E., Saucan, E., and Zeevi, Y.Y.
http://www.ee.technion.ac.il/people/eliap/Demos.html

[4] Caraman, P. *n-Dimensional Quasiconformal (QCf) Mappings*, Editura Academiei Române, Bucharest, Abacus Press, Tunbridge Wells Haessner Publishing, Inc., Newfoundland, New Jersey, 1974.

[5] Gehring, W. F. and Väisälä, J. *The coefficients of quasiconformality*, Acta Math. **114**, pp. 1-70, 1965.

[6] Gu, X. Wang, Y. and Yau, S. T. *Computing Conformal Invariants: Period Matrices*, Communications In Information and Systems, Vol. 2, No. 2, pp. 121-146, December 2003.

[7] Gu, X. and Yau, S. T. *Computing Conformal Structure of Surfaces*, Communications In Information and Systems, Vol. 2, No. 2, pp. 121-146, December 2002.

[8] Gu, X. and Yau, S. T. *Global Conformal Surface Parameterization* , Eurographics Symposium on Geometry Processing, 2003.

[9] Haker, S. Angenet, S. Tannenbaum, A. Kikinis, R. *Non Distorting Flattening Maps and the 3-D visualization of Colon CT Images*, IEEE Transauctions on Medical Imaging, Vol. 19, NO. 7, July 2000.

[10] Haker, S. Angenet, S. Tannenbaum, A. Kikinis, R. Sapiro, G. Halle, M. *Conformal Surface Parametrization for Texture Mapping*, IEEE Transauctions on Visualization and Computer Graphics, Vol. 6, NO. 2, June 2000.

[11] Hurdal, M. K., Bowers, P. L., Stephenson, K., Sumners, D. W. L., Rehm, K., Schaper. K., Rottenberg, D. A. *Quasi Conformally Flat Mapping the Human Crebellum*, Medical Image Computing and Computer-Assisted Intervention - MICCAI'99, (C. Taylor and A. Colchester. eds), vol. 1679, Springer-Verlag, Berlin, 279-286, 1999.

[12] Stephenson, K. *personal communication*.

[13] Sheffer, A. de Stuler, E. *Parametrization of Faceted Surfaces for Meshing Using Angle Based Flattening*, Enginneering with Computers, vol. 17, pp. 326-337, 2001.

[14] Surazhsky, T., Magid, E., Soldea, O., Elber, G. and Rivlin E. *A Comparison of Gaussian and Mean Curvatures Estimation Methods on Triangular Meshes*, Proceedings of the IEEE International Conference on Robotics and Automation. Taipei, Taiwan, pp 1021-1026, September 2003.

[15] Thurston, W. *Three-Dimensional Geometry and Topology, vol.1, (Edited by S. Levy)*, Princeton University Press, Princeton, N.J. 1997.

[16] Väisälä, J. *Lectures on n-dimensional quasiconformal mappings*, Lecture Notes in Mathematics 229, Springer-Verlag, Berlin - Heidelberg - New-York, 1971.

Bony Structure Suppression in Chest Radiographs

M. Loog[1] and B. van Ginneken[2]

[1] The Image Group, IT University of Copenhagen, Copenhagen, Denmark
marco@itu.dk
[2] Image Sciences Institute, University Medical Center Utrecht, Utrecht, The Netherlands

Abstract. Many computer aided diagnosis schemes in chest radiography start with preprocessing steps that try to remove or suppress normal anatomical structures from the image. Examples of normal structures in posteroanterior chest radiographs are bony structures. Removing these kinds of structures can be done quite effectively if the right dual energy images—two radiographic images from the same patient taken with different energies—are available. Subtracting these two radiographs gives a soft-tissue image with most of the rib and other bony structures removed. In general, however, dual energy images are not readily available.

We propose a supervised learning technique for inferring a soft-tissue image from a standard radiograph without explicitly determining the additional dual energy image. The procedure, called dual energy faking, is based on k-nearest neighbor regression, and incorporates knowledge obtained from a training set of dual energy radiographs with their corresponding subtraction images for the construction of a soft-tissue image from a previously unseen single standard chest image.

1 Introduction

One of the major difficulties in interpreting projection chest radiographs stems from the fact that many normal anatomical structures are shown superimposed on possibly abnormal structures. For this reason, many computer aided diagnosis (CAD) schemes in projection chest radiography may benefit from the suppression of as much of the normal structures as possible. In the ideal case this would mean that, after processing a chest radiograph, one obtains an image depicting only the abnormalities present in the original radiograph. In practice however, the output will be an image that contains less of the normal structures and hopefully stronger responses to the abnormalities.

Especially the suppression of the bony structures that overlay the lung fields, e.g. clavicles, ribs, and scapulae, is interesting because in many detection tasks it would lead to a reduction in the number of false positives. For instance, a recent study showed that most lung cancer lesions that are missed on frontal chest radiographs are located behind the ribs and that the inspection of a soft-tissue image can improve detection performance [1]. In addition, we note that obtaining a bone dual energy (DE) image would also be interesting in its own respect. It enables, for example, a better detection of calcified (benign) nodules [2].

In many digital chest units, it is technically feasible to acquire two radiographs with different energies (kVs) at the same time: The DE images (see Figure 1). These im-

R.R. Beichel and M. Sonka (Eds.): CVAMIA 2006, LNCS 4241, pp. 166–177, 2006.
© Springer-Verlag Berlin Heidelberg 2006

ages can then be used to obtain a subtraction image[1] in which bony structures are almost entirely invisible (see Figure 1, refer to [3] for more on the technical and physical background of this technique). However, most of the time, DE images are not readily available and one may attempt to construct such a subtraction image in a different way.

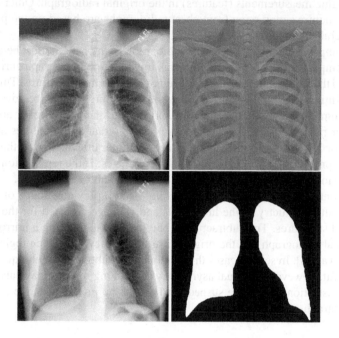

Fig. 1. Top row: An instance of DE images. On the left is the original PA chest radiograph and on the right the image containing the bony structures. Bottom row: The left image shows the soft-tissue image associated with the DE images which is obtained through subtraction. On the right is the corresponding manual lung field segmentation.

Here we propose the suppression of bony structures from the lung fields of standard posteroanterior (PA) chest radiographs by estimating a soft-tissue image using regression (see also [4]). This soft-tissue image should be similar to what would normally be obtained by subtracting a pair of DE images. Here, an attempt is made to infer the (high energy level) bone image from the original radiograph. The pair obtained can then be used to construct a subtraction image with much of the bony structures suppressed. This method is referred to as explicit dual energy faking (explicit DEf). A different approach pursued is the direct prediction of a soft-tissue image from a PA chest radiograph without explicitly determining the bone image. This method is referred to as implicit dual energy faking (implicit DEf).

The approach to the problem is supervised and uses a number of actual PA radiographs and their corresponding soft-tissue images. These training images are used to

---

[1] Although we refer to these kind of images as subtraction images, they are not necessarily obtained from the raw dual energy pair by mere subtraction. Pre- and postprocessing of the images may be needed for this, which makes it in fact a nonlinear operation.

model the mapping we are looking for, i.e, the one used to predict bone or soft-tissue subtraction images from conventional radiographs. The mapping is formulated in terms of a k-nearest neighbor regression (kNNR) in which a nonparametric k-nearest neighbor procedure is employed to predict the pixel values in the subtraction image from per-pixel gray value measurements (features) in the original radiograph. Other approaches to normal structure suppression from chest radiographs are based on temporal [5,6,7] or contralateral subtraction [8].

For the temporal technique, an earlier radiograph of the patient must be available. If there is, attempts can be made to register this image to the radiograph currently being analyzed and then subtract these images to remove the normal structures. This technique has the potential of not only removing the bony structures, but to remove all normal structures from the image. On the other hand however, if there are already abnormalities in the earlier radiograph, it is of course also possible that abnormalities are removed completely or in part in the subtraction image. Another crucial step in the procedure, also causing problems, is the registration of both images: If the registration is not done properly, we might even create suspect artifacts in the subtraction image.

For the contralateral technique, one does not need a previous image of the patient. In this case, the symmetry of the lung fields and rib cage are used for the removal of these normal structures. The subtraction is obtained by subtracting a mirrored version of the original radiograph and the original itself after they have been registered in the appropriate way [8]. In several cases this contralateral subtraction technique has proven to be powerful, however the actual asymmetry of the lung regions may cause problems and a misregistration may cause suspect artifacts in the image, as is the case with the temporal subtraction technique.

2   Materials and Methods

PA dual energy radiographs and JSRT data. The materials used for training the mapping are eight pairs of standard PA chest radiographs together with their corresponding DE and soft-tissue images. These images were obtained from the University of Chicago, IL, Department of Radiology. The images used in the tests have dimensions 512 by 512 and were obtained by linearly subsampling the original 1760 by 1760 images. See Figure 1 for an example of a PA and a soft-tissue image. The evaluation is carried out using the Chicago data as well as two radiographs taken from the JSRT (Japanese Society of Radiological Technology) database [9]. The latter images are used to inspect the performance of the scheme when training is performed on radiographs coming from one unit and used to infer soft-tissue images on radiographs coming from another unit (e.g. coming from a different manufacturer, using different post-processing methods, etc.). In addition, both these images contain a lung nodule enabling us to check how the system behave on such abnormalities.

Because we are interested in the performance of the scheme within the lung fields, in addition to the radiographs, manual delineations were obtained and employed in the experiments to indicate the regions of interest (see Figure 1 for an example). This step can be automated, see, for example, [10].

Processing prior to regression. The PA—both from the Chicago and the JSRT databases—and soft-tissue images are six times locally normalized on a very large scale σ equal to 128 pixels. This is done to remove possible image dependent near-global offsets and intensity variations.

A locally normalized form $\bar{L}$ of an original image L is defined as

$$\bar{L} = \frac{L - L_\sigma}{\sqrt{(L^2)_\sigma - (L_\sigma)^2}},$$

where L_σ defines a Gaussian blurred [11,12] version of L at scale σ. The DE images used in the training phase are constructed from the normalized PA and soft-tissue image by subtracting the one from the other (this latter image is what is actually depicted in the upper-right corner of Figure 1).

Additionally, the normalization also aids the possibility of inferring soft-tissue images from radiographs coming from a different unit. With respect to this point, we should remark that it is not clear that carrying out a local normalization multiple times makes it generally possible to switch between units and still use the same faking scheme for inferring soft-tissue or bone images from a standard PA image. In our current experiments, normalizing the images turns out to work reasonably well and so no additional image processing or unit-dependent feature transformations are applied. However, to finally make DEf schemes broadly applicable, it may be necessary to apply more elaborate processing techniques first.

k-*Nearest neighbor regression.* The method used for predicting a soft-tissue image from a standard chest radiograph is per-pixel k-nearest neighbor regression (kNNR) [13]. The most well-known method to perform regression is simple linear regression, which aims to optimally predict the output values in terms of a linear combination of its associated inputs [14]. However, for the current purpose, linear regression is too rigid to perform well and therefore the nonparametric k-nearest neighbor method is employed. This type of regression has a strong theoretical basis and many results are known concerning its convergence properties and consistency characteristics [13].

Finally, experiments were also conducted with kNNR in conjunction with the linear dimension reduction technique presented in [4].

3   Pilot and Leave-One-Out Experiments

In order to test the DEf techniques, leave-one-out experiments were conducted. That is, mappings based on kNNR were trained using seven pairs of images—which constitutes the training set, and tested on the remaining PA image. The performance of the DEf methods is measured by means of the standard correlation, i.e., Pearson's r [15], between the target image and the inferred image.

Predictors/features. Before one can actually perform kNNR, however, one has to decide on the features to use as predictor variables. In addition, it has to be decided if—and if so, which—linear dimension reduction should be performed. In order to do so for DEf, a small pilot experiment was run on a single fold from the leave-one-out procedure in which several combinations of Gaussian kernel-based n-jets [11,12] over several scales were examined. That is, at every pixel position, on several scales, features obtained using up to nth order derivatives of Gaussian filters are included. For implicit DEf, the final set of features used for every pixel position consists of all Gaussian kernel-based features up to order 3 at scales 1, 2, 4, 8, 16, and 32. In addition to these 60 features, the raw pixel value was included, resulting in 61 input variables. The features for explicit DEf are all Gaussian features up to order 2 at 6 scales logarithmically distributed between 1 and 64 plus the raw gray value which results in 37 features.

Dimension reduction. It should be noted that for the initial regression step, the exact choice of features appears not to be really critical. The system does not seem to behave significantly different over a range of settings. Most notable is that the order is more of an influence than the size and number of scales. Linearly transforming the input features using common techniques, like normalization (or standardization) of the features or global whitening of the input, did have a clear, but detrimental effect on the performance of the system. However, whitening the data in combination with nonparametric local linear dimension reduction (see [4]) seems to give a substantial improvement in case of performing explicit DEf. A dimension reduction, after whitening, also seems to give a moderately improved implicit DEf. Based on our findings in the pilot experiments, we decided to compare 4 different schemes in the leave-one-out experiments: Two implicit and two explicit schemes and two schemes with and two schemes without dimension reduction. Table 1 gives an overview of settings used in this comparison. Two of these schemes are also used in the additional experiments on the two JSRT radiographs.

Table 1. Settings employed in the regression schemes used for performing implicit and explicit dual energy faking. One implicit DEf scheme uses the full predictor vector, while the other employs an additional linear dimension reduction (LDR) for which the target dimension d and the k defining the neighborhood are also provided. The same holds for the explicit scheme.

	Gaussian predictors (features)	k	LDR d
implicit DEf	up to order 3, scales 1,2,4,8,16,32	51	— 15
explicit DEf	up to order 2, scales 1,2.30,5.28,12.13,27.86,64	51	— 18

k *(in the kNNR).* The number of neighbors used in the regression, k, was set to 51 for all schemes. Again, not much difference in performance was visible for a wide range of ks. Only when k becomes too low (e.g. $k < 10$) or to high (e.g. $k > 100$), the resulting soft-tissue image significantly deteriorates. In the former case it becomes much more noisy and in the latter case the output image tends to be oversmoothed.

4   Experimental Results

The Chicago data set. Table 2 gives the leave-one-out results over all eight images in the Chicago data set. The predicted image is compared to the soft-tissue image. Comparison is based on the standard parametric correlation, Pearson's r, of the gray values

Table 2. Average correlation over the eight instances from the Chicago data set obtained from the leave-one-out experiments are provided together with the p-values based on a paired t-test by which means the several schemes are compared to each other. Note the improvements obtained using the schemes employing dimension reduction. Note also the high correlation the unprocessed PA radiographs already attain with the soft-tissue images.

			implicit DEf		explicit DEf	
		PA	full	LDR	full	LDR
	average	0.965	0.983	0.985	0.983	0.987
PA		—	$2.8 \cdot 10^{-6}$	$3.4 \cdot 10^{-6}$	$4.5 \cdot 10^{-7}$	$4.3 \cdot 10^{-8}$
implicit full		$2.8 \cdot 10^{-6}$	—	$3.5 \cdot 10^{-3}$	$7.6 \cdot 10^{-1}$	$4.3 \cdot 10^{-4}$
implicit LDR	p-value	$3.4 \cdot 10^{-6}$	$3.5 \cdot 10^{-3}$	—	$2.8 \cdot 10^{-2}$	$2.5 \cdot 10^{-2}$
explicit full		$4.5 \cdot 10^{-7}$	$7.6 \cdot 10^{-1}$	$2.8 \cdot 10^{-2}$	—	$6.3 \cdot 10^{-6}$
explicit LDR		$4.3 \cdot 10^{-8}$	$4.3 \cdot 10^{-4}$	$2.5 \cdot 10^{-2}$	$6.3 \cdot 10^{-6}$	—

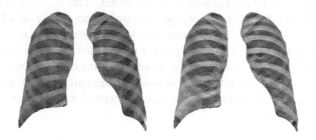

Fig. 2. On the left an example of a target bone image, which is also depicted in Figure 1. On the right is the explicitly faked bone image which is obtained using the explicit DEf scheme in combination with dimension reduction.

within the regions of interest, i.e., the lung fields. The same measure is determined between the soft-tissue image and the original PA radiograph. The latter is done to put the obtained correlations between soft-tissue and implicit DEf prediction in a better perspective. From the table it is clear that explicit DEf in conjunction with the dimension reduction scheme performs significantly better than the other schemes. Although in comparison with the implicit scheme in combination with LDR this significance is only moderate.

In addition to the results in the table, we report that for the full and the LDR-based explicit DEf schemes, the average correlations between the inferred bone image and the target bone image are 0.747 and 0.805, respectively (p-value for the difference equals $2.4 \cdot 10^{-4}$). Note that the difference in correlation, $5.8 \cdot 10^{-2}$ in this case, is considerably larger than when measured using the inferred soft-tissue images in which case it is $4.0 \cdot 10^{-3}$.

Clearly, the correlation between original PA radiograph and target soft-tissue image is generally already very large: Larger than 0.960 over all eight images. For this reason comparing of the outcomes of the experiments may not be obvious and, in addition, the improvements the schemes attain may not be well appreciated. Therefore, a second evaluation is provided in which for every image the correlation score between the PA image and the soft-tissue image was set to zero and perfect correlation was set to 1.

Table 3. Average normalized correlation over the eight instances from the Chicago data set obtained form the leave-one-out experiments are provided together with p-values based on a paired t-test by which means the several schemes are compared to each other. Note the improvements obtained using the schemes employing dimension reduction. The explicit DEf scheme using LDR provides the best performance overall.

		implicit DEf		explicit DEf	
		full	LDR	full	LDR
	average	0.513	0.558	0.518	0.621
implicit full		—	$1.8 \cdot 10^{-3}$	$6.1 \cdot 10^{-1}$	$8.4 \cdot 10^{-4}$
implicit LDR	p-value	$1.8 \cdot 10^{-3}$	—	$2.2 \cdot 10^{-2}$	$2.5 \cdot 10^{-2}$
explicit full		$6.1 \cdot 10^{-1}$	$2.2 \cdot 10^{-2}$	—	$4.6 \cdot 10^{-5}$
explicit LDR		$8.4 \cdot 10^{-4}$	$2.5 \cdot 10^{-2}$	$4.6 \cdot 10^{-5}$	—

Based on this the original correlations are 'normalized'. That is, if r_{PA} is the correlation between the PA and the soft-tissue image, the correlation score r of a DEf scheme is normalized to $(r - r_{\mathrm{PA}})/(1 - r_{\mathrm{PA}})$: 0 means no improvement with respect to the original PA chest radiograph, while 1 means a perfect reconstruction of the soft-tissue image. Table 3 gives the outcome in terms of this normalized measure. In this table the results when using explicit DEf for inferring soft-tissue images are included and compared to implicit DEf. Again, the results indicate that the explicit scheme using LDR is better than all other schemes.

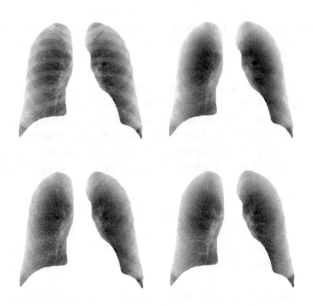

Fig. 3. In the top left-hand corner is the PA radiograph from Figure 1. In the lower right-hand corner its corresponding soft-tissue image, which is depicted in Figure 1 as well. The top right-hand image gives the implicit DEf image obtained employing dimension reduction and in the lower left-hand corner is the soft-tissue image obtained by subtracting the explicit DEf image from Figure 2 from the original PA chest radiograph in the top left-hand corner.

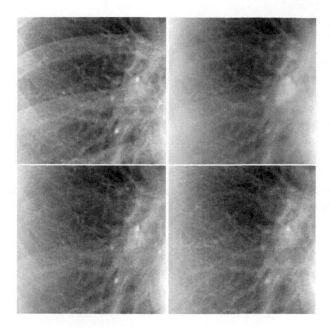

Fig. 4. Details taken from the images shown in Figure 3. The patch is taken from the right lung and contains part of the hilum. The figures are presented in the same order as in Figure 3. Top left-hand: PA, top right-hand: Implicit DEf, bottom left-hand: Explicit DEf, and bottom right-hand: Target soft-tissue. The explicit DEf scheme performs better than the implicit one. Furthermore, the image obtained using explicit DEf seems to be sharper than the actual ground, preserving non-bony details slightly better.

Figure 2 shows the target bone image and the inferred bone image using the best performing explicit DEf scheme. In Figures 3 and 4, the best performing implicit DEf and the best performing explicit DEf schemes are compared to the original PA radiograph and the target image. From these images it appears that explicit DEf performs better than implicit DEf. Moreover, using explicit DEf, detailed structures seem to be better preserved than in the target soft-tissue image. However, it is also obvious that ribs are also not completely filtered out using explicit DEf, leaving quite some room for improvement.

JSRT data. To see to what extent the trained DEf schemes can be used on PA chest radiographs obtained from other machines (which is, by the way, a nontrivial task), the performance of two best performing explicit and implicit schemes (see Table 2) is further examined using two radiographs from the JSRT database. Both images are shown in Figure 5. In both images a lung nodule is present in the lower part of the right lung. The training of the schemes is now carried out using all eight images from the Chicago data set.

Figures 6 and 7 present—going from left to right in the figures—the original image, the result obtained using implicit DEf, and the resulting soft-tissue image employing the explicit DEf scheme, both using dimension reduction.

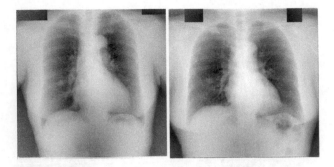

Fig. 5. Two chest radiographs from the JSRT database, both containing an obvious lung nodule in the right lung field

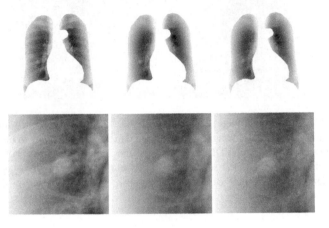

Fig. 6. Top row: Illustration of the results obtained using DEf on an image from the JSRT database. On the left is the original, in the center is the implicit DEf result, and the right image shows the result employing the explicit scheme. Bottom row: Details from the images in the top row: The nodule and an area surrounding it. On the left is a patch from the original PA radiograph, in the center is the implicit DEf result, and the right image shows the result employing the explicit scheme. (See also Figure 7.)

With respect to filtering out bony structures, both schemes perform rather well. Much of the rib structures present in the original PA image are completely filtered out or, at least, removed to a large extent. Again, the explicit scheme provides sharper images than the implicit one. On the other hand, the latter scheme seems to preserve nodules better than explicit DEf, which is most apparent from Figure 7.

5   Discussion and Conclusions

The methods proposed, tested, and exemplified in this paper—explicit and implicit dual energy faking—aim at filtering out bony structures from standard PA chest radiographs and attempts to infer a soft-tissue image from the latter. The main reason for developing such schemes is their applicability in computer-aided detection of abnormalities, e.g.

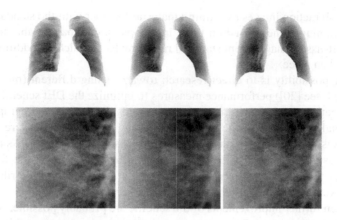

Fig. 7. Top row: Illustration of the results obtained using DEf on an image from the JSRT database. On the left is the original, in the center is the implicit DEf result, and the right image shows the result employing the explicit scheme. Bottom row: Details from the images in the top row: The nodule and an area surrounding it. On the left is a patch from the original PA radiograph, in the center is the implicit DEf result, and the right image shows the result employing the explicit scheme. (See also Figure 6.)

nodules or interstitial disease [16,17,18,19], as filtering out bony structures may result in significant performance improvement.

As illustrated by Figures 3 to 7, the method performs promising on data similar to the training data but also on radiographs taken from a different data set. The visibility of the ribs and the clavicle in the lung fields has been reduced considerably in most parts of the lung fields while other structures have been preserved to a large extent. Moreover, the correlation between the solutions obtained by kNNR and the soft-tissue images is very high: Around 0.985 on average (see Table 2). It is noted, however, that the correlation between the soft-tissue and the PA images is also rather high (0.965), but the increase in correlation using our technique is obviously significant.

The performance is more clearly illustrated in Table 3 in which the correlation scores are normalized per image, based on the original PA radiograph. The explicit DEf scheme which employs the dimension reduction technique is the overall best performing system, when measured in a leave-one-out experiment on the Chicago data. This latter scheme preserves image details to a great extent, surprisingly, even more that the target soft-tissue image. In an attempt to substantiate this observation, correlation scores between soft-tissue and slightly blurred explicit DEf images were calculated, which indeed led to a consistent, and (moderately) significant, improvement in average correlation over all eight Chicago radiographs (p-values around $3 \cdot 10^{-2}$ in a paired t-test for scales around 0.45). However, the tests on the JSRT data showed inferior performance on preservation of lung nodules in comparison with the best implicit scheme.

We notice that a drawback of soft-tissue images, and therefore also of the method presented, is that they are rather noisy [3]. However, a strong feature of the kNN method employed is that it could easily incorporate some form of denoising. One of the most powerful ways to accomplish this is to provide high-dose, and therefore less noisy, soft-tissue subtraction images as training material together with the standard PA chest images. If training is then based on these image pairs, one may be able to learn how to obtain soft-tissue images from standard radiographs in which, in addition, noise removal has taken place.

A further possibility is to direct research towards using different (more to human vision related, see [20]) performance measures to optimize the DEf schemes. Agreeing that in estimating a soft-tissue image from a standard PA chest radiograph, one will inevitably make errors, the basic idea behind using some other measure to optimize the schemes is that other errors than the current ones would be made. As an example, an error measure that would allow for a large amount of noise in the faked image, but penalizes the presence of large scale edges (i.e., coming from the ribs) might be preferable over the currently used correlation measure.

While even further improvements of the scheme are probably possible, we may conclude that the presented qualitative and quantitative results show that this approach is able to perform the highly nontrivial separation of bone and tissue components in chest radiographs. The method is completely automatic and yields satisfying results, even on data coming from a different source.

References

1. Shah, P.K., Austin, J.H.M., White, C.S., Patel, P., Haramati, L.B., Pearson, G.D.N., Shiau, M.C., Berkmen, Y.M.: Missed non-small cell lung cancer: Radiographic findings of potentially resectable lesions evident only in retrospect. Radiology 226(3) (2003) 235–241
2. Fischbach, F., Freund, T., Röttgen, R., Engert, U., Felix, R., Ricke, J.: Dual-energy chest radiography with a flat-panel digital detector: Revealing calcified chest abnormalities. American Journal of Roentgenology 181 (2003) 1519–1524
3. Warp, R.J., 3rd, J.T.D.: Quantitative evaluation of noise reduction strategies in dual-energy imaging. Medical Physics 30(2) (2003) 190–198
4. Loog, M.: Supervised dimensionality reduction and contextual pattern recognition in medical image processing. Ph.D. Thesis, Image Sciences Institute, Utrecht University, The Netherlands (2004)
5. Kano, A., Doi, K., MacMahon, H., Hassell, D., Giger, M.: Digital image subtraction of temporally sequential chest images for detection of interval change. Medical Physics 21(3) (1994) 453–461
6. Katsuragawa, S., Tagashira, H., Li, Q., MacMahon, H., Doi, K.: Comparison of quality of temporal subtraction images obtained with manual and automated methods of digital chest radiography. Journal of Digital Imaging 12(4) (1999) 166–172
7. Loeckx, D., Maes, F., Vandermeulen, D., Suetens, P.: Temporal subtraction of thorax CR images using a statistical deformation model. IEEE Transactions on Medical Imaging 22(11) (2003) 1490–1504
8. Li, Q., Katsuragawa, S., Ishida, T., Yoshida, H., Tsukuda, S., MacMahon, H., Doi, K.: Contralateral subtraction: A novel technique for detection of asymmetric abnormalities on digital chest radiographs. Medical Physics 27(1) (2000) 47–55
9. Shiraishi, J., Katsuragawa, S., Ikezoe, J., Matsumoto, T., Kobayashi, T., Komatsu, K., Matsui, M., Fujita, H., Kodera, Y., Doi, K.: Development of a digital image database for chest radiographs with and without a lung nodule: Receiver operating characteristic analysis of radiologists' detection of pulmonary nodules. American Journal of Roentgenology, 174 (2000) 71–74

10. Ginneken, B., Haar Romeny, B., Viergever, M.A.: Computer-aided diagnosis in chest radiography: A survey. IEEE Transactions on Medical Imaging **20**(12) (2001) 1228–1241
11. Florack, L.M.J.: Image Structure. Volume 10 of Computational Imaging and Vision. Kluwer, Dordrecht . Boston . London (1997)
12. Lindeberg, T.: Scale-Space Theory in Computer Vision. Kluwer Academic Press, Boston (1994)
13. Devroye, L., Györfi, L., Lugosi, G.: A Probabilistic Theory of Pattern Recognition. Springer-Verlag, New York . Berlin . Heidelberg (1996)
14. Edwards, A.L.: Multiple Regression and the Analysis of Variance and Covariance. W. H. Freeman, San Francisco (1979)
15. Rice, J.A.: Mathematical Statistics and Data Analysis. second edn. Duxbury Press, Belmont (1995)
16. Ginneken, B., Katsuragawa, S., ter Haar Romeny, B., Doi, K., Viergever, M.: Automatic detection of abnormalities in chest radiographs using local texture analysis. IEEE Transactions on Medical Imaging **21**(2) (2002) 139–149
17. MacMahon, H.: Clinical application of CAD in the chest. In: Computer-Aided Diagnosis in Medical Imaging. Volume 1182 of International Congress Series. (1999) 23–34
18. Schilham, A.M.R., Ginneken, B., Loog, M.: Multi-scale nodule detection in chest radiographs. In Ellis, R.E., Peters, T.M., eds.: Medical Image Computing and Computer-Assisted Intervention. Volume 2878 of Lecture Notes in Computer Science., Springer (2003) 602–609
19. Xu, X.W., MacMahon, H., Doi, K.: Detection of lung nodule on digital energy subtracted soft-tissue and conventional chest images from a CR system. In: Computer-Aided Diagnosis in Medical Imaging. Volume 1182 of International Congress Series. (1999) 63–70
20. Eskicioglu, A.M., Fisher, P.S.: Image quality measures and their performance. IEEE Transactions on Communications **43**(12) (1995) 2959–2965

A Minimally-Interactive Watershed Algorithm Designed for Efficient CTA Bone Removal

Horst K. Hahn, Markus T. Wenzel, Olaf Konrad-Verse, and Heinz-Otto Peitgen

MeVis, Center for Medical Diagnostic Systems and Visualization,
Universitaetsallee 29, 28359 Bremen, Germany
wenzel@mevis.de

Abstract. We introduce a novel minimally-interactive watershed algorithm that needs no initial parameterization, but lets the user refine the automatic segmentation close to real-time. In contrast to previous proposals, our algorithm encapsulates all time consuming calculation in a processing step executed only once. Thereby, a hierarchical subdivision of the incoming image data is generated. This subdivision serves as a basis for computing automatic segmentation results according to a given multi-dimensional classification scheme as well as for interactive refinement according to local markers. We have successfully applied our algorithm to efficiently removing bone structures from computed tomography angiography data, which is among the very challenging segmentation problems in medical image analysis.

1 Introduction

In medical image analysis, an especially challenging problem is the efficient removal of bone structures from large CTA (Computed Tomography Angiography) image volumes [1,3,5,9,10,11,13,14]. The motivation is to yield an unhindered view on the vascular structures and inner organs for diagnostic purposes such as detecting stenoses or aneurysms. The difficulty of the bone removal problem lies partly in the fact that both osseous and vascular structures show patterns of highly variable shape and contrast. For example, bone marrow and cortical bone structures strongly differ in contrast, with bone marrow contrast being close to average vessel contrast. Vessels, on the other hand, may also exhibit high intensity patterns resembling those of bone, partly due to high concentrations of contrast agent or calcified vessel plaque. Further segmentation problems are due to metallic endovascular stents, aneurysm clips etc. Moreover, the close proximity of bone and vessels, e.g. at the skull base, complicates automated segmentation. Manual bone segmentation is impractical due to the large number of bones contained in routine CT examinations.

Our general research objective is to provide an algorithmic framework capable of efficiently segmenting large image volumes with none or minimal user input based on a set of regional features plus spatial connectivity. Our specific objective is to provide a software assistant for CTA bone removal being intuitively usable and moreover being fast and reliable enough for routine clinical applications. Hence requirements to meet in design and implementation are:

R.R. Beichel and M. Sonka (Eds.): CVAMIA 2006, LNCS 4241, pp. 178–189, 2006.

- *applicability* to large data sets in full resolution (current scanners deliver data sets with, e.g., $512 \times 512 \times 2{,}000$ voxels for runoff studies),
- high degree of *automation* in removing osseous structures from CTA images,
- *speed* with max. one minute computation time for a complete automatic segmentation at the above resolution, and
- *intuitive* user control with full undo/redo functionality.

In this paper we present a modified watershed algorithm that executes the computationally expensive steps only once. After a short introduction into the watershed transform (WT) and its application to segmentation in image processing (Sec. 2), we propose a novel algorithm with improved capabilities (Sec. 3). We will show how to efficiently collect data for automatic classification during the WT. The accompanying data structures are explained in Section 3.1. The reconstruction phase and a simple, yet successful classification schemes based on the collected data are then delineated (Sec. 3.2) with a prospect of possible extensions that will improve the classification. Thereafter, we describe the realization of user-interactive refinement by manual markers and their interplay with the classification result (Sec. 3.3). Experimental results give a good impression on the performance of our proposal. We detail this in Section 4 and close our contribution with some prospects of the ongoing research.

2 Related Work

The watershed transform (WT) is today among the most widely used tools for image segmentation. Originally proposed as an image analysis tool within the framework of mathematical morphology by DIGABEL and LANTUÈJOUL [2], it was comprehensively recapitulated by ROERDINK and MEIJSTER [12].

An n-dimensional grayscale image is interpreted as an $n+1$-dimensional topographic relief where the gray value at any image position $x = [x_1, \ldots, x_n]^T$ is interpreted as the elevation at this position. For a two-dimensional image the interpretation as a relief is shown in Figure 1, where the gray values are either interpreted as height or depth information. The most important notions are *minima, catchment basins* (or simply *basins*), and *watersheds* separating basins. In this nomenclature, the WT applied to an image results in a set of basins plus a set of watersheds.

Standing out in the considerable body of scientific work on the WT is the 1991 TPAMI paper of VINCENT and SOILLE [15], who suggest an algorithm that allows for extremely fast implementations. Their algorithm follows the idea of immersion—as opposed to calculation of steepest slope and topographical distance—of the landscape. The impacts on the segmentation result are for example discussed in [5,12].

Only since then the WT yielded practical applicability to the solution of problems in processing large images. Recently, ROERDINK and MEIJSTER published an excellent overview on definitions, algorithmic implications, and parallelization strategies [12]. But still are there little, if any, approaches to deal with its major shortcoming, namely the oversegmentation of images, from *within* the algorithm.

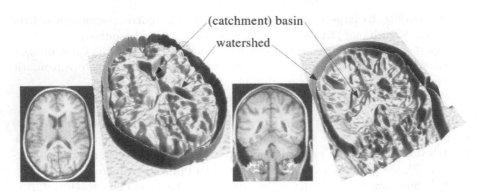

Fig. 1. Interpretation of a 2D grayscale image as a 3D topographic landscape. Left: Axial view, interpretation of gray value as altitude information. Right: Same image, but coronal view; gray level interpreted as depth information.

Commonly, makers are defined *before* the WT to avoid oversegmentation. Moreover, image enhancement techniques may be used to preprocess the image, e.g. to reduce noise, but will lead to a loss of information and/or generality besides the required computational efforts.

In contrast, our algorithm postpones the handling of noise. During the WT it builds up a tree-like data structure according to the immersion scenario. Based on this data structure, noise reduction can then be implemented as a cheap operation that can be interactively influenced by the user. Furthermore, it provides the possibility to propagate both a priori and user provided knowledge, defined only on a small number of basins, to other basins. The idea to perform bone segmentation by applying the WT directly to the original CT data interpreted as depth information, as opposed to computing image gradients beforehand, was risen during a study where the individual segmentation of all carpal bones of the human wrist was required [5,7].

Other contributions to automated bone segmentation in medical imaging include automated techniques, e.g. [1,3,10,13,14], as well as user interactive ones, e.g. [1,8,9,11]. The results of fully automated approaches are often modest [10,13], and the interactive ones are often rather simple by design, such as the one described by ALYASSIN and AVINASH that allows the user to steer global thresholds [1]. Those techniques, which excel in segmentation performance, often achieve their specificity at the expense of computation time and/or a restricted range of applications [8,9]. Most approaches apply manual placing or computation of regional markers before the WT (e.g. [4]), meaning that the transform must be recalculated upon each marker change, or they implement costly multiresolution strategies.

Probably the closest approach to the one proposed in this paper is the one of RAMAN *et al.* [11], where the user has to point and click on each bone and vessel only once to segment them. In contrast to [11], our approach contains an automatic bone classification scheme only requiring a single click by the user if a bone has not been marked correctly.

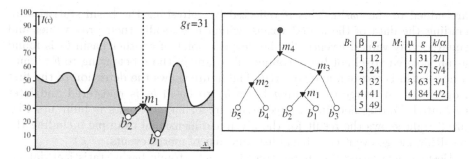

Fig. 2. Left: Depicting the *hierarchical* WT. The landscape is flooded from bottom to top. At gray value $g_f = 31$ a ridge point is detected. A merge event candidate m_1 is registered. Right: Final tree structure of merge events after flooding the landscape.

3   Minimally-Interactive Watershed Transform

Classical watershed transform (WT) algorithms allow user interaction only before the actual WT starts. This severely limits interactivity and is prohibitive in large images, when refinement by alteration of certain parameters would require the whole transform to be calculated from scratch.

In contrast, we propose to extend the Interactive Watershed Transform [7], which provides full user interactivity if desired, but can deliver good results also without. It comprises a hierarchical Fast Watershed Transform (FWT) and a user interaction mechanism that works on the data provided by the FWT. The underlying thought is to transform the image without any beforehand noise suppression and thereafter to provide mechanisms of automatically or interactively adapting the reconstruction to deal with image noise. This is pursued by employing a tree-like data structure that is built up during the WT process. Only in a second step—the reconstruction phase—the user may interfere by varying global parameters and placing markers to influence the segmentation result. To avoid the necessity of extensive interaction, a classification scheme places initial automatic markers according to basin statistics gathered during the WT step on a per-basin basis.

In the subsequent section we will outline the FWT algorithm. In two further subsections we will detail the automatic basin classification procedure as well as the reconstruction phase including the interplay of automatic and manual markers.

3.1   The Fast Watershed Transform

The novelty of the employed Fast Watershed Transform is in the computation of a hierarchical representation of the basins found by immersion of the $n + 1$-dimensional landscape [7]. Figure 2 shows this for the 1-dimensional case. Consider incrementally flooding the depicted landscape. Initially, basin b_1 is found. When flooding continues, voxels to the left and to the right of the basin are added to the basin. This is reflected by refreshing the basin statistics including the data of the added voxels, which is basically their gray values and squared gray values. Eventually the deepest point of another basin b_2 is found as an isolated voxel not being connected to any of those belonging to b_1. Thus, a new basin is created, and so forth. The figure shows the detection of the first ridge point. A merge event *from* basin b_2 *to* basin b_1 is registered and later evaluated. During flooding, a tree structure of merge events is built up. Figure 2 right shows the result for the given 1-dimensional example including the resulting merge event tree, basin list, and list of merge events.

Besides generating the merge tree, for each atomic basin statistical data is collected. In detail, besides the gray value at the deepest point g_{seed} (in HU), we record per basin the following data (HU: Hounsfield units):

- mean gray value g_{mean} (in HU),
- gray value standard deviation σ (in HU),
- gray value coefficient of variation $CV = \sigma/g_{mean}$ (in %), and
- volume V (in ml).

All basins are stored in a vector data structure that is naturally sorted by ascending g_{seed} values and that allows fast index access.

Whenever a ridge point is reached, neighborhood considerations tell that this voxel is connected to more than a single basin and must thus be part of a watershed. In our implementation, we do not explicitly encode the watershed voxels but rather add the voxel to the basin of highest priority. Here, priority is simply associated to the absolute basin depth, which has already shown excellent results within another field of application [6]. Thereafter, a merge event with the basin of highest priority is recorded for any further neighboring basin containing information on the two basins merged by the event and on the gray level g_{merge}, at which the merge occurs. Moreover, an index is generated on all merge events and sorted by ascending g_{merge} values.

A specialty of the employed WT algorithm is that on each processing step it only requires information on isolated voxels plus their direct neighbors with one processing step thus being in complexity class $\mathcal{O}(1)$. The WT algorithm as a whole is therefore in $\mathcal{O}(n)$ with n being the number of voxels in the volume. If only a small subset of the voxels are of interest for the given segmentation problem—and this is the case regarding the high intensity voxels for the CTA bone removal problem—we therefore propose to use a sparse sampling of these voxels, resulting in a dramatic image compression. Commonly, one can assume to find about 2% to 5% of voxels representing bright vessel or bone structures, easily justifying a compression of image data to 25% the original size.

In the following, the WT will work on the sparse representation of bright image elements that fall above a given threshold. The input threshold for our problem has a 175 HU default value but could changed for specific applications. This choice is motivated by the experience that cortical bone structures that hinder the view on vascular structures will usually show up in CT with at least 175 HU, while a huge amount of soft tissue that can be disregarded here shows up at less than 175 HU. Of course, a further compression and speed-up could, e.g., be effectuated by simply downsampling the incoming data by a factor of two for each slice before processing, which is often acceptable based on the high in-plane resolution of current CT scanners.

3.2 Automatic Pre-classification and Reconstruction

The basin statistics collected during the FWT suffices to provide an initial segmentation that can be later refined by the user. Our objective was to satisfy the following criteria with respect to the employed classification scheme:

- be *fast*: use the collected data per basin efficiently,
- be *modular*: allow for arbitrary classification algorithms, and
- be *extendable*: allow for new per-basin or higher-order features.

Our experiments regarding CTA bone removal showed that—given the basin statistics described above—even a simple classification scheme operating on the statistical data performs considerably well for *inside* (i.e. *bone*) as well as for *outside* (i.e. *non-bone*) classification. Before actually classifying voxels as bone or none bone, simple thresholding on basin size models the assumption that bone structures will not tend to be smaller than a minimum volume (default: $V_{min} = 0.5$ ml). Our classification scheme is then best depicted by two ellipses in the feature space spanned by CV vs. g_{max} (cf. Fig. 3 right for an illustration of the ellipse used for bone labeling). All feature points that fall between the inner (bone) and the outer (non-bone, not shown) ellipses will initially remain unlabeled. The use of CV as a derived basin feature was motivated by visual inspection of a plot of σ vs. g_{mean} (Fig. 3 left).

The incorporation of new features can be performed in a straightforward manner and is only limited by memory constraints. Each per-basin feature has to be stored within the basin data structure, and since all basin data is kept in main memory for interactive rework, one should think carefully before adding new features. Given that the feature is incrementally computable during the FWT computation, the increase in computation time can be neglected. Also, features that are related to merge events, final basin depths etc. may be considered and are subject to our ongoing research.

Moreover, in our current experiments we substituted the simple elliptic classification scheme by a support vector machine that was trained on expert segmentation results. With this classification the results ameliorated, but as thorough exploration is pending, a more detailed analysis is left to our future research.

Whatever classification utilized, it will store markers in a number of basins, for which the feature vector falls within the *inside/bone* or *outside/non-bone* region of the decision function. Note that an arbitrary number of basins may be marked by the classification scheme. Neither are all basins required to be marked, nor is there an upper limit to the number of marked basins. In the following discussion, denote the marker of a basin by b^{marker}. Markers can be either of include, exclude or explicitly none of the previous, denoted m_{in}, m_{out}, and m_{no}, respectively.

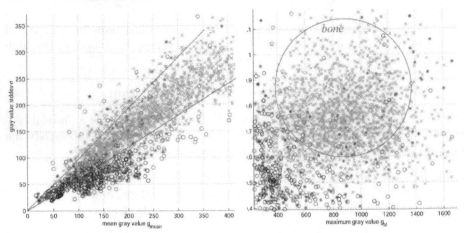

Fig. 3. Left: Comparing g_{mean} to σ for all basins larger than V_{min} from 14 data sets, the (green) crosses representing bone, all other symbols representing non-bone. Right: Classification scheme region (ellipse) for generating automatic bone markers. Only 47 false positives are inside the ellipse.

3.3   Marker-Based Interactive Segmentation

The markers provided by the classification scheme alongside those given by the user are employed to construct the segmentation result. Therefore, the treelike structure of basins is traversed by ascending gray levels of merge events as they were recorded during the watershed transform.

The markers are propagated to adjacent basins on behalf of the following algorithm. Let $\mathsf{Base}(b)$ be a function returning the deepest basin connected to b, initially returning the basin itself. Think of a merge event as a ridge point, at which a directed slopping over of fluid from one basin into another occurs. The direction is defined to come *from* the shallower basin and flow *to* the deeper one.

Denote with b_{from} the basin, from which the fluid flows, and with b_{to} the target basin. Then, the marker propagation works as described by Algorithm 1., which, however, is a condensation in that in the actual implementation works only on those basins not already merged according to a user defined preflooding level. The concept of preflooding within the WT was introduced in [6].

The reconstructed image is presented to the user who may refine it interactively. Practically, this means clicking on image positions that are segmented false positive or false negative, thereby assigning include or exclude markers to the respective basins. Another option for the user is to modify global classification parameters, whereafter the classification step is repeated for all basins. In case the user places one or more markers manually, Algorithm 2. helps to reconstruct the image for both manual and automatic markers. When evaluating manual markers, basins without explicit manual markers are filled with automatic markers, if present (lines 5–6).

With this provided, the calculation of all markers is done by a simple call of COMPUTELABEL(basin_i) in a loop over all basins. Additionally, to obtain full undo/

Algorithm 1. MERGEALL(): Propagation of inside and outside markers in basin list.

```
 1. for all mergeevent_i ∈ mergelist, i ∈ [1...m] do
 2.     if (b_from)^marker ≠ m_no then      /* Marker present in b_from. */
 3.         if (b_to)^marker = m_no then      /* No marker present in b_to. */
 4.             Base(b_from) := Base(b_to)      /* Merge and propagate marker. */
 5.             Base(b_to)^marker := Base(b_from)^marker
 6.         else if Base(b_from)^marker = Base(b_to)^marker then      /* Markers identical. */
 7.             Base(b_from) := Base(b_to)      /* Merge only. */
 8.         end if
 9.     else      /* No marker in b_from. */
10.         Base(b_from) := Base(b_to)      /* Merge only. */
11.     end if
12. end for
```

redo functionality is suffices to simply keep track of all user input, i.e. marker placement/deletion and parameter changes. Reverting to a previous state only involves re-evaluation of the comparably inexpensive COMPUTELABEL(basin$_i$) with the list of markers and parameters of the respective state.

4 Results

To show the speed during interaction we evaluated the performance on six real-world data sets of different size from various multidetector CT scanners. In order to qualitatively assess the results of our segmentation, Figure 4 shows two of these data sets using direct volume rendering of the original data, of the removed bone structures, and of the data after bone removal (from left to right). Table 1 lists the data sets in terms of slice thickness and image size and provides timing results. We would like to focus the attention on the rightmost column giving the time in seconds required to transform a user input, i.e. any marking of image regions as bone or non-bone, into a new segmentation result.

In the table, column 2 lists the initial size of the data set. After compression, the sparse volume representation of the data sets consist of a maximum of roughly 10 000 000 voxels. From these voxels, a number of basins are formed (column 3, ♯basins). The number of basins depends on image characteristics and is not linear in the image size. The time for setting/unsetting an arbitrary number of markers (column 7, t_{marker}) depends on the number of basins.

From Table 1 note that all interaction time is well below 1 s, even for data sets as large as 430 MVoxels (*Runoff*). Also note, that neither the number of basins found in a particular image is a function of image size, nor is the time for interaction. The number of basins depends on a variety of image characteristics, whereas the time for interaction depends on the number of basins only and is thus related to image characteristics as well.

Algorithm 2. COMPUTELABEL(mode $\in \{\texttt{auto}, \texttt{manu}\}$): Determination of automatic and manual markers for one basin.

1. $l := b^{\text{marker}}$
2. **if** $l = m_{\text{no}}$ **then**   /* No marker set yet. */
3.   **if** Base$(b) \neq b$ **then**   /* Recurse until self-reference. */
4.   COMPUTELABEL(Base(b))
5.   **else if** mode $= \texttt{manu} \wedge b^{\text{automarker}} \neq 0$ **then**
6. $l := b^{\text{automarker}}$ /* Copy automatic marker to manual. */
7.   **else**
8. $l := m_{\text{out}}$ /* Assign *outside* marker */
9.   **end if**
10. $b^{\text{marker}} := l$
11. **end if**
12. **return** l

For example, two almost equally large images (*Extremity* and *Cup*) lead to the biggest and the smallest number of basins, respectively, and as a consequence to quite different interaction times. Conversely, *Runoff* as the biggest data set by number of voxels does not stand out in any particular way.

Contrasting this result, it is obvious, that compression time (column 5, t_{comp}) mainly depends on the size of the data set, which is discernible by the data given. The deviations from linearity are mainly due to the number of voxels stored above the threshold. Finally, the segmentation time (column 6, t_{seg}) depends on the number of voxels after compression and on their spatial compactness.

In Table 2, we explore the impact of the number of basins on user interactivity in more detail. The algorithm was forced to deliver decreasing numbers of basins by altering an input threshold on the image. For ease of reading we provide relative measures for number of basins and number of merges with respect to the number of voxels in the compressed volume (3rd and 5th column, respectively). Also, we scaled the time measured for marker setting and resetting to a value corresponding to 1,000,000 input voxels (rightmost column, $\varrho = \frac{t_{\text{marker}} \cdot 10^6 \text{voxels}}{\sharp \text{voxels}}$ in ms). It is discernible that all measured parameters are roughly linear with respect to the number of voxels (3rd, 5th, and 7th column).

Table 1. Dependence of interaction time on number of basins. Table sorted by number of basins. d is the slice thickness in mm.

Id.	d	Size	$\sharp$basins	t_{comp}	t_{seg}	t_{marker}
Heart	0.4	$512 \times 512 \times 368$	112,221	10.39 s	16.32 s	0.08 s
Patient III	2.4	$512 \times 512 \times 210$	285,566	4.99 s	9.93 s	0.22 s
Runoff	0.9	$512 \times 512 \times 1637$	292,462	42.37 s	17.96 s	0.21 s
Thorax	1.2	$512 \times 512 \times 559$	308,982	12.87 s	14.72 s	0.24 s
Cup	1.5	$512 \times 512 \times 763$	450,631	14.58 s	18.68 s	0.32 s
Extremity	1.5	$512 \times 512 \times 790$	752,445	13.55 s	17.84 s	0.57 s

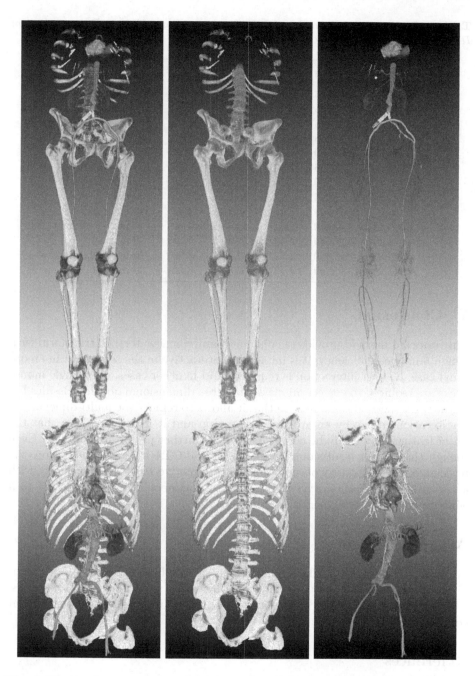

Fig. 4. Direct volume rendering of data sets *Runoff* (top) and *Thorax* (bottom). From left: Original data; bone structures; soft tissue (i.e. original data after bone removal). Note that stents in the top image series are correctly not segmented as bone, but are shown in the soft tissue image. Even a novice user was able to segment the whole 1637 slices CTA scan in about two minutes.

Table 2. Performance measured against different numbers of basins. Data set *Patient III* with a size of $512 \times 512 \times 210 = 55,055,240$ voxels.

♯voxels	♯basins	$\frac{\text{♯basins}}{\text{♯voxels}}$	♯merges	$\frac{\text{♯merges}}{\text{♯voxels}}$	t_{marker}	ϱ
5,208,879	285,566	5.48	278,433	5.35	220 ms	42.2 ms
4,885,864	277,215	5.67	266,619	5.46	210 ms	43.0 ms
4,543,215	266,898	5.87	256,983	5.66	220 ms	48.4 ms
4,149,390	256,958	6.19	245,955	5.93	200 ms	48.2 ms
3,669,954	244,160	6.65	229,456	6.25	190 ms	51.8 ms
3,117,635	223,086	7.16	201,422	6.46	160 ms	51.3 ms
2,600,122	189,320	7.28	160,827	6.19	130 ms	50.0 ms
1,319,828	82,214	6.23	66,453	5.03	50 ms	37.9 ms
1,136,652	64,149	5.64	53,932	4.74	40 ms	35.2 ms
1,006,119	50,660	5.04	43,484	4.32	40 ms	39.8 ms
925,170	41,649	4.50	37,132	4.01	20 ms	21.6 ms
872,831	36,860	4.22	34,173	3.92	20 ms	22.9 ms
831,960	34,349	4.13	32,656	3.93	30 ms	36.1 ms

5   Conclusion

The proposed method provides a coherent hierarchical watershed transform with a high numerical efficiency. It is minimally-interactive in the sense that in an optimal case, no user interaction is required, and in other cases, only single mouse clicks are required to correct misclassified three-dimensional objects. Besides being fast, the method is modular in that it allows to replace the multi-dimensional classification engine by an arbitrary algorithm and it is extendable in that the set of features can easily be complemented by further per-basin statistics. Even though the current results only cover the field of CTA image segmentation, the basic algorithmic strategy of combining the interactive watershed transform with a trainable classification scheme is generic and expected to be applicable to a wide range of image segmentation problems.

Acknowledgments

We would like to thank Clara Soulié (Siemens Medical Solutions, Forchheim) for providing the CT data. In addition, this work would not have been possible without the valuable discussions with and indispensable support of our colleagues.

References

1. Alyassin, A. M., Avinash, G. B.: Semiautomatic bone removal technique from CT angiography data. Med Imaging, Proc. SPIE **4322** (2001) 1273–1283
2. Digabel, H., Lantuèjoul, C.: Iterative algorithms. In Chermant, J. L., editor Proc. 2nd European Symp Quantitative Analysis of Micro-structures in Material Science, Biology and Medicine (1978) 85–99

3. Fiebich, M., Straus, C. M., Sehgal, V., Renger, B. C., Doi, K., Hoffmann, K. R.: Automatic bone segmentation technique for CT angiographic studies. J Comput Assist Tomogr **23(1)** (1999) 155–161
4. Grau, V., Mewes, A. U. J., Alcañiz, M., Kikinis, R., Warfield, S. K.: Improved watershed transform for medical image segmentation using prior information. IEEE Trans Med Imaging **23(4)** (2004) 447–458
5. Hahn, H. K.: Morphological Volumetry Theory, Concepts, and Application to Quantitative Medical Imaging. Ph.D. thesis, University of Bremen (2005)
6. Hahn, H. K., Peitgen, H.-O.: The skull stripping problem in MRI solved by a single 3d watershed transform. MICCAI—Medical Image Computing and Computer-Assisted Intervention, LNCS **1935** (2000) 134–143
7. Hahn, H. K., Peitgen, H.-O.: IWT—Interactive Watershed Transform: A hierarchical method for efficient interactive and automated segmentation of multidimensional grayscale images. Med Imaging, Proc. SPIE **5032** (2003) 643–653
8. Kang, Y., Engelke, K., Kalender, W. A.: A new accurate and precise 3-D segmentation method for skeletal structures in volumetric CT data. IEEE Trans Med Imaging **22(5)** (2003) 586–598
9. Moore, E. A., Grieve, J. P., Jäger, H. R.: Robust processing of intracranial CT angiograms for 3D volume rendering. Eur J Radiol **11(1)** (2001) 137–141
10. Mullick, R., Avila, R., Knoplioch, J., Mallya, Y., Platt, J. Senzig, R.: Automatic bone removal for abdomen CTA: A clinical review. Proc. RSNA (2002)
11. Raman, R., Raman, B., Hundt, W., Stucker, D., Napel, S., Rubin, G. D.: Improved speed of bone removal in CT angiography (CTA) using automated targeted morphological separation: Method and evaluation in CTA of lower extremity occlusive disease (LEOD). Radiology **225(P)** (2002) 647
12. Roerdink, J. B. T. M., Meijster, A.: The watershed transform: Definitions, algorithms, and parallelization strategies. Fundamenta Informaticae **41** (2000) 187–228
13. Suryanaranayanan, S., Mullick, R., Mallya, Y., Wood, C., McCullough, C., Thielen, K.: Automatic bone removal for head CTA: A preliminary review. Proc. RSNA (2003)
14. van Straten, M., Venema, H. W., Streekstra, G. J., den Heeten, C. B. L. M., G. J., Grimbergen, G. A.: Removal of bone in CT angiography of the cervical arteries by piecewise matched mask bone elimination. Medical Physics **31 (10)** (2004) 2924–2933
15. Vincent, L., Soille, P.: Watersheds in digital spaces: An efficient algorithm based on immersion simulations. IEEE Trans Pattern Analysis Machine Intel **13(6)** (1991) 583–598

Automatic Reconstruction of Dendrite Morphology from Optical Section Stacks

S. Urban[1], S.M. O'Malley[1], B. Walsh[1], A. Santamaría-Pang[1],
P. Saggau[2], C. Colbert[3], and I.A. Kakadiaris[1]

[1] Computational Biomedicine Lab, Dept. of Comp. Sci., U. of Houston, Houston, TX
[2] Div. of Neuroscience, Baylor College of Medicine, Houston, TX
[3] Dept. of Biology & Biochemistry, U. of Houston, Houston, TX

Abstract. The function of the human brain arises from computations that occur within and among billions of nerve cells known as neurons. A neuron is composed primarily of a cell body (soma) from which emanates a collection of branching structures (dendrites). How neuronal signals are processed is dependent on the dendrites' specific morphology and distribution of voltage-gated ion channels. To understand this processing, it is necessary to acquire an accurate structural analysis of the cell. Toward this end, we present an automated reconstruction system which extracts the morphology of neurons imaged from confocal and multiphoton microscopes. As we place emphasis on this being a rapid (and therefore automated) process, we have developed several techniques that provide high-quality reconstructions with minimal human interaction. In addition to generating a tree of connected cylinders representing the reconstructed neuron, a computational model is also created for purposes of performing functional simulations. We present visual and statistical results from reconstructions performed both on real image volumes and on noised synthetic data from the Duke-Southampton archive.

1   Introduction

Brain function is based on the computation that occurs concurrently within and among nerve cells, where information from thousands of synaptic inputs is received at the dendritic spines and processed by the dendrites' specific morphology and distribution of voltage-gated ion channels. In order to analyze dendritic interaction, we require computational models of the neuron which incorporate relevant morphological features (i.e., dendritic structure). Building such models has been difficult in the past as technical considerations have dictated that neuronal structure and function be acquired separately. However, recent advances in optical imaging allow us to image the structure of living nerve cells and perform multi-site recording of neuronal function during a single experiment. Nevertheless, the choice of sites for functional imaging must still be made. Ideally, the operator would be able to choose recording sites based on an online simulation of the nerve cell under study; this would enable the selection of optimal sites for further hypothesis testing. Such a simulation requires that structure be imaged, a morphological reconstruction be performed, and a compartmental model of

R.R. Beichel and M. Sonka (Eds.): CVAMIA 2006, LNCS 4241, pp. 190–201, 2006.

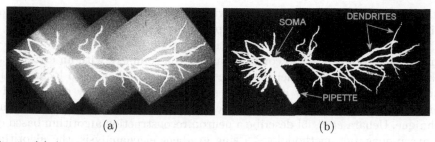

(a)   (b)

Fig. 1. (a) A set of overlapping image stacks comprising one volume and (b) a volume denoised using our method, with typical features labeled

the neuron be created, all during the short time frame of an acute experiment. Unfortunately, the current state-of-the-art in this area is far from capable of generating the necessary reconstruction within this time limit: manual reconstructions may take days to weeks to produce accurately (and still suffer from inter- and intra-observer variability) while most automated or computer-aided methods take many hours.

In this paper, we describe our contributions toward a rapid, fully automated system [1]. In addition to describing the overall framework, we will introduce novel methods including (1) an automated pipette[1] remover and soma picker that eliminates the need to manually delineate the soma, (2) a fast skeletonization algorithm that obviates the need for user-selected seed points or other initialization, and (3) a module that interacts with the *NEURON* [2] software package to allow an operator to select dendrites from the resulting reconstruction in 3-D in order to view functional simulations for particular branches.

The remainder of this paper is organized as follows. Section 2 presents an overview of previous work, Section 3 describes the data to be processed and the methods we use to accomplish reconstruction, and Section 4 discusses our results and validation.

2   Previous Work

Manual Reconstruction Methods: The vast majority of reconstructions are currently performed by computer-aided, but still inherently manual, measuring systems such as *Neurolucida*™. With such a system, a single neuron reconstruction may require ~6-8 hours of manual effort without accurate dendrite diameters and over a week otherwise. Consequently, such methods are almost prohibitively tedious while still being subject to user error and bias.

Full Reconstruction Algorithms: Al-Kofahi *et al.* [3] describe a reconstruction scheme which uses an adaptive exploratory search at the voxel intensity level. This method uses directional filters which assume no preprocessing and

---

[1] Used to inject fluorescent dye, this appears as a connected "part" of the neuron that can create erroneous reconstruction results if not carefully removed.

is thus well-suited mainly for images with minimal noise or other acquisition artifacts. Dima *et al.* [4] present an approach to neuron segmentation using a 3-D wavelet transform to perform a multiscale validation of dendrite boundaries. This segmentation is used to construct a skeleton complete with an estimate of local axial directions and their variances, which are then used to locate bifurcations. Their results show gaps in the skeleton, for which they plan to add a manual correction option. No timings are provided to gauge the efficiency of this technique. Uehara *et al.* [5] describe a neuron reconstruction algorithm based on a wave propagation methodology. Using gradient eigenanalysis, the algorithm generates a field indicating the probability of each voxel belonging to a cylindrical structure (assumed to be dendritic). A digital wave is then propagated through this field to provide dendrite paths. However, the multi-scale gradient analysis used here is prohibitively expensive for large volumes.

3   Materials and Methods

Acquisition: The data are obtained using confocal or multi-photon microscopes through optical serial sectioning along the optical axis. Cells are either loaded with Alexa Fluor 555 or 488 dyes or are taken from a line expressing enhanced green fluorescent protein. The acquired stack of images have a resolution of $\sim 0.3\ \mu m^2$ in-plane, a voxel aspect ratio of about $1:1:3$ when considered as a volume, and dimensions of around $1024 \times 1024 \times 200$ voxels. A complete neuron volume is comprised of three or more such overlapping stacks (Fig. 1(a)). The current cells of interest are CA1 pyramidal cells from mouse or rat hippocampus, though we plan on reconstructing other cell types in the future. The salient features of our volumes are illustrated in Fig. 1(b). For the remainder of this paper, the z-axis will refer to the axis parallel to the optical axis, while the x-y plane will refer to the imaging plane.

The major challenges posed by these datasets are: the 3-D point spread function imposed by the optics of the microscope, variable contrast due to uneven dye distribution within the cell, thermal noise, photon shot noise, the presence of a prominent (but irrelevant) pipette in the image volume, and the fact that many features of interest (i.e., thin dendrites) are at the limit of imaging resolution. These issues will be discussed further where appropriate.

Algorithm Overview: The algorithm is executed sequentially using the steps below; a detailed description of each step follows.

Step 1: Register and combine the multiple image stacks into a single volume.

Step 2: Deconvolve and denoise the volume.

Step 3: Select a grey-level threshold which segments the neuron.

Step 4: Remove the pipette from the neuron object.

Step 5: Skeletonize the neuron object to extract its medial axis tree.

Step 6: Convert the medial axis tree to a tree of tapered cylinders.

Step 7: Output (i) neuron morphology statistics, (ii) data representing the tree structure of the neuron, (iii) a simulation model understood by the simulation software *NEURON*, and (iv) a polygonal 3-D model.

Step 1: In order to obtain adequate resolution over the entirety of the neuron, the cell is scanned in multiple segments and stored in several image volumes. These volumes are registered and combined into a single volume before further processing. To accomplish this, first, the experimenter supplies estimated x, y, and z offsets between each stack; these are obtained when the microscope's area of acquisition is translated from one region of interest to the next. Maximum intensity projections along the x- and z-axes of each stack are then computed.[2] Next, 2-D registration is performed on the mutually-overlapping regions of these images for each pair of stacks, where registration on the x-axis projections provides the needed y and z offsets and registration on the z-axis projections provides x offsets. Finally, these transformations are applied to each image volume as they are placed into the single large volume used for further processing.

To measure the similarity of the projections during registration, we use the mean squared difference metric. This is minimized using limited-memory Broyden Fletcher Goldfarb Shannon (BFGS) minimization with simple bounds [6,7]. This algorithm is designed to solve large, non-linear optimization problems when the objective function gradient is available. It uses a limited-memory BFGS matrix [8] to approximate the Hessian of the objective function, thereby eliminating the need to calculate second derivatives for large-scale problems. Additionally, it allows for translations as well as rotations, both of which are bounded here using parameters set by the experimenter.

We have noted that the pipette may appear to be in slightly different positions between stacks as a result of parallax effects due to the differing orientation of the microscope and subject between stack recordings. As this effect may skew the registration results, the experimenter is given the option to review the registration results: a projection of the aligned stacks is presented and, if necessary, the stacks may be registered again with a smaller search space.

Step 2: Due to the 3-D point spread function (PSF) imposed on the data by the optics of the microscope, our image volumes are inherently blurred, especially along the z-axis where the image is distorted (elongated). To alleviate this effect, an experimental PSF is estimated by performing an imaging experiment on a volume of sparsely-scattered latex beads (diameter: $\sim 0.2\ \mu$m) which are absorptive of the fluorescent dye used in these experiments. These beads simulate ideal point light sources; by averaging many of them (~ 15), a robust estimate of the microscope's PSF may be obtained (Fig. 2). This PSF is then used to deconvolve the 3-D image using a standard maximum-likelihood method.

Due to the poor signal-to-noise ratio of confocal imagery, one of the steps necessary to accomplish an accurate segmentation is a denoising that can effectively remove high frequencies associated with noise while preserving the details of fine structures. To accomplish this, we have developed a non-separable 3-D Parseval frame based on a 1-D piecewise linear spline tight frame. Our frames-based approach operates by a statistical analysis of an ensemble of thresholds associ-

---

[2] Use of the x-axis projections assumes that the stacks align along the y-axis. If they align horizontally, the y-axis projections are used instead.

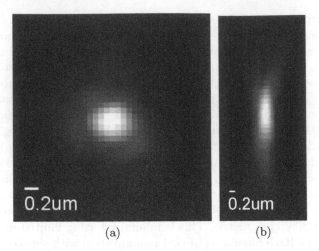

(a)   (b)

Fig. 2. Experimental PSF derived from bead data: (a) x-y plane and (b) x-z plane

ated with frame coefficients. Our approach to denoising differs from the classical wavelet approach in the following ways. First, unlike wavelets, the frames transform allows some redundancy in the signal since the 3-D Parseval frame is not a basis for the set of 3-D digital signals. Hence, when frame coefficients associated with noise are removed, their information content is not entirely lost, providing a more accurate signal reconstruction. Second, the frame transform is undecimated; there are no sampling operations to decompose the signal. This leads to more reliable localization of high-frequency components compared to wavelets, where the size of the signal is subject to change. Finally, the same frame used to decompose the signal is used to reconstruct it [9,10].

Step 3: Following denoising, we employ the grey-level thresholding technique of Otsu [11] to binarize the denoised data. In this context, the frames-based denoising is essential to producing the reliably bimodal histogram which many thresholding methods, including Otsu's, require.

Step 4: The two brightest features in the neuron image stack are the soma and the pipette through which dye is injected during the imaging process. Because these two features are in direct contact with each other, it is necessary to first segment the combined soma/pipette object from the volume and then separate these objects from each other. These steps are performed as follows.
Soma/Pipette Extraction: We calculate an additive projection P_{xy} with respect to the x-y plane of the image volume. An initial estimation of the soma/pipette region is found by applying a threshold T_{xy} to P_{xy}, where T_{xy} is proportional to $max(P_{xy})$. The extreme brightness of the soma/pipette object guarantees that the segmentation contains our object of interest. We fit an ellipse to the resulting segmentation to robustly estimate a bounding box containing the soma/pipette object. The bounding volume by default always contains the entire z-axis.

Soma/Pipette Separation: Given the subvolume bounding the soma and pipette, it is necessary to determine a cutting plane with which to separate the two objects. This plane ideally transects the "neck" or narrowing between the soma and pipette (Fig. 3(a)). Following this we also aim for complete removal of the pipette from the binary volume containing the segmented neuron; hence, in this section we operate solely on the binary representation of the soma/pipette subvolume.

Given the matrix containing the coordinates for the voxels representing the combined soma/pipette object, $\mathbf{A} = \begin{pmatrix} x_1 \ y_1 \ z_1 \\ . \quad . \quad . \\ x_n \ y_n \ z_n \end{pmatrix}$, where each row represents the coordinates of one voxel, we find its 3×3 covariance matrix, $\mathbf{C_A}$. The principal eigenvector of $\mathbf{C_A}$, $\mathbf{v_1}$, indicates the direction of the medial axis of the combined soma/pipette object while the columnwise mean of $\mathbf{A}$, $\mathbf{G_A}$, indicates its center of gravity. The medial axis may then be parametrized by $\mathbf{M}(t) = \mathbf{G_A} + t\mathbf{v_1}$. Scanning the binary subvolume along $\mathbf{M}(t)$, we find the bounds, t_α and t_β, of t such that these delineate the bounds of the soma/pipette object along $\mathbf{M}(t)$. Since the vector $\mathbf{v_1}$ may point in either direction along the object, we must then find the direction from the pipette base toward the soma. The distance transform (DT) is applied to the binary object, which indicates the minimum distance from any point in the soma/pipette object to its boundary. The DT values along $\mathbf{M}(t)$ are extracted, giving the scalar function $D(t) = \mathrm{DT}[\mathbf{M}(t)]$. An outlier-rejecting least-squares fit is applied to $D(t)$; the slope of this fit indicates in which direction along the pipette the line $\mathbf{M}(t)$ points, as $D(t)$ decreases toward the narrow end of the pipette. Next, t_α and t_β are exchanged if necessary to provide the bounds for $\mathbf{M}(t)$ and $D(t)$ such that $\mathbf{M}(t_\alpha)$ is at the pipette base (i.e., its thickest point) and $\mathbf{M}(t_\beta)$ is where the soma/pipette object terminates (i.e., on the side of the soma opposite the pipette). The function $D(t)$ is then used to determine the location of the neck, as it produces a peak near the soma and a gradual slope along the length of the pipette. In particular, the function is smoothed with an approximating spline to eliminate aliasing, and the linear fit computed previously is subtracted to accentuate the location of the neck and soma. Finally, the neck is located at the trough with the highest gradient to its right, in the parametrization of Fig. 3(b). The location of the neck is $\mathbf{M}(t_\gamma)$, where $t_\gamma \in [t_\alpha, t_\beta]$ (though we can usually expect that $|t_\gamma - t_\beta| < |t_\gamma - t_\alpha|$).

Once the neck-centered voxel is found, the two eigenvectors perpendicular to $\mathbf{v_1}$, along with the point $\mathbf{M}(t_\gamma)$, will define a cutting plane. Using this plane, the voxels representing the pipette are removed from the binary volume (i.e., they are set to zero).

Step 5: To extract the medial axis of our segmented neuron, we employ a DT-based skeletonization method inspired by the penalized-distance algorithm of Bitter *et al.* [12]. This algorithm produces a skeleton that is guaranteed to be tree-structured: one of the requirements for neuron reconstruction. Our implementation includes three modifications to the original method. Firstly, the algorithm was not designed for thin objects, yet most of the dendrites we are

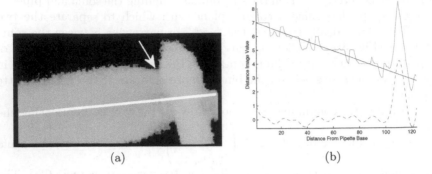

Fig. 3. (a) Binary soma/pipette object with detected medial axis line and arrow indicating "neck;" (b) raw distance signal $D(t)$ with linear fit (solid lines) and smoothed fit-adjusted signal (dotted line). The peak in (b) represents the soma location.

interested in are of low apparent width due to their being near the limits of our imaging resolution. To alleviate the problems this induces, the voxel flagging portion of the algorithm was modified to include a larger number of potential centerline candidates before the DT vector field tracing begins.

Secondly, the various intermediate penalized-distance and "sphere rolling" fields are updated on an iterative, local basis, reducing the time needed to maintain these fields.

Thirdly, we use information from the skeletonization process to intelligently cull false dendrites from the neuron. In particular, it may be possible that long false-positive dendrites are detected which merely originate from surface noise, while at the same time there may exist short dendrites which belong to legitimate branches. Many reconstruction algorithms cull false-positive branches in the post-skeletonization stage based solely on their length. However, by using intermediate information from the skeletonization process, we are able to obtain a measure of saliency related to how much a branch contributes to the volume of the object. That is, if the neuron is represented by its "skeletal reconstruction" (i.e., the object generated by rolling over the skeleton a sphere whose diameter varies by the DT function), a dendrite's saliency is defined as the length of the dendrite that lies outside the skeletal reconstruction produced by *all other* dendrites. Once a branch is marked to be culled, it is culled only if it has no children; hence the culling process is multi-pass as children are culled, their parents checked for saliency and culled, etc. This process is rapid as all necessary information is gathered during the skeletonization process.

Step 6: The skeletonization process returns a tree of paths representing the medial axes of the salient branches in the binarized neuron volume. In addition, a distance transform (DT) volume is generated as a byproduct. Due to the aliasing inherent in the generated voxel-resolution paths, an approximating spline is fit to each path before further processing. The only information now lacking to create a complete cylinder-tree representation of the neuron is a function describing dendrite widths along each spline. Given a single spline path, $P(t)$ parametrized with $t \in [0,1]$, this width function is determined as follows. A series of small (e.g., 5-15 voxel) planes are sliced from the DT volume at multiple sample points along P, where the planes' normals are the tangent of P at each point. From each slice i, the width function, $w(i)$, is defined as the maximal DT value in the slice by gradient ascent from the center of the slice image. (Gradient ascent accounts for slight deviations from the medial axis due to the aliasing correction.) To provide a more accurate and higher-resolution width estimate, a least-squares linear fit[3] is then made to w to give function w'. Finally, the curve P is discretized adaptively (i.e., to a greater extent in areas of high curvature and to a lesser extent elsewhere) to generate a line-segment description of each path. At each line segment start and end point, the continuous function w' is sampled to provide radii for the start and end caps of the tapered cylinder representing that segment.

Step 7: The outputs of a complete reconstruction include morphology statistics, a geometric model, and a simulation model. The morphology statistics describe the following properties: branch angle, or the angle by which each branch deviates from its parent; branch radius, or the number of branch points in the neuron versus their radial distance from the soma (e.g., Fig. 6(a)); and dendrite length, or the number of branch points in the neuron versus their path-length distance from the soma (e.g., Fig. 6(b)) [13]. Also included are Rall's ratio versus branch order and Rall's ratio versus branch thickness [14].

A polygonal 3-D model is output in the standard Autocad DXF format. In addition, a cylinder-based description is output in a variation of the Duke-Southampton SWC format [15] which allows the representation of tapered cylinders. A simulational model is output in the HOC format expected by the simulation package *NEURON* [2].

4 Results

Figure 4 depicts a synthetic volume, its skeleton, and its cylindrical reconstruction, along with detailed views of each. Figure 5 displays the user interaction window for the results of a reconstruction performed on a real dataset, along with a figure displaying voltage and calcium current versus time for a particular branch. Figure 7 illustrates real data at four different points in the processing pipeline. Denoising is also illustrated in Fig. 1.

Reconstruction accuracy is determined using synthetic volumes created with SWC morphology data from the Duke-Southampton archive [16]. Each of these datasets encodes the cylinder-tree structure of a single neuron. Our ground-truth volumes are created as follows. A binary volume is generated from the SWC file

---

[3] The assumption made here is that dendrites either remain the same thickness or thin consistently toward their extremities; they cannot, e.g., thicken and thin repeatedly.

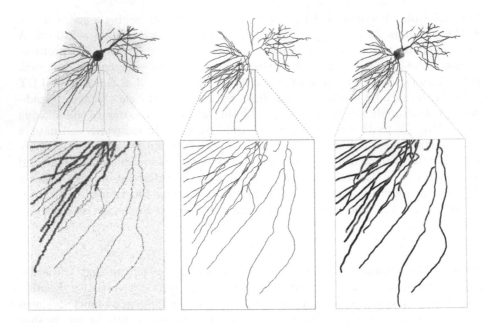

Fig. 4. From left to right: synthetic data reconstructed from an SWC file (with added noise), the extracted skeleton, and the 3-D cylindrical reconstruction

Table 1. Maximum and mean voxel error for four representative test cases

Cell Name	A_{max}	A_{mean}	B_{max}	B_{mean}
n125	6.325	0.680	3.606	0.136
n142	3.317	0.448	5.477	0.368
n414	3.162	0.183	3.000	0.324
n418	3.162	0.295	5.385	0.346

and artificially corrupted by additive Gaussian noise ($\sigma = 10$) and uniformly-distributed multiplicative noise ($\sigma = 20$). Reconstructions are then compared as follows. Given the ground truth volume A and our reconstruction B, we measure both (a) the volume of the object in A unaccounted for by the object in B (false negatives) and (b) vice-versa (false positives). Due to the sparsity of the binary neuron volumes, a global voxel-by-voxel comparison provides meaningless statistics. Instead, we report the maximum deviation between the objects in cases (a) and (b) (A_{max} and B_{max} in Table 4) and the average deviation over the extent of the objects in cases (a) and (b) (A_{mean} and B_{mean}). In all cases, distances are measured in voxels.

Our software requires 7-10 min to complete a reconstruction on volumes of the order 10^6-10^7 cubic voxels using a standard Windows™ workstation. In addition, we have reconstructed volumes of up to $1100 \times 3100 \times 220$ voxels ($\sim 7.5 \times 10^8$ cubic voxels) on an 8-way Linux™ cluster with 32 Gb of physical memory.

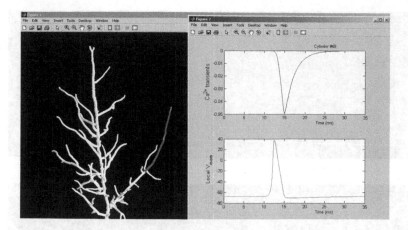

Fig. 5. Simulation viewer displaying voltage and calcium current versus time for the highlighted branch

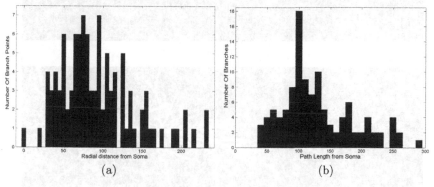

Fig. 6. (a) Branching radius and (b) dendrite lengths from one test case

5   Discussion

We have presented a tool implementing a suite of algorithms tuned specifically for rapid, robust, and automated reconstruction of dendrite morphology from optical section stacks. The output provides statistics about the neuron's structure as well as models that can be used for simulation and visualization. The tool presents a significant improvement over previous methods as well as a major step toward *online* reconstruction of dendrite morphology (i.e., during the lifespan of the cell being imaged): a critical capability for future functional experimentation.

We plan to expand our denoising framework to handle apparent dendrite gaps in order to alleviate the "missing branches" problem that plagues many (if not all) existing reconstruction algorithms. This problem is induced by uneven distribution of fluorescent dye within the neuron and can lead to the truncation of dendrites within the reconstructed model.

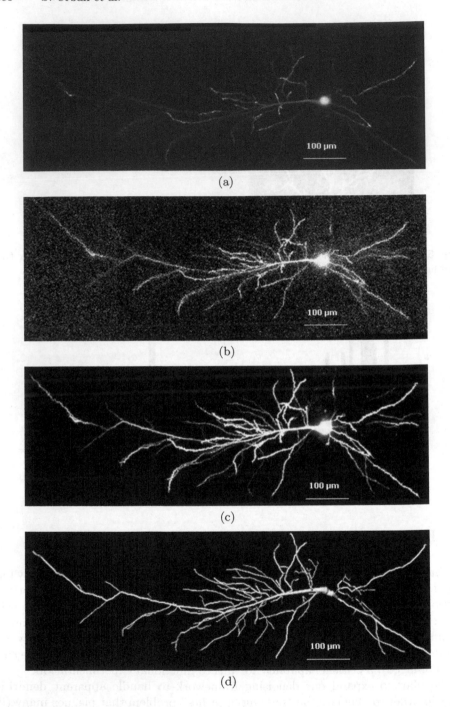

Fig. 7. Real data (a) immediately following acquisition, (b) following deconvolution, (c) following denoising, and (d) following reconstruction (i.e., the final cylinder-tree representation)

Acknowledgements. We would like to thank B. Losavio and T. Hoogland for valuable assistance. This work was supported in part by NIH 1R01EB001048, NIH 1R01AG027577, and a NSF Graduate Research Fellowship (SMO).

References

1. Urban, S.: Automatic reconstruction of dendrite morphologies from optical sections of living fluorescently-labeled neurons. Master's thesis, Univ. of Houston (2005)
2. NEURON: http://www.neuron.yale.edu/neuron (2005)
3. Al-Kofahi, K., Lasek, S., Szarowski, D., Pace, C., Nagy, G.: Rapid automated three-dimensional tracing of neurons from confocal image stacks. IEEE T Inf Technol B **6** (2002) 171–187
4. Dima, A., Scholz, M., Obermayer, K.: Automatic segmentation and skeletonization of neurons from confocal microscopy images based on the 3-D wavelet transform. IEEE T Image Process **11** (2002) 790–801
5. Uehara, C., Colbert, C., Saggau, P., Kakadiaris, I.: Towards automatic reconstruction of dendrite morphology from live neurons. In: Proc IEEE EMBS. (2004)
6. Byrd, R., Lu, P., Nocedal, J.: A limited memory algorithm for bound constrained optimization. SIAM J Sci Stat Comp **16** (1995) 1190–1208
7. Zhu, C., Byrd, R., Nocedal, J.: Algorithm 778: L-BFGS-B, FORTRAN subroutines for large scale bound constrained optimization. ACM T Math Software **23** (1997) 550–560
8. Byrd, R.H., Nocedal, J., Schnabel, R.B.: Representation of quasi-Newton matrices and their use in limited memory methods. Math Program **63** (1994) 129–156
9. Konstantinidis, I., Santamaría-Pang, A., Kakadiaris, I.A.: Frames-based denoising in 3D confocal microscopy imaging. In: Proc IEEE EMBS. (2005)
10. Santamaría-Pang, A., Bildea, T.S., Konstantinidis, I., Kakadiaris, I.A.: Adaptive frames-based denoising of confocal microscopy data. In: Proc IEEE Intl Conf Acoust Speech (ICASSP). (2006)
11. Otsu, N.: A threshold selection method from gray-level histograms. IEEE T Syst Man Cyb **9** (1979) 62–66
12. Bitter, I., Kaufman, A., Sato, M.: Penalized-distance volumetric skeleton algorithm. IEEE T Vis Comput Gr **7** (2001) 195–206
13. Famiglietti, E.: New metrics for analysis of dendritic branching patterns demonstrating similarities and differences in ON and ON-OFF directionally selective retinal ganglion cells. J Comp Neurol **324** (1992) 295–321
14. Rall, W.: Core conductor theory and cable properties of neurons. In: Handbook of Physiology: The Nervous System. Volume 1. Williams and Wilkins (1977) 39–98
15. Cannon, R.C., Turner, D.A., Pyapali, G.K., Wheal, H.V.: An on-line archive of reconstructed hippocampal neurons. J Neurosci Meth **84** (1998) 49–54
16. Duke-Southampton Archive: http://neuron.duke.edu/cells/ (2005)

Modeling the Activity Pattern of the Constellation of Cardiac Chambers in Echocardiogram Videos

Shahram Ebadollahi[1], Shih-Fu Chang[2], and Henry Wu[3]

[1] IBM T.J. Watson Research Center, Hawthorne, NY, USA
ebad@us.ibm.com
[2] Department of Electrical Engineering, Columbia University, New York, NY, USA
sfchang@ee.columbia.edu
[3] College of Physicians and Surgeons, Columbia University, New York, NY, USA
hdw1@columbia.edu

Abstract. A novel approach is presented for modeling the complex activity pattern of the heart in echocardiogram videos. In this approach, the heart is represented by the constellation of its chambers, where the constellation is modeled by pictorial structure at each instance in time. Pictorial structure is then extended to the temporal domain to simultaneously capture the evolution pattern of the appearance of each chamber, the evolving spatial relationships between them, and the topological transformations in their constellation due to phase transitions. Inference and learning algorithms are presented for the model. The problem of correspondence is solved at each stage of the inference process, by matching the evolving model of the complex activity pattern to the observed constellations. The model, which is trained using examples of normal echocardiogram videos is shown to be efficient in temporal segmentation of the content of echocardiogram videos into different phases during one cycle of heart activity.

1 Introduction

Figure 1 illustrates a typical activity pattern of the collection of cardiac chambers during one cycle of the operation of a normal heart in *apical four chamber* view [1]. Each phase corresponds to a different state of the heart function determined by the collective state of the cardiac valves. At phase boundaries, certain valves either open or close, which result in a change in the topology. Within each phase, the appearance characteristics of the chambers evolve, for example, in the first phase *right ventricle* gradually contracts.

In this paper, our goal is to provide a novel approach for the analysis and modeling of such activity patterns. This is motivated by the need for efficient tools for automatic indexing of the archived echocardiogram videos for better content management. In our earlier work [2], we presented an approach for automatic view recognition in echocardiogram videos, which provided access to the content of these videos at the view level. Here, we would like to provide the capability to access the content of the echocardiograms at the level of cardiac phase boundaries. In addition to the video indexing motivation, models created from the normal patterns of the heart activity could be leveraged for classifying cycles of different echocardiograms into normal and abnormal cases, based on the collective behavior of the cardiac chambers throughout one cycle of the heart activity. This forms the basis of our future work.

R.R. Beichel and M. Sonka (Eds.): CVAMIA 2006, LNCS 4241, pp. 202–213, 2006.

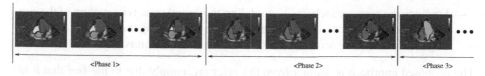

<Phase 1>   <Phase 2>   <Phase 3>

Fig. 1. Sequence of echocardiogram frames showing three phases of heart operation in *apical four chamber* view. (Note: Chambers are color coded for illustration purposes.)

In our description of the activity pattern of the heart (Figure 1), we alluded to the representation of the heart by the collection of its chambers. There is a broad consensus for representing classes of objects using the assembly of their *parts* [3,4], where parts can be either image patches or features. In the example above, parts are blobs corresponding to cardiac chambers. *Pictorial structures* [4] is a popular way to model classes of objects represented by the constellation of their parts with a single flexible template, which captures both the appearance characteristics of each individual part and the geometrical characteristics of their assembly.

Activity as described above, when applied to an instance of an object class modeled by pictorial structures translates into 1- deformations in the spatial relationships between the parts (*geometrical*), 2- change in the number of parts throughout the activity (*topological*), and 3- metamorphosis of the appearance of the individual parts during the course of the activity. We propose here the extension of the notion of pictorial structures to the temporal domain for modeling the complex activity pattern of the constellation of cardiac chambers.

In this model, we assume that during each phase of the activity, parameters of the pictorial structure pertaining to individual parts and their spatial relationships evolve according to a Gauss-Markov process. We also assume that at phase boundaries, pictorial structure experiences a topological transformation, due to merging or splitting of the the the parts according to pre-defined semantics. No assumptions are made regarding the availability of specialized part detectors, or labels of the parts, such as the ones available in motion capture data sets. At each time instance, the evolved pictorial structure is used to find the correspondence information for an observed constellation of parts in the image.

A dynamic Bayesian network (DBN) in the form that is a variation of the *switched linear dynamic system* (SLDS) [5] is used to capture the causal relationships among the characteristics of the evolving model of the object, the observations, and the correspondence information. Learning the parameters of this model and therefore the model of the activity pattern of the object is done using the expectation-maximization [6] procedure. The expectation step or equivalently the inference is performed using a modified form of the Viterbi algorithm.

The contributions of this paper are:

– Extending the notion of pictorial structures to the temporal domain,
– Solving the correspondence problem at each step of the algorithm in a holistic approach by matching the evolved model of the object to the observed constellation of parts,

– Applying the proposed scheme to modeling the complex activity pattern of the constellation of cardiac chambers, for the purpose of indexing the content of echocardiogram videos at the level of their constituent temporal units.

The proposed approach is distinct from the prior art, mainly due to the fact that it allows topological transformations in the model of the constellation and more importantly
solves the correspondence problem on the fly using the model of the evolving constellation.

Hamid *et al.* [7] separately track each part (object) using *particle filters* based on
its appearance and shape models extracted from the initial state of the activity. After
the correspondence information has been established, characteristics of the spatial relationships between the agents at each image of the sequence is derived and used as the
feature vector representing the constellation of agents. The sequence of the features for
the duration of the activity are then quantized into discrete states with the help of an
HMM model. In this method the appearance of the agents are assumed to be constant
with time.

The main difference of the proposed model to the SLDS model of Pavlovic *et al.* [5],
is that we do not assume the availability of parts labels and automatically infer them in
the process of learning the model.

The most similar approach is that of Wang and Zhu [8], which proposes a method
for modeling *video texture*, through modeling the evolving attributed graphs obtained
from applying *primal sketch* to the frames of the video. However, that method does not
take into account the evolution of the appearance characteristics of the parts.

We submit that our approach is effective in modeling the evolution pattern of the
constellation of parts. As reported in section 4 an average precision of 87.3% is obtained
for automatic phase tracking in echocardiogram videos.

2   Time-Varying Pictorial Structures

We denote the model of an object category $\mathcal{O}$ represented by the constellation of the
parts with a relational structure (we follow the notation of [9]), $\mathcal{G}' = (\mathcal{L}, \mathcal{N}', \Theta)$, where
$\mathcal{L} = \{l_1, \ldots, l_M\}$ denote the labels of the parts of the object, $\mathcal{N}'$ represents the spatial
dependencies between those labels, and $\Theta = [\Theta^{(1)}, \Theta^{(2)}, \ldots, \Theta^{(K)}]$ stands for the
parameters of the models of the attributes of the cliques [9] of sizes $\{1, 2, \ldots, K\}$ of the
relational structure, which define the constraints on the possible values of the attributes
in the instances taken from the object class. Note that $\Theta^{(1)} = \{\theta_1^{(1)}, \ldots, \theta_M^{(1)}\}$, where
each $\theta_m^{(1)}$ is the parameter defining the attribute of the m-th part in the object. The
parameters of the other cliques can be defined in a similar fashion.

For example, if we assume that the attributes of the cliques of size one are their *areas*,
and those of cliques of size two are the *distance* and *angle* between the centers of the
two parts in the clique, and if we assume that those attributes are Gaussian random
variables, then their corresponding $\theta^{(1)}$ and $\theta^{(2)}$ specify the mean and covariance of
their probability distributions.

When the object category $\mathcal{O}$ undergoes an activity pattern α, *i.e.* $\alpha(\mathcal{O})$, the constraints on the features of the relational structure modeling the object category change

with the progress of time to reflect the effect of the activity pattern. In this case, we can write the evolving model of the object as: $\mathcal{G}'_\alpha(t) = (\mathcal{L}, \mathcal{N}', \Theta_\alpha(t))$. Note that the identity of the parts in the constellation and their spatial dependencies do not change with time throughout the duration of the activity phase.

We assume that the evolution of the parameters of the model of the object are governed by a *Gauss-Markov* process, *i.e.* the probability distribution of the parameters of the model at each time step is Gaussian given the values of the parameters for the previous time step. We use the generic notation $x_{(.)}(t)$ to denote the mean and $W_{(.)}(t)$ to denote the covariance of the clique potentials of any size at time t, where $(.)$ should be filled with the appropriate term for those cliques. We also assume that at the beginning of the *simple* activity the probability distribution of a clique potential is Gaussian, *i.e.* $\mathcal{N}(x_0, W_0)$. According to the Gauss-Markov assumption we have the following equations. Note that $H(.)$ will be considered to be identity in the rest of the work.:

$$x_{(.)}(t) = A(.) \times x_{(.)}(t-1) + H(.) \times w_{(.)}(t)$$
$$w_{(.)}(t) \sim \mathcal{N}(0, W(.)) \tag{1}$$

2.1   Correspondence

An observed instance of the activity $\alpha(\mathcal{O})$ at time t could also be represented by a relational structure, $\mathcal{G}(t) = (\mathcal{R}(t), \mathcal{N}(t), \mathbf{d}(t))$, where $\mathcal{R}(t) = \{r_1, r_2, \ldots, r_{N_t}\}$ are the regions observed in the scene at time t, $\mathcal{N}(t)$ is their neighborhood structure, and $\mathbf{d}(t) = [\mathbf{d}^{(1)}(t), \mathbf{d}^{(2)}(t), \ldots, \mathbf{d}^{(K)}(t)]$ are the features obtained from the constellation for cliques of size $\{1, 2, \ldots, K\}$, where $\mathbf{d}^{(k)}(t) = \{d^{(k)}(r_1, \ldots, r_k, t) | r_i \in \mathcal{R}(t), \forall i \in \{1, \ldots, k\}\}$. Note that some of the observed regions correspond to the actual parts of the object, whereas some are just false parts and some of the parts of the object may be missing from $\mathcal{R}$.

Correspondence is then defined as the best match, $f_t^* : \mathcal{G}(t) \mapsto \mathcal{G}'_\alpha(t)$, between the labels of the object parts ($\mathcal{L}$) and the observed regions at time t ($\mathcal{R}_t$). The problem of finding the optimal match is posed as finding the optimal configuration of a Markov random field (MRF) [9] defined on the set of observed parts $\mathcal{R}_t$, where each random variable takes values in the set of labels $\mathcal{L}$.

$$\mathbf{f}_t^* = \underset{\mathbf{f}_t \in \Omega_t}{argmin}(U_t(\mathbf{f}_t | \mathbf{d}(t)))$$
$$= \underset{\mathbf{f}_t \in \Omega_t}{argmin}(U_t(\mathbf{d}(t) | \mathbf{f}_t) + U_t(\mathbf{f}_t)) \tag{2}$$

U_t is the time-varying version of the Gibbs energy function [9]. $\Omega_t = \mathcal{L}^{N_t}$ is the *configuration space* of the random field, where it is assumed that the random variables defined on the sites in $\mathcal{R}(t)$ all take values in the time-independent label set $\mathcal{L}$. Note that correspondence is found here through a holistic approach by matching the snapshot at time t of the evolving model of the object ($\mathcal{G}'_\alpha(t)$) to the observed constellation of parts at that instance in time ($\mathcal{G}(t)$). The time-varying posterior energy function in 2 can be decomposed into the *prior* and *likelihood* energies:

$$U_t(\mathbf{f}_t) = \sum_{r \in \mathcal{R}(t} \phi_1^t(f(r)) \quad +$$

$$\sum_{r \in \mathcal{R}(t), r' \in \mathcal{R}(t) - \{r\}} \phi_2^t(f(r), f(r'))$$

$$U_t(\mathbf{d}(t)|\mathbf{f}_t) = \sum_{r \in \mathcal{R}(t)} \phi_1^t(d^{(1)}(r, t)|f(r)) \quad +$$

$$\sum_{r \in \mathcal{R}(t), r' \in \mathcal{R}(t) - \{r\}} \phi_2^t(d^{(2)}(r, r', t)|f(r), f(r')) \tag{3}$$

where, $\phi_1(.)$ and $\phi_2(.)$ are the *potential functions* defined on cliques of size one and two respectively [9]. We only consider the local features of each site in the constellation and its relationships with all its neighbors. However, one can consider contextual dependencies of higher orders as well.

The *prior potential* functions $\phi_1^t(f(r))$ and $\phi_2^t(f(r), f(r'))$ encode our prior belief on the form of the configurations at each time instance t by associating a penalty value to certain configurations. We assume here, that those penalty values remain constant with time to show that the prior belief in the form of the configurations do not change with time throughout the activity. Therefore we have $\phi_1^t = \phi_1 = cst.$ and $\phi_2^t = \phi_2 = cst.$

Likelihood potentials on the other hand capture the temporal variations in the constraints imposed on the elements of the random field by the model of the activity. We represent the variations in the likelihood potentials with *dynamic kernels*, where both the center and the bandwidth of the kernels vary according to the specifications of the activity as determined by the model.

$$\phi_1^t(d^{(1)}(r, t)|f(r)) = $$
$$\Phi(\| d^{(1)}(r, t) - x_{f(r)}(t) \|)$$
$$\phi_2^t(d^{(2)}(r, r', t)|f(r), f(r')) = $$
$$\Phi(\| d^{(2)}(r, r', t) - x_{f(r), f(r')}(t) \|) \tag{4}$$

In these equations, $x_{(.)}(t)$ is the estimated center of the kernel, or equivalently the true value of the attributes of the cliques as predicted by the Gauss-Markov model of the activity according to equation 1, and $d_n(.)$ is the *actual* observed value of the clique in the observation sequence. Φ is the Gaussian kernel employed here to reflect the fact that the attributes of the observed sites in the constellations at each time instance are noise corrupted versions of the actual values.

We employ the *Highest Confidence First (HCF)* method proposed by Chou and Brown [10] to find the optimal labeling f_t^*. This is a deterministic algorithm for inferencing in random fields with discrete configuration spaces.

Having found the labeling of the parts f_t^* in the observed constellation, we can now obtain the observed values corresponding to each clique in the model $\mathcal{G}_\alpha'(t)$. If we use the generic notation $y_{(.)}(t)$ for these observed values of the cliques, we can write the following relationship:

$$y_{(.)}(t) = C(.) \times x_{(.)}(t) + v_{(.)}(t)$$
$$v_{(.)}(t) \sim \mathcal{N}(0, V(.)) \tag{5}$$

We assume $C = I$, so that value of the clique at any time is just a noise corrupted version of the true state of the clique as projected by the pattern of the activity.

The combination of equations 1 and 5 for all the cliques constitute a linear dynamic system. However, in this system the correspondence between the state of the system and the observations are not available a priori and are obtained as described above. The following provides a description of the mechanics of this process.

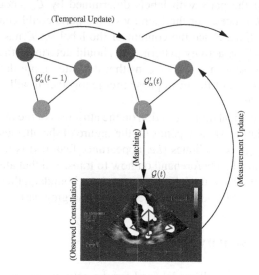

Fig. 2. Mechanics of the *filtering* process. The evolved pictorial structure $(\mathcal{G}'_\alpha(t-1) \to \mathcal{G}'_\alpha(t))$ is used to find correspondence $(f_t^* : \mathcal{G}(t) \mapsto \mathcal{G}'_\alpha(t))$. Parameters of the model are then updated.

We can picture the interaction of the evolving model of the constellation with the observation at each instance of time as a linear dynamic system extended to relational structures (Figure 2). Assuming the constraints on the formation of the constellation at time $(t-1)$ are already known, we can estimate those constraints on the features of the different cliques for the next step at time t (*time update*). Using the predicted model at time t, labeling of the parts in the observed constellation at time t could be established as described above. Having access to the correspondence information, we can now obtain the measurements corresponding to each clique in the model and use them to correct our estimate of the model of the constellation (*measurement update*) previously obtained through the *time update* stage.

2.2 Phase Transitions

It was mentioned earlier that the object experiences topological transformations, such as split and merge, at phase boundaries. The semantics of the part-based representation change due to such transformations, *e.g.* new parts with different identities and characteristics emerge as the result of a split. If we denote the sequence of activity phases with: $\alpha_1 \to \alpha_2 \to \ldots \to \alpha_P$, then at phase boundary $\alpha_m \to \alpha_n$, at time t, the model of the evolving constellation of parts changes according to: $\mathcal{G}'_{\alpha_m}(t) \to \mathcal{G}'_{\alpha_n}(t+1)$, where $\mathcal{G}'_{\alpha_p}(t) = (\mathcal{L}_{\alpha_p}, \mathcal{N}'_{\alpha_p}, \Theta_{\alpha_p}(t)), \forall p \in \{1, 2, \ldots, P\}$

This transformation entails transforming the semantics of the collection of the parts of the object, and the corresponding transformation in the constraints imposed on the observed constellations by the model: $\mathcal{L}_{\alpha_m} \to \mathcal{L}_{\alpha_n}$ and $\Theta_{\alpha_m}(t) \to \Theta_{\alpha_n}(t)$. Note that since we consider the neighborhood structure $\mathcal{N}'$ to be fully connected in each phase, we are not concerned with the transformation in the neighborhood structure, because it is automatically determined by the number of part labels after the transformation.

The collection of the parts with labels determined by $\mathcal{L}_{\alpha_n}$ could change in size (through *birth/death* process) or the identity of the parts could change or both could happen at the same time. Since the content of the label set $\mathcal{L}$ has to do with the associated semantics of the activity pattern, one should determine the label set for each possible phase of the sequence. This means that it has to be pre-defined that if for example parts $l_i^{\alpha_m}$ and $l_j^{\alpha_m}$ of the m-th phase merge together it will result in part $l_k^{\alpha_n}$ in phase n of the activity.

The effect of topological transformation on the attributes of the model of the evolving constellation , to a large extent depends on the nature of the attributes. For example, if the attribute of a single-site cliques (*i.e.* appearance features) is its area, then certain rules have to be established beforehand on how to transform that attribute at the phase-boundary. If two parts in the model merge at a phase boundary, then we can obtain the area of the resulting part by adding the areas of the merging parts, for example.

3   Multi-phase Activity Model

Figure 3 illustrates the overall model used for the activity pattern of the constellation of parts. Activity is decomposed into a sequence of segments $\{\alpha_1, \alpha_2, \ldots, \alpha_P\}$ each corresponding to a phase. We assume that the distribution of the phases satisfies a first-order Markovian dynamics governed by transition matrix $\psi_{i,j} = Pr(\alpha_p = j | \alpha_{p-1} = i)$. In phase p, activity progresses according to the continuous dynamics determined by the parameters of the model λ_{α_p}, in that phase.

Note that λ_{α_p} stands for the all parameters of the time-varying pictorial structure $\mathcal{G}'_{\alpha_p}(t)$ of phase p. Also note that unlike *segmental models* [11], where the linear models in the consecutive discrete phases are unrelated, in the case here, the initial condition for the evolving pictorial structure model in each phase depends on its final state in the previous one. Its topology and initial characteristics also depend on the pair (α_{p-1}, α_p).

3.1   Inference and Learning

Figure 4 displays a dynamic Bayesian network, that captures in compact form the causal relationship between the variables depicted in figure 3. For an activity sequence of duration T, the sequence of discrete states $\{S_0, S_1, \ldots, S_T\}$ is a rolled-out version of the sequence of phases $\{\alpha_1, \alpha_2, \ldots, \alpha_P\}$ shown in Figure 3. At each time instance, the state S_t corresponds to a phase of the activity, *i.e.* $\{S_t | t = \{1, 2, \ldots, T\}, S_t \in \{\alpha_1, \ldots, \alpha_P\}\}$. The transition between the states is determined by the phase transition matrix Ψ and is defined as: $\psi_{i,j} = Pr(S_t = \alpha_i | S_{t-1} = \alpha_j)$. Activity starts in state S_0 with probability $P(S_0) = \pi_0$. $\mathcal{F}_{0:T} = \{\mathbf{f}_t | t = 0, \ldots, T\}$ are the correspondence information for the observed constellations.

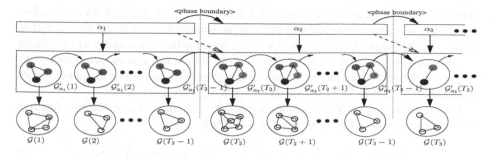

Fig. 3. Non-linear dynamic model of the multi-phase activity pattern of an object represented by the constellation of parts

In the joint probability distribution of the variables of the DBN $P(\mathcal{S}_{0:T}, \mathcal{G}'_{0:T}, \mathcal{G}_{0:T}, \mathcal{F}_{0:T})$, $(\mathcal{S}_{0:T}, \mathcal{G}'_{0:T}, \mathcal{F}_{0:T})$ are the hidden variables, which need to be inferred from the sequence of observations $\mathcal{G}_{0:T}$ by finding the posterior probability $P(\mathcal{S}_{0:T}, \mathcal{G}'_{0:T}, \mathcal{F}_{0:T} |\mathcal{G}_{0:T})$.

Following the work of Pavlovic *et al.* [5] we employ the Viterbi approximation to obtain the most likely sequence of discrete states $S^*_{0:T}$. As a by product and due to the step-by-step nature of the Viterbi algorithm we find the approximation to the sequence of correspondence information $\mathbf{f}^*_{0:T}$ as well, using the procedure described in section 2.1. In essence, instead of finding the posterior probability $P(\mathcal{S}_{0:T}, \mathcal{G}'_{0:T}, \mathbf{f}_{0:T}|\mathcal{G}_{0:T})$, we obtain the mode $P(\mathcal{G}'_{0:T}|\mathcal{G}_{0:T}, \mathcal{S}^*_{0:T}, \mathbf{f}^*_{0:T})$.

Given the correspondence information at each step of the Viterbi approximation, we transform $\mathcal{G}_t$ and $\mathcal{G}'_t$ at each time $t = 1, \ldots, T$ into the set of variables corresponding to the cliques of size one and two, *i.e.* $\mathcal{G}_t \mapsto \mathbf{Y}_t$, and $\mathcal{G}'_t \mapsto \mathbf{X}_t$. Therefore, the logarithm of the joint probability distribution can be re-written as:

$$P(\mathcal{S}_{0:T}, \mathcal{X}_{0:T}, \mathcal{Y}_{0:T}) = P(S_0)\prod_{t=1}^{T}P(S_t|S_{(t-1)}) \quad +$$

$$P(\mathbf{X_0}|S_0)\prod_{t=1}^{T}P(\mathbf{X_t}|\mathbf{X_{(t-1)}}, S_t, S_{(t-1)}) \quad +$$

$$\prod_{t=0}^{T}P(\mathbf{Y_t}|\mathbf{X_t}, S_t) \tag{6}$$

Using the Gauss-Markov assumptions and employing equations 1 and 5 we can write:

$$\left(\mathbf{X}_t|\mathbf{X_{(t-1)}} = \mathbf{x}_{(t-1)}, S_t = \alpha_i, S_{(t-1)} = \alpha_j\right) \sim$$
$$\begin{cases} \mathcal{N}(A_i\mathbf{x}_{(t-1)}, \mathbf{W}_i) & \text{, if } i = j \\ \mathcal{N}(\beta_{i,j}(\mathbf{x}_{(t-1)}), \mathbf{W}_i) & \text{,otherwise} \end{cases}$$
$$(\mathbf{Y}_t|\mathbf{X}_t = \mathbf{x}_t, S_t = \alpha_i) \sim \mathcal{N}(\mathbf{x}_t, \mathbf{V}_i)$$
$$(\mathbf{X}_0|S_0 = \alpha_i) \sim \mathcal{N}(\mathbf{x}_{0,i}, \mathbf{W}_{0,i}) \tag{7}$$

In these equations, $\beta_{i,j}(.)$ is a non-linear function, which depends on the specific topological transformation applied to $\mathbf{X}_{(t-1)}$ to obtain $\mathbf{X_t}$ and is defined by the pair of states $(S_{(t-1)}, S_t)$ as described in section 2.2. Note that if the phase of the system does not change at a given time t, the dynamics of the continuous state of the system will be defined by the regular Gauss-Markov process, which is the characteristics of the linear dynamic systems. Also, at the start of the activity, we assume that the properties of the cliques of the part-based representation of the object have a normal distribution with parameters $(\mathbf{x}_{0,i}, \mathbf{W}_{0,i})$ for the case that the activity start in phase α_i.

For implementing the Viterbi approximation the definition of a *partial cost* function $\delta_t(i)$ is necessary, which is defined as the following:

$$\delta_t(i) = \min_{\mathcal{S}_{0:t}, \mathcal{X}_{0:t}} \{-logP[\{\mathcal{S}_{0:(t-1)}, S_t = \alpha_i\}, \mathcal{X}_{0:t}, \mathcal{Y}_{0:t}|\lambda]\} \tag{8}$$

The innovation cost $\delta_{t,(t-1)}(i,j)$ could be defined as the incremental error incurred in finding the true state of the dynamic system by the process of filtering as just described for a specific transition $j \rightarrow i$. This cost can be written as the following:

$$\delta_{t,(t-1)}(i,j) = \frac{1}{2}[(y_t - C_i\tilde{x}_{t|t-1,i,j})' \times (C_i\Sigma_{t|t-1,i,j}C_i' + V_i)\times$$
$$(y_t - C_i\tilde{x}_{t|t-1,i,j})] + \frac{1}{2}log|C_i\Sigma_{t|t-1,i,j}C_i' + V_i| - log\psi_{i,j}$$

As the result of the multi-stage inferencing described above, the following sufficient statistics becomes available: $E[s_t]$, $E[s_t s'_{(t-1)}]$, $E[x_t s_t]$, $E[(x_t s_t)(x_t s_t)']$, $E[(x_t s_t)(x_{(t-1)} s_{(t-1)})']$. Using these sufficient statistics the parameters of the segmental linear dynamic systems corresponding to each single phase of activity could be estimated by the maximization step as described by Ghahramani in [12] to obtain: A_i^{new}, W_i^{new}, C_i^{new}, V_i^{new}, and the phase transition $\Psi_{i,j}$ for all phases $\alpha_i, i = 1, \dots, P$.

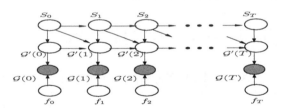

Fig. 4. DBN for modeling the relationships between the elements of the non-linear dynamic model. (Note: Empty nodes represent hidden variables.)

4   Experiments and Results

The effectiveness of the model is demonstrated here in the context of automatic phase tracking and identification in echocardiogram videos. Samples in the corpus are taken from the activity pattern of the normal heart in the *apical four chamber* view [1] of the heart. The corpus contains a total of 21 sample activity sequences from 10 different echocardiograms. Experiments are conducted in a leave-one-out fashion, namely for 21 different rounds, each time an activity sequence was left out and a model for the activity

pattern was learned from the remaining 20 samples. The resulting model was then used
to segment the left-out activity sequence. The final results of the temporal segmentation
performance were averaged over all 21 rounds.

Activity of the heart throughout one heart-cycle in *apical four chamber* view consists
of 3 distinct phases. It always starts in phase 1 and then progresses to the other phases.
The set of labels of the parts for each phase is as following [1]:

$$
\begin{aligned}
\text{phase 1:} \quad \mathcal{L}_{\alpha_1} &= \{\text{LV,RV,RA,LA}\} \\
\text{phase 2:} \quad \mathcal{L}_{\alpha_2} &= \{\text{RC, LC}\} \\
\text{phase 3:} \quad \mathcal{L}_{\alpha_3} &= \{\text{RC, } LV, LA\}
\end{aligned}
\tag{9}
$$

where RC is the result of merging between RA and RV and LC is produced by merging
LA and LV.

Nature of the transitions are defined a priori, which is consistent with introducing
the expert knowledge into the model of the activity. Note that pre-defining these rules,
by incorporating the expert knowledge, for the topological transformations is to limit
the number of all possible transitions that should be considered in the process of inferring the variables of the model. However, if such expert knowledge is not available
in a certain problem, then one should consider all the possible forms of topological
transformations in the process of inferencing.

The form of the translations between the parameters of the dynamic relational structures in different phases, *i.e.* the mean of the dynamic kernels specifying the evolution
of the constraints on the object in each phase, at the phase boundaries should also be
defined a priori. This means that, if for example one of the appearance characteristics
is the *size* of a part, how does that characteristic change, when the part splits in two or
merges with some other part. In this experiment, local characteristics of the parts are
their locations and areas and the relational characteristics are the distance and angle
between two neighboring parts.

At a phase boundary if a split occurs, then the initial mean area after the boundary for
the two new parts will be half of the splitting part before the boundary. Mean location
of the two new parts will be located equidistantly from the center of the splitting part
on a line on either side. The new distances and angles will be calculated from the new
set of parts' locations. For a merge an inverse operation will be in effect. Note that the
specifics of the transformations made to the characteristics of the relational structures
at the phase boundaries are very specific to the type of characteristics defined for the
objects and is different in different settings.

Having defined the nature of the topological transformations at the phase boundaries,
the goal is to learn the set of parameters of the model $\{\{\lambda_{\alpha_1}, \lambda_{\alpha_2}, \lambda_{\alpha_3}\}, \varPsi\}$, where
$\lambda_{\alpha_i} = \{A_i, W_i, C_i, V_i, x_{0,i}, W_{0,i}\}$ is the parameters of the LDS under phase i of the
activity, and $\varPsi$ is the phase transition matrix, which determines the probability of the
transition between the different phases and therefore the *geometric* distribution of the
length of stay in each phase before making a transition.

Boundaries of the heart chambers are manually traced for the 21 sequences in the
corpus. The reason for this requirement is that we want to make sure that perfect foreground part detection is available, due to the fact that total number of parts in heart

---

[1] LV=Left Ventricle, LA=Left Atrium, RV=Right Ventricle, RA=Right Atrium.

sequences is low. For example, in phase 2 which consists of only 2 parts if either parts is missed, we will get a degenerate constellation, which will be very unreliable for any correct activity model learning. If for another application, the number of parts are higher, then the tolerance for missing parts will correspondingly be higher as well, and there won't be any need for the assumption of correct foreground part detection. Note that in this work our focus is on modeling the activity pattern of the constellation of parts and not perfect part detection. In order to make the experiments realistic, few false parts are added to the constellations. The appearance attributes of the added false parts are sampled from the distribution of those attributes for the true parts, which make the false parts similar to the foreground ones. These parts are then randomly positioned in the image. Care is taken not to make them overlap with the foreground parts.

The inference algorithm was initialized with the mean and covariance of the constellation of the cardiac chambers at the start of the activity sequences in the corpus in order to obtain a better result. It is well-know that the Viterbi approximation is susceptible to initialization.

Figure 5 depicts the average result of applying the model in each round of experiment (total of 21), to the test sequence of that round. As shown in the figure, the automatic phase detection matches the ground truth well most of the time, specifically 87.73% on average over all sequences.

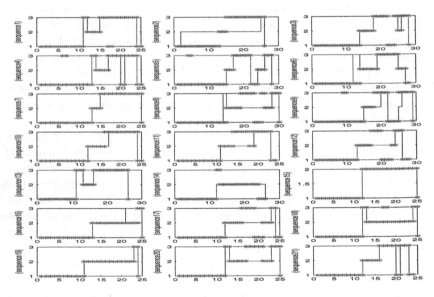

Fig. 5. From left to right and top to bottom, each panel show the phase tracking results for rounds 1 to 21. *'Blue'* line stands for the automatically detected phase, and *'red'* shows the ground truth.

5   Discussion and Conclusion

We proposed an approach for modeling the complex activity pattern of objects represented by the constellation of their parts. The approach extends the notion of *pictorial structure* to the temporal domain. The resulting model is able to capture the pattern of the variations in the appearance of the individual parts, the dynamics of the geometry of the constellation of parts, and topological transformations in the constellation. Inference and learning algorithms are provided for the model.

The approach was applied to modeling the *multi-phase* activity pattern of the constellation of cardiac chambers in echocardiogram videos during one cycle of heart operation. The model was learned from exemplars taken from *normal* echocardiogram videos, and then successfully applied for decomposing the video of each heart cycle into its constituent *phases*.

Several important issues need to be addressed in the future. First and foremost, is dealing with the problem of simultaneous chamber detection and modeling the activity pattern of the constellation of chambers in echocardiogram videos. Second, it is valuable to use the proposed scheme in learning the pattern of the normal heart and using it for classification of test sequences into normal and abnormal cases. Finally, we would like to apply the proposed approach to other domains to further assess its efficiency and accuracy.

References

1. Feigenbaum, H.: Echocardiography. LeaFebiger(1993)
2. Ebadollahi, S., Chang, S.F., Wu, H.: Automatic View Recognition in Echocardiogram Videos Using Parts-Based Representation. In: Proceeding of IEEE International Conference on Computer Vision and Pattern Recognition. (2004) 2–9
3. Fergus, R., Perona, P., Zisserman, A.: Object Class Recognition by Unsupervised Scale-Invariant Learning. In: Proceeding of IEEE Conference on Computer Vision and Pattern Recognition. (2003)
4. Felzenszwalb, P., Huttenlocher, D.:Efficient Matching of Pictorial Structures.In: IEEE Conference on Computer Vision and Pattern Recognition. (2000) 66–73
5. Pavlovic, V., Rehg, J.M., MacCormick, J.: Learning Switching Linear Models of Human Motion. In: Proceedings of the Advances in Neural Information Processing Systems (NIPS). (2000) 981–987
6. Dempster, A., Laird, N., Rubin, D.: Maximum likelihood from incomplete data via the em algorithm. Journal of the Royal Statistical Society, Series B **39**(1) (1977) 1–38
7. Hamid, R., Huang, Y., Essa, I.: ARGMode-Activity Recognition using Graphical Models. In: Proceedings of the 2nd IEEE Workshop on Detection and Recognition of Events in Video, Madison, Wisconsin. (2003)
8. Wang, Y., Zhu, S.C.: Modeling Complex Motion by Tracking and Editing Hidden Markov Graphs.In: Proceedings of IEEE Computer Society Conference on Computer Vision and Pattern Recognition (CVPR04). Volume1. (2004) 856–863
9. Li, S.Z.: Markov Random Field Modeling in Image Analysis. Springer-Verlag (2001)
10. Chou, P.B., Brown, C.M.: The Theory and Practice of Bayesian Image Labeling. International Journal of Computer Vision **4** (1990) 185–210
11. Li, Y., Wang, T., Shum, H.Y.: Motion texture: a two-level statistical model for character motion synthesis. In: Proceedings of the 29th annual conference on Computer graphics and interactive techniques, ACM Press (2002) 465–472
12. Ghahramani, Z., Hinton, G.E.: Parameter Estimation for Linear Dynamical Systems. Technical Report CRG-TR-96-2 (1996)

A Study on the Influence of Image Dynamics and Noise on the JPEG 2000 Compression Performance for Medical Images

Peter Michael Goebel[1], Ahmed Nabil Belbachir[2], and Michael Truppe[1]

[1] Karl-Landsteiner Institute for Biotelematics, A-1010 Vienna, Austria
{pgoebel, mtruppe}@landsteiner.org
http://www.landsteiner.org
[2] ARC, Seibersdorf Research GmbH
A-1220 Vienna, Austria
belbachir@ieee.org

Abstract. This paper addresses two questions concerning JPEG2000 compression - firstly - how much has noise influence on compression performance - secondly - can compression performance be improved by applying a new complementary conception with introducing a denoising process before the application of compression? Indeed, radiographic images are a combination between the relevant signal and noise, which is per definition not compressible. The noise behaves generally close to a mixture of Gaussian and/or Poisson statistics, which generally affects the compression performance. In this paper, the influence of noise on the compression performance of JPEG2000 images with investigating the parameters signal dynamic and spatial pattern frequency are considered; and the JPEG2000 compression scheme combined with a denoising process is analyzed on simulated and real dental ortho-pan-tomographic images. The test images are generated using Poisson statistics; the denoising utilizes a Monte Carlo noise modeling method. A hundred selected images are denoised and the compression ratio, using lossless and lossy JPEG 2000, is reported and evaluated.

1 Introduction

Trends in medical imaging are developing increasingly digital; meanwhile the amount of images captured per year is in the range of hundred petabytes[1] and still on the rise. The aim of image compression is to reduce the amount of data to be coded by removing redundant information. Therefore, relevant information of diagnostic demand is selected in the image and the coding process is reorganized so that, on the one hand relevant information is emphasized, and on the other hand noise and non-meaningful data are dropped. To achieve this, one can focus on the region of interest; filter out noise; and quantize information accordingly to adaptive perceptual thresholds to satisfy constraints given by Weber-Fechner's law [7]. The law defines just noticeable differences (JND) that are mediated by medical expertise to prevent relevant information loss.

---

[1] $1 peta = 1000 tera$.

R.R. Beichel and M. Sonka (Eds.): CVAMIA 2006, LNCS 4241, pp. 214–224, 2006.

1.1 Background

Compression have become a valuable technology by introducing the standards JPEG [14], Lossless JPEG (LJPEG)[14], and recently JPEG2000 [18] for widespread use. Special fields are Teleradiology, Telemammography and Telepathology, where the full diagnostic information is transferred digitally. Generally, a compression concept consists of a transform stage, a quantization stage and an entropy coder. Each of those stage can be tuned to satisfy the needs of the application at hand.

In general, two types of compression schemes - lossless and lossy - are known. The term lossless [6] means a reversible scheme that achieves modest compression rates by allowing exact reconstruction of the original image. Controversy, a lossy compression scheme is irreversible and cannot achieve exact reconstruction. Roughly speaking, a lossy scheme differs from a lossless in applying an additional quantization stage. This stage provides parameters to enable a balance between compression rate and induced artifacts.

To achieve visually lossless compression [13], a contrast sensitivity function (CSF), which is the visual ability to see objects that may not be outlined clearly or that do not stand out from their background, can be made adaptive to the human visual system (HVS) [10,2] to regulate the quantization step-size and therefore to minimize the visibility of artifacts. Therefore, image quality can be classified into five general categories:

1. Original data, as a "gold standard".
2. Data lossless compressed, as a "silver standard"; finite numerical precision causes small errors that are detectable mathematically.
3. Visually lossless, thus an observer cannot detect compression noise nor artifacts.
4. Diagnostically lossless, the artifacts are detectable but do not impact accuracy.
5. Artifacts put an substantially impact onto the diagnostic image content. The image gets useless from point of view of the medics'.

In current clinical practice lossy schemes are not often being used, because of legal questions and regularity policies. New clinical testing can develop reasonable policies and acceptable standards for the use of lossy schemes. The performance of human observers can have additional impact on the assessment quality. The ideal observer approach (IOA) can be used for benchmarking, and represents a Bayesian method to perform detection tasks. Investigations show human performance limited by suboptimal sampling efficiency and by additive internal noise [16].

Many compression techniques have been developed since the formalization of data compression by Shannon. Clunie [6] tested seventeen lossless schemes with over three-thousand different images from multiple anatomical regions and came to the conclusion that newer lossless compression techniques perform better than older, and predictive schemes with statistical modeling and with transform based coding perform better than dictionary based coding. Belbachir et al. [3] proposed a hybrid compression scheme by extending the wavelet transform (JPEG2000), adopting anisotropy and smooth boundaries, in applying the Contourlet transform, for the processing of the fine detail coefficients scales. This scheme shows less artifacts in the image and achieves better compression rate at high resolution (i.e. larger $\geq 1024^2$) medical images. Al-Shaykh [1] et al. studied the effect of noise on image compression using the JPEG lossy image processing standard, where it was found that at higher compression rates the coders filtered out most of the noise, but also degraded the image quality measured by peak signal to noise ratio (PSNR). Slone et al. [17] assessed twenty posteroanterior chest radiographs by five observers and concluded on one hand that lossless compression provides an inadequate reduction of the data amount, and on the other hand lossy compression artifacts may be detectable, but their presence does not affect diagnostic performance. A recently published work [15] assessed JPEG competing with JPEG2000 schemes and came to the conclusion that JPEG could perform better than JPEG2000 for low compression rates. Herein, an open question arises in how one may compare the results from different investigations, concerning perceived image quality.

Subjective quality ratings, utilizing usual mean opinion scale (MOS) statistics, built from averaging observations, done by medical experts considering compression artifacts, can prove lossy compression to be usable. Although, objective quality ratings, calculated by classical metrics, like the Peak Signal Noise Ratio (PSNR) or the Root Mean Square Error (RMSE) that can exactly determine any loss of signal, are not sufficient to predict differences between images as perceived by a human observer. Several CSFs [11] that are determined by a measure of the limit of visibility for low contrast patterns, were proposed (e.g. Campbell & Robson, Movshon, Barten, Daly, etc.).

Wang et al. [19] described the decomposition of the distortion between two images into a linear combination of components by the structural similarity index measure (SSIM), which separates out non-structural luminance and contrast distortions that are less important to the degradation impression of diagnostic information. Measures stemming from spatial autocorrelation[2], which consider the neighborhood relations between pixels, can cope better with the classification of artifacts, without affecting the diagnostic content [5].

However, in particular – questions are – how much has noise influence on the compression performance – is it possible to increase compression efficiency by the application of an accurate denoising method?

1.2   The Contribution of This Work

This work improves the compression performance by embedding a denoising process in the JPEG2000 compression scheme. The assessment for the investigation of compression efficiency of the JPEG2000 algorithm is performed on noisy simulated and real dental ortho-pan-tomographic (OPT) images. The influence of the noise on the compression efficiency as a function of the signal dynamics is simulated, rather than shown by other assessments, where the noise consists of a fraction of the signal by means of a back-projection method. The approach can be exploited to every field of application, which utilizes an appropriate noise model. The quality of the images are compared by means of a MSSIM algorithm proposed by Wang et al. [19] and the usual PSNR. Although the results are validated on radiographic medical images, this work can be extended to other medical images like mammograms, where compression is also of interest, and the dedicated noise model has to be deduced in the same way as it was performed for x-ray images.

---

[2] i.e. Moran I statistics.

The paper is organized as follows: in Section 2, the compression scheme JPEG2000; and OPT image reconstruction is revised as prerequisites. Section 3 focuses on the assessment of compression efficiency. In section 4, the conclusions and thoughts on prospective further work are given, and section 5 lists the bibliography references.

2   Preliminary Notions

Within medical diagnostics alongside medical expertise intuitive decisions are often made solely, based on experience. Therefore, appropriate reconstruction methods have to be able to detect small, low contrast image details, frequently situated side by side, often hardly differing in gray-level-means, while maybe just exhibiting a slightly distinct variance. Herein an affinity to image compression is given, where similar objectives are considered. With this in mind this paper is motivated.

2.1   Ortho-pantomographic Radiography

This is a technique where the entire dentition is projected onto a sensing device by means of the photons of a poly-energetic x-ray beam. The x-ray source and the detector are in opposition, rotating around the patients head, where the focus zone of the x-ray beam describes a planar curve, which is standardized for the human teeth and jaw.

2.2   JPEG2000

JPEG 2000 [18] may produce a lossless compressed image, which means, no data will be lost during compression and the entire data set can be recreated. Since 2001, JPEG2000 support is added to the standard of Digital Imaging and Communications in Medicine (DICOM).

Lossless compression ratios of 2:1 to 5:1 are possible. Visually lossless compression ratios can go much higher, theoretically to over 100:1, depending on the image characteristics. JPEG2000 supports more than the 3 bands, like JPEG and other compression schema accept, and so it can easily handle hyper-spectral and multi-spectral imagery. Hyper-spectral imaging is the simultaneous acquisition of images in many narrow, contiguous, spectral bands. For example, most satellites today measure energy at many wavelengths, thus this is called multi spectral imaging.

Regions of Interest (ROI) allow greater image quality in the foreground, while other parts of a huge image may receive aggressive compression. That means, features of interest are maintained at source level of detail, and the rest of the image is only provided for contextual purpose. JPEG2000 specifies a 9/7 wavelet for ordinary lossy compression, and a 5/3 wavelet for lossless compression. The 8x8 blocking artifacts of JPEG compression are prevented by the allowance of pixel blocks of much higher size.

3   The Methodology: OPT Image Reconstruction Revisited

Goebel et. al. have recently shown in [9] that the noise statistics of dental OPT images follow a mixture of two generalized Gamma distributions, rather than pure Poisson distributions, where one of them stems from photon attenuation scatter (i.e. the absorbed photons) and the other from the photon scatter-glare (i.e. photons whose traveling paths have changed, and have not been absorbed), which is accountable to the noise contribution. An image model

$$x = As \tag{1}$$

was presented by adopting an idea stemming from blind source separation (BSS) [4][3], with x the observation vector, A the mixing matrix, and s the hidden original signal source vector. Utilizing an inverse BSS model, one may find a matrix

$$B = A^{-1} \tag{2}$$

which reformulates to

$$\hat{s} = Bx \tag{3}$$

that yields the solution

$$\hat{s} = i - \widehat{\kappa}(s) \tag{4}$$

with i the image, and the noise estimate

$$\widehat{\kappa}(s) = \widetilde{N} \tag{5}$$

The noise estimate $\widetilde{N}$ is generated by an empirical Bayesian backward scatter projection method. The noise is then modeled by an finite realization of an infinite field of locally Gaussians with mean zero and variance one $N(0,1)$, scaled by an spatially varying noise coherence factor ξ, yielding

$$\widetilde{N} = \xi_{[x,y,\sigma(x,y)^2]} N(0,1) \tag{6}$$

Thus, although the variance of the noise in radiography follows per definition the image value by some function, one can treat an acquired image i as an additive mixture from the diagnostic source image s contaminated by an independent noise function n. For example, if one is assuming a Poisson process the noise model can be written as:

$$i = s + \kappa(s) \tag{7}$$

where i is the observed image, s is the "source" signal without noise, and the noise function is proportional to:

$$\kappa(s) \propto \sqrt{s} \tag{8}$$

In particular, in the utilized denoising approach, the noise function is modeled by the Generalized Nakagami-m (GND) [12] distribution

$$f(x|m, \Omega, \lambda) = \frac{2\lambda}{\Gamma(m)} \left[\frac{m}{\Omega}\right]^m x^{(2m\lambda-1)} e^{-\frac{m}{\Omega}x^{2\lambda}} \tag{9}$$

In Equ. 9, λ is the shape adjustment parameter, which controls the heaviness of the distribution tail. For $\lambda < 1$ there are heavy tails, which vanish for $\lambda > 1$ to a tight

---

[3] BSS in general is the separation of a set of n statistically independent signals $s = [s_1 \ldots s_n]$ from a set of m observed signals $x = [x_1 \ldots x_m]$, tied together by a mixing matrix A, leading to $x = As$.

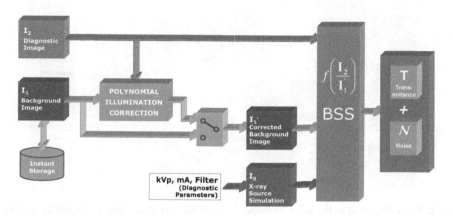

Fig. 1. The acquisition part of the approach, which is using three images, the diagnostic image I_2, a background image I_1, and a Monte Carlo simulation of the x-ray source image I_0. Nonlinearities from the x-ray source can be compensated by polynomial illumination correction. The background image I_1 may be stored for instant use.

density function. For $m = \lambda = 1$ the GND becomes the Rayleigh density function; for $m = 1, \lambda \neq 0$ the function becomes the Weilbull density function; and for $m = 1$ and $\lambda = \frac{1}{2}$ it becomes a simple exponential density function.

The result of the noise estimation approach was used by Goebel et. al. in [8] for OPT image restoration. Fig. 1 shows the acquisition part of the approach. This concept makes possible neglecting the inherent dependence of the noise variance on the diagnostic image values. The OPT projection process is supported by a GND for the forward projection modeling of the photon scatter distribution, which is simulated by a Monte Carlo method. A backprojection yields a solution for the photon scatter-glare distribution, which is causing the noise contribution. Stressing Plancherel's Theorem, the energy of the noise estimate is then subtracted from the noisy transmittance[4] image in the wavelet domain (see Fig. 2). The reconstructed estimate of the transmittance $\widetilde{T}$ getting reduced noise by preserving diagnostic details. The approach was tested against classical wavelet hard- and soft-thresholding methods. It was shown that it performed substantially better than the former in terms of modulation transfer function (MTF) and signal to noise ratio (SNR). Within this paper, the denoising of the real radiographic images is supported by the model.

Since early stages of the HVS are optimally "tuned" to sine-wave gratings, synthetic test patterns are often used in tests of acuity. Therefore, the assessment deploys sine-wave gratings as test images with smooth increasing frequencies from 0.10 lines per mm (lpmm) to the upper bound frequencies of 0.5, 1 and 2.5 lpmm. In image processing the lpmm is an useful unit for images, but not for humans. Spatial frequency in visual psychophysics is measured in cycles/deg visual angle (c/deg). If an observer views the image at 57 cm, then 10 mm=1deg, and therefore 1mm=0.1 deg; the spatial frequencies would be: 1cd/deg (0.1lpmm), 5cd/deg (0.5lpmm) and 25cd/deg (2.5lpmm) [16]. This

---

[4] The transmittance is calculated by the fraction $T = I_2/I_1$, as shown in Fig. 2.

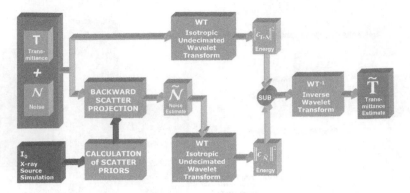

Fig. 2. The subtraction of the noise estimate $\widetilde{N}$ from the diagnostic image mixture by utilizing the conservation of energy within the wavelet space. The model exploits an empirical Bayesian approach for the auto-calculation of the backward scatter projection. The transform used is the isotropic undecimated a-trous wavelet transform.

range indeed is the optimal range for vision, and therefore it is used for the investigations in this paper.

Fig. 3 shows one of the set of test patterns that are duplicated and perturbed by Poisson noise $\widetilde{N}$ to test the behavior of common noise simulation methods.

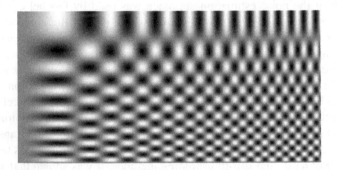

Fig. 3. A synthetic test pattern deployed by sine-wave gratings, which are optimally tuned to the HVS. The test images are perturbed by Poisson noise for the assessment.

4 Experimental Results and Evaluation

One-hundred test images per set, with logarithmic amplitude stepping from set to set were generated to study the influence of changing dynamic range, resolution and scatter noise onto the compression factors. Thus, six sets of test images were generated: – an original set – an original set with Poisson noise added – and then – a copy of both sets compressed by lossless compression – and again – another copy of both sets compressed by lossy compression (Q=40).

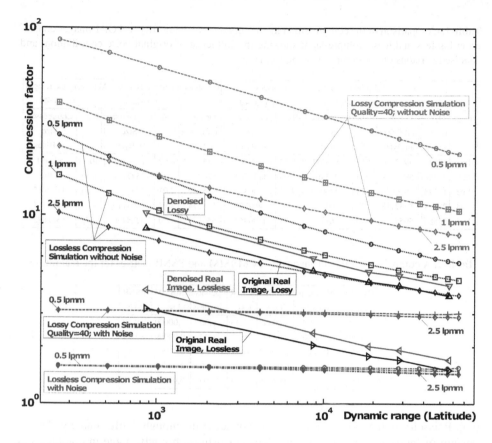

Fig. 4. The dependency of the compression factor on the dynamic range for smooth noisy images. There are four groups, each showing the three lines-per-millimeter frequencies 0.5, 1 and 2.5 lpmm, for lossless, lossy, lossless with noise and lossy with noise images. Additionally, results from the original real radiologic images of Table 1 are shown; performing closely to the noiseless simulation.

Fig. 4 shows the simulation results of the dependency of the compression factor on the dynamic range for the smooth, noisy images. There are four groups, each showing the three lines-per-millimeter frequencies 0.5, 1 and 2.5 lpmm, for lossless, lossy, lossless with noise and lossy with noise. Additionally, results stemming from a set of original real radiologic images, listed in Table 1, are shown. The results are plotted for five real image examples, with different dynamic ranges 1:N.

In the noise free cases, the graphs from the simulation results show a nearly linear behavior between logarithmic dynamic range and logarithmic compression factors. The lines-per-mm frequency produces a practically parallel shift of the curves. The noise added cases behave nearly constant, regardless of the dynamic value. Compared this to the graphs of the real diagnostic images, there is a different behavior – the real images compete like the simulation images, without noise, in both, the lossless and the lossy cases. Therefore, the usual method of just adding noise, bound by some function

Table 1. Comparison of the compression ratio results for five out of fifty real OPT images considering lossless and lossy compression; showing the influence of original noise contribution; and denoised versions on the compression performance

Image	Dyn. Range 1:N	Original TIFF Size in Bytes	Ratio	Compressed Size in Bytes	Ratio	Compressed Size in Bytes	Original TIFF Size in Bytes	Ratio	Compressed Size in Bytes	Ratio	Compressed Size in Bytes
		Compression of the Original Images					Compression of the Denoised Version of the Images				
			Lossless		Lossy Q=40			Lossless		Lossy Q=40	
Im1	859	5953770	3,19	1865511	8,53	697955	5554802	4,02	1381881	10,23	542991
Im2	8598	5956778	2,04	2913467	5,08	1171541	5541896	2,36	2347144	5,87	944041
Im3	18598	5956926	1,78	3346022	4,42	1346354	5551302	2,01	2759379	5,01	1109115
Im4	28598	5957118	1,70	3504326	4,34	1409780	5553742	1,92	2894115	4,77	1164495
Im5	56553	5958622	1,50	3968786	3,73	1596354	5551738	1,70	3264450	4,23	1311882

Table 2. A comparison of the image quality by MSSIM and PSNR metrics for the real images

Dyn. Range	Original MSSIM lossless	lossy	PSNR lossy	Denoised MSSIM lossless	lossy	PSNR lossy
859	1,00	1,00000	95,43	1,00	1,00000	101,01
8598	1,00	0,99997	79,12	1,00	0,99999	82,89
18598	1,00	0,99992	74,62	1,00	0,99996	77,57
28598	1,00	0,99982	71,11	1,00	0,99993	74,66
56553	1,00	0,99966	68,04	1,00	0,99981	69,94

(e.g. Poisson) on the image values, seems not accurate enough. Unfortunately, the denoising of the real diagnostic images does not bring a big advantage in compression performance alone. Table 2 compares the quality measures achieved. The denoised images perform better in both metrics', the PSNR and MSSIM. Therefore, utilizing the denoising method, one achieves higher compression together with better image quality. The higher the dynamic of the image, the more there is a limitation stemming from the quantization stage of the compression. Therefore, the dynamic range of the image should not be spread by extra contrast enhancement prior to compression.

5   Conclusion and Outlook

This paper studied the improvement potential of the JPEG 2000 codec performance for medical images while including a denoising process. The additional denoising improved image quality; and the compression performance for $\approx 13\%$. Although the improvement is found not very significant, the better image quality exhibits viewing with enhanced contrast. This is only true if the denoising is appropriately tuned to the type of images.

An improved compression, satisfying legal thoughts by aggressively using the ROI concept in JPEG2000 and a denoising step, seems to have potential for the compression of radiographic images. The scheme can use a noise estimate, exploited by a Monte

Carlo simulation for determination of an importance map– as shown in Fig. 5, proposed in [9] – that spatially defines the regions of interest for fidelity compression. The remainder of the image can be compressed more aggressively. In particular for dental use, the importance map can focus on the teeth and their surrounding neighborhoods that having fine detail, rather than other areas.

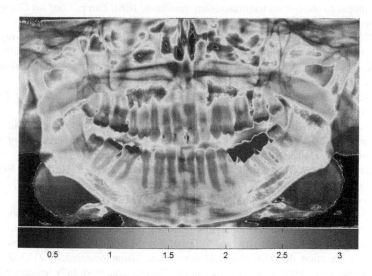

Fig. 5. The dedicated noise coherence factor $\xi(x, y, \sigma^2)$ image. In the areas of interest, the factors are below 1, which causes softer denoising.

A combination of a recently proposed hybrid compression scheme by exploiting the Contourlet- and Wavelet-transform [3], may reduce artifacts for the lossy portion of the image furthermore. As a perspective, this procedure will be validated for mammograms as compression is highly solicited and the dedicated noise model should be deduced. It is also intended, as a next investigation focus, to improve the JPEG2000 compression, utilizing the hybrid contourlet/wavelet transform [3] and Monte Carlo noise modeling [9].

References

1. K. O. Al-Shaykh and R. M. Mersereau. Lossy compression of noisy images. *IEEE Trans. on Image Proc.*, 7(12), 1998.
2. A. N. Belbachir and P. M. Goebel. Color image compression: Early vision and the multiresolution representations. *DAGM 2005, LNCS 3663 Springer.*, 3663:25–32, Sep. 2005.
3. A. N. Belbachir and P. M. Goebel. The contourlet transform for image compression. *PSIP'05 Physics in Signal and Image Proc.*, Jan. 2005.
4. J. F. Cardoso. Blind signal separation: statistical principles. *Proceedings of the IEEE*, 9(10):2009–2025, 1998.
5. T. J. Chen, K. S. Chuang, J. Wu, S. C. Chen, I. M. Hwang, and M. L. Jan. A novel image quality index using moran i statistics. *Physics in Medicine and Biology.*, 48:131–137, Apr. 2003.

6. D. A. Clunie. Lossless compression of grayscale medical images - effectiveness of traditional and state of the art approaches. *SPIE Med. Imaging*, Feb. 2000.
7. J. M. Degroot, E. L. Hall, R. N. Sutton, G. S. Lodwick, and S. J. Dwyer. Perception of computer simulated pulmonary lesions in chest radiographs. *Proceedings of the ACM Annual Conference*, pages 146–151, Aug. 1972.
8. P. M. Goebel, A. N. Belbachir, and M.Truppe. Background removal in dental panoramic x-ray images by the a-trous multiresolution transform. *IEEE Europ. Conf. on Circuit Theory and Design, ECCTD05*, Aug. 2005.
9. P. M. Goebel, A. N. Belbachir, and M. Truppe. Noise estimation in panoramic x-ray images: An appl. analysis approach. *IEEE Workshop on Stat. Signal Proc., SSP05*, July 2005.
10. X. Kai, Y. Jie, Z. Y. Min, and L. X. Liang. HVS-based medical image compression. *Europ. Journal of Radiology*, 55(1):139–145, July 2005.
11. M. J. Nadenau, J. Reichel, and M. Kunt. Wavelet-based color image compression: Exploiting the contrast sensivity function. *IEEE Trans. on Image Proc.*, 12(1), Jan. 2003.
12. M. Nakagami. The m-distribution, a general formula of intensity of rapid fading. *In W. G. Hoffman, editor, Statistical Methods in Radio Wave Propagation: Proceedings of a Symposium held at the University of California, Pergamon Press*, pages 3–36, 1960.
13. M. Rabbani and P. W. Jones. *Digital image compression techniques*. SPIE Press, Bellingham WA., 1991.
14. K. Sayood. *Introduction to Data Compression*. Morgan Kaufmann, 2000.
15. K. M. Siddiqui, J. P. Johnson, B. I. Reiner, and E. L. Siegel. Discrete cosine transform jpeg compression vs. 2d jpeg2000 compression. *Proc. of SPIE Medical Imaging*, Feb. 2005.
16. W. A. Simpson, H. K. Falkenberg, and V. Manahilov. Sampling efficiency and internal noise for motion detection, discrimination, and summation. *Vision Research*, 43:2125–2132, 2003.
17. R. M. Slone, D. H. Foos, B. R. Whiting, and al. Assessment of visually lossless irreversible image compression: Comparison of three methods by using an image-comparison workstation. *Radiology*, 215:543–553, 2000.
18. D. Taubman, E. Ordentlich, M. Weinberger, and G.Seroussi. Embedded block coding in JPEG 2000. *Signal Proc. Image Comm.*, 17(1):49–72, Jan. 2002.
19. Z.Wang and E. P. Simoncelli. An adaptive linear system framework for image distortion analysis. *IEEE Int. Conf. on Image Proc.*, Sep. 2005.

Fast Segmentation of the Mitral Valve Leaflet in Echocardiography

Sébastien Martin[1], Vincent Daanen[1],
Olivier Chavanon[1,2], and Jocelyne Troccaz[1]

[1] TIMC Lab, CAMI Team,
Institut d'Ingénierie d'Information de Santé (IN3S)
Faculté de Médecine - 38706 La Tronche cedex - France
{Sebastien.Martin, Vincent.Daanen, Jocelyne.Troccaz}@imag.fr
http://www-timc.imag.fr/gmcao/index.html
[2] Grenoble University Hospital, Cardiac Surgery Department,
38043 Grenoble - France
OChavanon@chu-grenoble.fr

Abstract. This paper presents a semi-automatic method for tracking the mitral valve leaflet in transesophageal echocardiography. The algorithm requires a manual initialization and then segments an image sequence. The use of two constrained active contours and curve fitting techniques results in a fast segmentation algorithm. The active contours successfully track the inner cardiac muscle and the mitral valve leaflet axis. Three sequences have been processed and the generated muscle outline and leaflet axis have been visually assessed by an expert. This work is a part of a more general project which aims at providing real-time detection of the mitral valve leaflet in transesophageal echocardiography images.

Keywords: Medical Image Analysis, Tracking and Motion, Active Contours, Ultrasound Imaging.

1 Introduction

The mitral valve is one of the four valves of the heart; its function is to keep the blood flow in the physiological direction when the heart contracts. Due to various pathological factors, a mitral regurgitation can occur. The work presented in this paper belongs to a more general project of robot assisted surgery which aims at repairing a pathological mitral valve in a context of microinvasive beating heart surgery. The control of the robot is performed under ultrasound imaging guidance and required robust and real time algorithms to segment the valve. This project called GABIE is supported by the CNRS program ROBEA, and involves 4 laboratories (LIRMM, TIMC, LRP and CEA) and 2 University Hospitals (APH Paris and University Hospital of Grenoble).

Although transesophageal echocardiography is the classical imaging technique for mitral valve surgery, there is no satisfactory method allowing an automated segmentation of the valve.

R.R. Beichel and M. Sonka (Eds.): CVAMIA 2006, LNCS 4241, pp. 225–235, 2006.

The tracking of the myocardial border of the left ventricle (LV) is a very active research area that makes intensive use of deformable models, ([1],[2]), Markov random fields [3] or optical flow methods ([4],[5]). Data processed are either in 2D+T or 3D+T ([6], [7], [8], [9] [10]). [11] propose to use information fusion to track the LV in echocardiography in real-time. His algorithm requires a statistical shapes analysis of the LV, obtained by principal component analysis (PCA) on a large number of LV shape. We think, these methods will not work for the segmentation of the mitral valve leaflet, because of the high inter-patient variability. Mikic [12] uses active contours to segment either the left ventricle or the mitral valve leaflet. The method requires a manual segmentation on a image of the sequence at the beginning of the procedure and estimation of the optical flow field along the sequence. It takes about 20 minutes to process one complete cardiac cycle (i.e ≃ 25 to 30 images). [13] processes an image sequence using wavelet packet decomposition (in 2D + T) and then selects the sub-bands (in the wavelet domain) which preserve most of the energy of the target structure with an acceptable *Signal to Noise Ratio*. These sub-bands are then recombined to create the feature footprint ; this footprint is then used to analyze an image sequence. Although this method seems to process an image sequence fast, the analyzed sequences must not differ markedly from the data used to construct the filters.

In this paper, we present a semi-automatic method (a manual initialization is required) to segment the axis of mitral valve leaflet in transesophageal ultrasound images. The proposed approach uses 2 active contours. The method is designed to be fast and to achieve the segmentation in near real-time.

This work is intended to be the pre-operative step of the surgery scenario and should provide semi-automatic segmentation of several mitral cycles. In an intra-operative second step which is actually under development, the set of segmentation obtained during the pre-operative step will be used to detect the valve in real time. Therefore only near real time capability are required for the pre-operative algorithm, in order to make it usable in a surgical context and to achieve the repeatability condition of the mitral valve motion needed by the intra-operative step (more details are provide in conclusion).

2   Material and Method

2.1   Context

The mitral valve is a left-sided valve located between the left atrium and the left ventricle, made up of two fibrous membranes which are attached to the left ventricle muscle through the mitral annulus. On the free edges of the two leaflets, there are multiple strong cords (like parachute cords), in turn attached to papillary muscles (reinforcement of the left ventricle wall). When the heart contracts, the two leaves billow up to close off the opening between the left atrium and the left ventricle. The closure mechanism is mainly passive according to the pressure gradient between each side of the leaflet. During the contraction of the left ventricle there is also a geometrical modification of the shape of the annulus. Although the cardiac muscle motion resulting of the heart contraction is non rigid, it appear close to a rigid motion in one dimensional echocardiography images. Therefore two major kinds of movements can be shown in these images:

- the leaflet movement (main component) which is non rigid but relatively close to a rotation around a point based on the muscle-leaflet junction area called junction point,
- the muscle movement which is approximately rigid with essentially translational components and small rotational components;

These movements can be used as an a priori knowledge in order to facilitate the semi-automatic segmentation of the mitral valve in echocardiography.

2.2   Method

The proposed method relies on the use of two active contours (Figure 1) to track the leaflet efficiently : one tracks the cardiac muscle and the other tracks the mitral valve leaflet. The tracking method can be chronologically divided in 2 times:

1. the segmentation of the cardiac muscle,
2. the segmentation of the mitral valve leaflet

  Each segmentation is realized in two steps :

1. rough segmentation using a curve fitting algorithm.
2. refinement using active contours.

This method allow us to solve two reluctant problems of the mitral valve tracking:

- the ability to track very fast motions.
- the ability to separate the valve snake of the muscle during the opening valve phase.

The curve fitting algorithm providing rough segmentations, use measurements along curves normals. Therefore some 1D image processing techniques are required to detect feature points on curves normals.

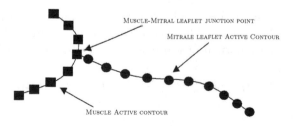

Fig. 1. The two contours

This paper is organized as follows: section 3 describes the method used to build a rough segmentation of both mitral valve and cardiac muscle. Section 4 presents the proposed method to refine rough segmentation using snakes. Figure 2 presents the pipeline of our method, and sets up briefly the connection between different section of the paper.

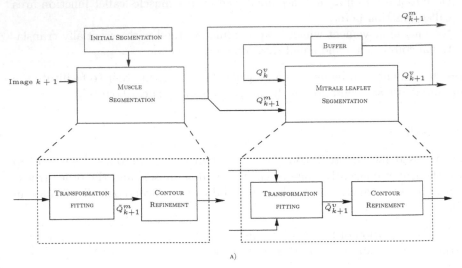

Fig. 2. Synoptics of the proposed method

3   Rough Segmentation

In this section, we explain how a rough segmentation of the cardiac muscle (resp. mitral valve leaflet) in the kth image is computed using the final segmentation of the $(k-1)^{th}$ image.

3.1   Curve Fitting Algorithm

The problem is to estimate the parameters of a transformation which minimizes the distance between two curves. Making the assumption that curves are defined by points stored in vectors: $Q = [x(s), y(s)]$, then the relation between two curves can be written as follows:

$$Q_f = WX + Q_i \tag{1}$$

where Q_f is the target curve and Q_i is the initial one. W is the transformation matrix and X the vector of the transformation parameters. The distance used is the sum of square normal measurements that can be approximated by:

$$\| Q_f - Q_i \|_n^2 = \frac{1}{N} \sum_{k=1}^{N} [(Q_f(k) - Q_i(k)).\boldsymbol{n}(k)]^2 \tag{2}$$

$$\approx \sum_{k=1}^{N} m(k)^2 \tag{3}$$

where $\| \cdot \|_n$ denotes the norm based on normal measurements, $n(k)$ is the normal vector to the curve at the abscissa k, $m(k)$ is the normal measurement computed from 2D operator on normal profiles. Robustness to noise can be obtained by using a regularization term so that the problem can be expressed as:

$$\hat{X} = \arg\min_{X}(\alpha \parallel X - \overline{X} \parallel^2 + \parallel Q_f - Q_i \parallel_n^2) \tag{4}$$

Solving Eq 4 in the least-squares sense is equivalent to a classical curve fitting problem. Blake has proposed a recursive algorithm to solve this problem in [14].

3.2 Rough Segmentation of the Muscle

As explained in section 2 the cardiac muscle motion appears close to a rigid motion in one dimensional images. Therefore, the rough contour position of the cardiac muscle is estimated from the initial template (manual segmentation on the first image) by translating it.

The rough contour for the image k is given by:

$$\tilde{Q}_k^m = W^m X_k^m + Q_0^m \tag{5}$$

where X_k^m is the transformation estimated (i.e. a translation) and

$$W_0^m = \begin{pmatrix} x_0^m & \mathbf{0} \\ \mathbf{0} & y_0^m \end{pmatrix} \tag{6}$$

with $\mathbf{0} = (0, 0, \ldots, 0, 0)^T$

The curve fitting algorithm requires feature detections on the curve normals. Therefore it is necessary to process the gray-level profiles corresponding to these directions in order to get the normal measurements.

A canny edge detector approximated by the derivative of the Gaussian kernel ($\sigma = 1.4$) is used for this purpose.

3.3 Mitral Valve Leaflet Transformation Estimation

In this section, the abscissa of the junction point on the muscle curve at time $k - 1$ is supposed to be given. It will be used as a rough estimate of the current abscissa of the junction point. Given that the leaflet motion is close to be a rotation around the junction point, this point must be invariant to the involved transformation. For this purpose, the previous segmentation of the leaflet (after refinement) is first translated on the junction point and then an affine transformation without translations components is used for fitting. All computation are made in a coordinate system centered on the junction point. In this way the junction point is a fixed point (invariant to the involved transformation). The computation of $\tilde{Q}_k^v$ is then given by:

$$\tilde{Q}_k^v = W_{k-1}^v . X_k^v + \underline{Q_{k-1}^v} \tag{7}$$

where:

$$W_{k-1}^v = \begin{pmatrix} x_{k-1}^v & 0 & 0 & y_{k-1}^v \\ 0 & y_{k-1}^v & x_{k-1}^v & 0 \end{pmatrix} \qquad (8)$$

and represents a 2D affine transformation matrix ; and Q_{k-1}^v represents the mitral valve leaflet contour of the $k-1^{th}$ image translated to the rough junction point of the kth image.

The presence of the mitral valve leaflet is characterized by a ridge in the image, that corresponds to a local maximum in the gray-level profiles along the normal directions. The second order derivative of a 1D Gaussian kernel is used to detect the valve on normal curves. In fact this operator is a good measurement of the contrast between two regions.

4   Refinements

4.1   Need for a Refinement

At the end of the previous step, the contours are in a neighborhood of feature structures. Thus we have to bring them closer to the cardiac muscle (resp mitral valve leaflet) ; This is done by using active contours.

Snakes has been originally introduced by Kass and al [15]. A snake contour is described parametrically by $v(s) = (x(s), y(s))$ where $x(s), y(s)$ are x, y coordinates along the contour (the so-called *snaxels*) and $s \in [0, 1]$ is the normalized parametrization. The snake model defines the energy of a contour $v(s)$, as:

$$E_{snake} = \int_{s=0}^{1} \lambda E_{Int}(s) + E_{Ext}(s) ds \qquad (9)$$

where E_{Int} is the internal energy of the contour, imposing continuity and curvature constraints, and where E_{Ext} is the image energy allowing the snake to move to the feature points in the image. λ is the regularization parameter governing the compromise between adherence to the internal forces and adherence to the external forces. An initial contour evolves by minimizing of the Equation 1.

4.2   Muscle Snake Energy Definition

The energy of the muscle snake is composed of two terms related to the internal energy and one term related to the external energy.

Internal Energies. The 1st term is related to the length of the curve. It penalizes curves where the distance between two successive snaxels is far to a distance d_m which is computed at the beginning of the algorithm. This energy keeps the length curve close to the initial one, and prevents the snake to segment the whole cardiac muscle. This 1st term is written:

$$E_{Int_1}^m(s_i) = \alpha_1^m(|s_{i-1} - si| - d_m)^2 \qquad (10)$$

where α_1^m is a weighting parameter.

The 2nd internal energy term approximates the 2nd order derivative of the curve. This term is computed from the 'cardiac muscle' control points s_i^m by using the finite differences:

$$E_{Int_2}^m(s_i) = \alpha_2^m \mid s(i-1) - 2s(i) + s(i+1) \mid \tag{11}$$

where α_2^m is a weighting parameter.

External Energy. The external energy term is related to the modulus of the gradient image. It allows the contour to move toward the cardiac muscle appearing as an edge in the image. This energy term is given below:

$$E_{Ext}^m(s_i) = - \parallel \Delta I(s_i) \parallel^2 \tag{12}$$

4.3 Mitral Snake Energy Definition

Because the movement of the mitral valve leaflet is a bit more complex than the movement of the cardiac muscle, we introduce different energy terms.

Internal Energies. The internal energy is composed of the same energy terms that for the muscle snake with weighting parameters α_1^v and α_2^v respectively for the length constraint and the curvature constraint.

External Energy. The image of the leaflet corresponds to a local maximum of intensity. Reasoning about the image intensity map as a surface in $\mathbf{R}^3$, features corresponds to areas where one of the principal curvatures is high (Figure 3). The image of the higher principal curvature allows us to build a robust external energy function:

$$E_{Ext}^v(s_i) = K^+(s_i) \tag{13}$$

where $K+$ is the higher principal curvature.

In the actual implementation, principal curvatures are computed from eigenvalues of the Hessian matrix of the image intensity map.

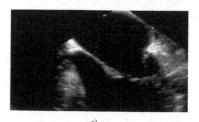 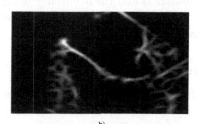

a)   b)

Fig. 3. a) Ultrasound image b) K^+ of the image

4.4   Dynamic Programming Minimization (DP)

The problem of energy snake minimization is solved using dynamic programming (DP). Amini has proposed this method [16] in order to overcome the limitations of classical variational methods like instability or non optimality and to allow the use of stronger constraints without falling into a local minimum. When an energy functional can be written as:

$$E_{snake} = \sum_{i=1}^{N-2} E_i(s_{i-1}, s_i, s_{i+1}) \tag{14}$$

the minimization can be obtained using Dynamic programming as described in [16].

The algorithm is iteratively applied to the contour. At each iteration, a snaxel can move in a previously defined neighborhood (search area). DP allows us to correctly minimize the energy function and provides a way to locate the junction point on the muscle curve. The search-area for each snaxel of the muscle snake is defined by a 8-neighborhood around the snaxel. We define the same search-area for all snaxels of the mitral snake, except for the one (junction point) which is connected to the muscle snake. For this one, the search area is defined by a region of 8 pixels around its previous estimate and on the muscle snake curve. We do not define an external energy term for this point. In this way, the junction point will be only driven by its internal energy according to the position of the two next snaxels and will be correctly adjusted to the muscle curve by continuity of the leaflet curve.

5   Results and Discussion

5.1   Algorithm Initialization

The algorithm is initialized by the manual segmentation of both the muscle and the mitral valve leaflet and by the specification of the junction point. The algorithm then computes d_m (resp d_v) the mean distance between two successive points of the muscle curve (resp of mitral curve). Manual segmentations influences the robustness and the accurency of segmentations. We have observed that segmenting a large part of the cardiac muscle during the initialization improve the robustness of the algorithm.

5.2   Results

The described method has been implemented using Matlab© (and in Matlab language). Dynamic programming algorithms has been coded in C using mex. Snakes requires the tuning of some parameters : (α_1^m, α_2^m) for the *muscle snake* and (α_1^v, α_2^v) for the *mitral snake*.

The processing time of our algorithm depends on the number of snaxels used. In a general rule to obtain accurate segmentations, the mean processing time is less 0.5 s and the number of iteration for the DP algorithm less than 10.

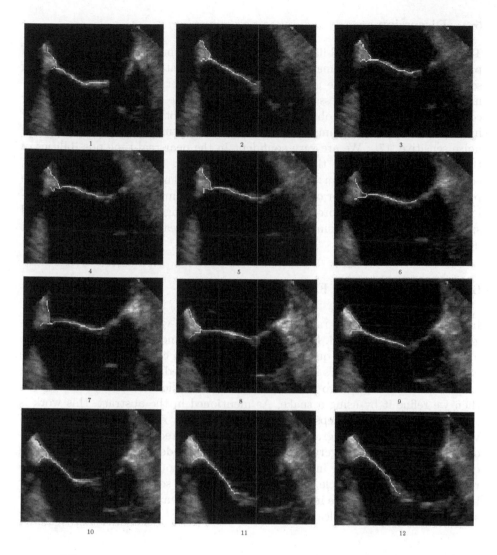

Fig. 4. Processing of a sequence. Segmentation of the biggest leaflet.

The validation of the method is based on the visual assessment of an expert. We have processed 4 sequences of 250 to 300 images. For each one, the medical expert is asked to segment the cardiac muscle, the mitral valve leaflet and to point the junction point. The sequence is then processed with the proposed method. The medical expert is then asked to give his opinion about the segmentation proposed by the method. Most of the time (about 90% of the images), the expert is very confident in the segmentation provided by the method. In the remaining 10%, although the segmentation is "bad" (and not absolutely false !), the snake re-converges to a good contour in the next 3-to-6 images.

5.3 Discussion

The proposed method still has some drawbacks. The main one is the tunning of parameters. However the main objective of our algorithm is to provide a set of segmentations that will be used during the intra-operative step where no tunning of parameters is necessary. So, we could imagine trying several parameter configurations in order to obtain a good tunning. Another point which could be improved is the way we compute the principal curvatures which is known to be noise sensitive [17] ; We are very confident in the near real-time possibilities of this algorithm needed for the surgical scenario (sec. 1). From our experience, converting algorithms from Matlab language to 'C' language should divide the processing time by a factor of 10. Other 'coding' optimizations such the dynamical selection of a ROI to process (instead of processing the whole image) should speed up the image processing and thus allow a near real-time mitral valve leaflet detection.

6   Conclusion and Future Work

In this paper, a method to rapidly segment the mitral valve leaflet in echocardiography has been presented. Due to the fact that the motion of the valve and the motion of the muscle are quite different, we use two contours to capture these motions. For each contours segmentations are realized in two step: first we use a curve fitting technique to provide rough segmentation of the tracked contour then we refine it by using a snake. As mentioned in the abstract, this work is the first step of a two-steps procedures which aims at segmenting the mitral valve leaflet in echocardiagraphic images. The presented method will be the pre-operative step of the surgery scenario and will provide segmentation of several cardiac cycles. During the intra-operative step, we should be able to segment in real time the cardiac muscle and the mitral leaflet by searching the more similar image in the pre-operative images and then applying a refinement to accurately segment the mitral valve leaflet.

References

1. Cootes, T., Taylor, C.: Active shape models - smart snakes. Proceedings of the British Machine Vision Conference" (1992) 266–275
2. Chalana, V., Linker, D.T., Haynor, D.R., Kim, Y.: A multiple active contour model for cardiac boundary detection on echocardiographic sequences. IEEE Trans. Med. Imag 15 (1996) 290–298
3. Mignotte, M., Meunier, J., Tardif, J.C.: Endocardial boundary estimation and tracking in echocardiographic images using deformable templates and markov random fields. Pattern Analysis and Applications 4 (2001) 256–271
4. Mailloux, G.E., Langlois, F., Simard, P.Y., Bertrand, M.: Restoration of the velocity field of the heart from two-dimensional echocardiograms. IEEE Trans. Med. Imag 8 (1989) 143–153

5. Adam, D., Hareuveni, O., Sideman, S.: Semiautomated border tracking of cine echocardiographic ventricular images field of the heart from two-dimensional echocardiograms. IEEE Trans. Med. Imag **6** (1987) 266–271
6. Jacob, G., Noble, J., Behrenbruch, C., Kelion, A., Banning, A.: A shape-space-based approach to tracking myocardial borders and quantifying regional left-ventricular function applied in echocardiography. IEEE Trans. Med. Imag **21** (2002) 226–238
7. andY. Chen, A.A., Elayyadi, M., Radeva, P.: Tag surface reconstruction and tracking of myocardial beads from spamm-mri with parametric b-spline surfaces. IEEE Trans. Med. Imag **20** (2001) 94–103
8. Lorenzo-Valds, M., Sanchez-Ortiz, G.I., Mohiaddin, R.H., Rueckert, D.: Atlas-based segmentation of 4d cardiac mr sequences using nonrigid registration. (2002)
9. Mitchell, S., Lelieveldt, B.P., van der Geest, R., Bosch, H.G., Reiber, J.H., Sonka, M.: Time-Continuous Segmentation of Cardiac MR Image Sequences Using Active Appearance Motion Models. Volume 4322 of SPIE Medical Imaging., Tokyo, Japan (2001) 249–256
10. Montillo, ., Metaxas, D., Axel, L.: Automated Segmentation of the Left and Right Ventricles in 4D Cardiac Spamm Images. Medical, Image Computing and Computer Assisted Intervention (MICCAI), Tokyo, Japan (2002) 620–633
11. Comaniciu, D., Zhou, X., andY. Chen, S.A., Elayyadi, M., Radeva, P.: Robust Real-Time Myocardial Border Tracking for Echocardiography : An Information Fusion Approach. IEEE Trans. Med. Imag **20** (2001) 94–103
12. Mikic, I., Krucinski, S., Thomas, J.D.: Segmentation and tracking in echocardiographic sequences: active contours guided by optical flow estimates. IEEE Trans. Med. Imag. **17** (1998) 274 – 284
13. Jansen, C., Arigovindan, M., Sühling, M., Marsch, S., Unser, M., P., H.: Multidimensional, multistage wavelet footprints: A new tool for image segmentation and feature extraction in medical ultrasound. In Sonka, M., Fitzpatrick, J., eds.: Progress in Biomedical Optics and Imaging, vol. 4, no. 23. Volume 5032 of Proceedings of the SPIE International Symposium on Medical Imaging: Image Processing (MI'03)., San Diego CA, USA (2003) 762–767 Part II.
14. A, B., M, I.: Active Contour. Springer-Verlag, Berlin Heidelberg New York (1998)
15. Kass, M., Witkin, A., Terzopoulos, D.: Snakes : Active contour models. International Journal of Computer Vision **1** (1988) 321331
16. Amini, A.A., Weymouth, T.E., Jain, R.C.: Using dynamic programming for solving variational problems in vision. IEEE Trans. Pattern Anal. Mach. Intell. **12** (1990) 855–867
17. Lachaud, J.O., Taton, B.: Deformable model with a complexity independent from image resolution. Computer Vision and Image Understanding (2005) Accepted. To appear.

Three Dimensional Tissue Classifications in MR Brain Images

Runa Parveen[1], Cliff Ruff[2], and Andrew Todd-Pokropek[1]

[1] Department of Medical Physics and Bioengineering, University College London, London
WC1E 6BT, United Kingdom
{runa, atoddpok}@medphys.ucl.ac.uk
[2] Department of Medical Physics, University College London Hospitals, London
NW1 2PQ, United Kingdom
cfr@medphys.ucl.ac.uk

Abstract. This paper presents an algorithm for classifying different tissue types in T1-weighted MR brain images using fuzzy segmentation. The main aim in this study is to compensate for the blurring effect on tissue boundaries due to partial volume effects. This paper is organized as follows: first, an adaptive greedy contour model has been developed to separate the intracranial volume (ICV) from the scalp and skull. Second, in order to deal with the problem of the partial volume effect, an algorithm for fuzzy segmentation is presented which has integrated fuzzy spatial affinity with statistical distributions of image intensities for each of the three tissues – cerebrospinal fluid, white matter and grey matter. This algorithm is tested on well-established simulated MR brain volumes to generate an extensive quantitative comparison with different noise levels and different slice thicknesses ranging from 1mm to 5mm. Finally, the results of this algorithm on clinical MR brain images are demonstrated.

1 Introduction

The advantages of magnetic resonance imaging (MRI) over other diagnostic imaging modalities are its good tissue contrast and its non-invasive nature. Accurate classification of MR images according to tissue type, white matter (WM), grey matter (GM) and cerebrospinal fluid (CSF) at the voxel level is important in many neuroimaging applications: multimodality image correlation, visualization, and quantification, and their clinical uses such as in tumour and lesion detection. Changes in the composition of tissues in the whole volume or within specific regions can be used to characterize physiological processes as well as pathological states [1]. In addition, the total brain volume has been shown to be correlated to various measures of disease severity, a reduction in grey matter volume may be particularly relevant in schizophrenia and Alzheimer's disease. Many automated or semi-automated approaches for tissue segmentation in single echo MR brain images or multi-spectral MR data have been reported [2].

Approaches to segmentation may be classified into different categories: edge-based detection, which represents the boundaries of objects where signal changes occur, while region-based methods [3] grow connected regions, which are homogenous

R.R. Beichel and M. Sonka (Eds.): CVAMIA 2006, LNCS 4241, pp. 236–247, 2006.
© Springer-Verlag Berlin Heidelberg 2006

according to some measure of gray level or texture. Automatic thresholding and morphological operations have also been used in many segmentation techniques. Each of these groups may be further divided into subgroups: hard and fuzzy – depending on whether the defined voxels are described with a binary value of 1 or 0 (known as hard) or the amount of tissue belonging to the given tissue class of the voxel (known as fuzzy) [2]. The soft tissue contrast enables complex and subtle brain structures to be clearly visualized. However, a unique correspondence of grey level ranges to different tissue types does not exist. The limited spatial resolution of MR imaging and the complex shape of the tissue interfaces in the brain imply that a large portion of voxels are affected by partial volume (PV) voxels [4], i.e., voxels that contain a mixture of two or more tissue types, and not a single tissue. Leemput et al [5] have applied a statistical framework to the problem of partial volume effects. In this study, we present a three-dimensional brain tissue segmentation which modifies the methodology of Udupa et al [6] to take into account the statistical distributions of the image intensities of each tissue element integrated with their fuzzy spatial affinities.

2 Materials and Methods

2.1 Digital Head Phantom and Simulated Data

Realistic, high resolution, digital, volumetric phantoms of the human brain were created using an MRI simulator [7]. The volumes contain $181 \times 217 \times 181$ voxels and cover the brain completely. The brainweb MRI simulator allow users to independently control a wide range of conditions, e.g., different levels of noise, image resolution including various MR acquisition parameters. This data consists of a partitioning of the head volume into 10 fuzzy tissue membership volumes (GM, WM, CSF, skull, fat, muscle/skin, skin, connective tissue, glial matter, and other), all of which are downloadable from http://www.bic.mni.mcgill.ca/brainweb. The voxel values in these fuzzy volumes reflect the proportion of tissue present in that voxel in the range [0, 1]. Note that the glial matter that occurs subcortically around the ventricles is not separable from the GM, therefore, in this calculation, glial matter tissue volumes are taken into account in GM volume estimation. The following parameters have been selected from this site: T1-weighted MR volume data with slice thicknesses of 1mm, 3mm and 5mm and different noise levels ranging from 0% to 7%.

2.2 Clinical MRI Data

Ten coronal (6 males and 4 females) MR scans acquired at the Centre for Morphometric Analysis (CMA), Massachusetts General Hospital (MGH) using a three-dimensional T1-weighted spoiled gradient echo MRI 3D-CAPRY sequence on an 1.5T General Electric Signa MR system with the following parameters: TR = 50msec, TE = 9msec, flip angle = 50°, field of view = 24 cm, slice thickness = contiguous 3.0 mm, matrix = 256×256, number of averages = 1 and number of slices between 60 – 65.

Ten MR (4 males and 6 females) head scans acquired on a 1.5T Siemens Magnetom MR system (Iselin, NJ) with the following parameters: TE = 40 msec, TE = 8 msec, flip angle = 50°, field of view = 30 cm, slice thickness = contiguous 3.1 mm, matrix = 256×256, number of averages = 1 and number of slices between 60 – 65.

These data sets and their manual segmentations were provided by the CMA, MGH and are available at http://neuro-www.mgh.harvard.edu/cma/ibsr. Results from all 20 data sets from MGH are presented in this paper. In addition, three sets of T1-weighted brain MR data are also tested in this study obtained from UCL volunteers.

2.3 Methods

In this study, a deformable contour model was developed to separate the intracranial volume (ICV) from the scalp and skull. The main aim of developing this deformable contour model was to facilitate the delineation of anatomical structures whilst reducing operator time and measurement variability. Next, a modified version of Udupa's algorithm was developed for the segmentation and analysis of brain structures in MR images. We validated each stage of our approach using real and simulated MRI data.

2.4 Deformable Contour Model

Active Contour Models (ACM) [8] provide a promising framework for boundary detection through the solution of energy minimization using variational calculus. The energy function is an integral sum of different weighted energy constraints. Williams et al [9] modified the ACM with the greedy algorithm to make it more stable and flexible. The original contour model was attracted to contours with large image gradients and in the greedy algorithm, the location that gives the smallest energy value is chosen. In this study, a deformable model has been developed based on this modified version to delineate the volumetric brain structures, full details can be found in Parveen et al [10] and a short description is presented here.

The three-dimensional deformable model is composed of a set of control points that are connected both in a two-dimensional plane and between slices. $v_{xy}(i)=\{x(i), y(i)\}$ and $v_{xyz}(i)=\{x(i), y(i), z(i)\}$ represent a section of contour in the xy plane and connected contours with components in xyz, where x, y and z are the spatial coordinates and i is the length along the contour. The total energy can be represented by equation (1):

$$E_{total} = \left[E_{dcm}\left[v_{xy}(i)\right] + E_{dcm}\left[v_{xyz}(i)\right]\right]$$
$$where \; E_{dcm}\left[v_{xy}(i)\right] = \alpha \, E_{int}\left[v_{xy}(i)\right] + \beta \, E_{ext}\left[v_{xy}(i)\right]$$
$$and \; E_{dcm}\left[v_{xyz}(i)\right] = \alpha \, E_{int}\left[v_{xyz}(i)\right] + \beta \, E_{ext}\left[v_{xyz}(i)\right]$$

(1)

where, E_{int} represents the internal spline energy, E_{ext} represents the energy from image features. α and β are the weighting parameters to control the internal energy and the image energy, respectively.

In MR brain images, the non-brain tissues, such as fat, bone marrow, are not distinctly separate from CSF, therefore, the energy functions were reparameterised so that the neighbourhood matrices contain comparable values. Therefore, the desired regions were obtained by normalizing the energy values for internal and external energies.

2.5 Relative Fuzzy Classification with Spatial Affinity

The main aim in this study is to compensate for the blurring effect of tissue boundaries due to the partial volume effect. To overcome this effect, the statistical distributions of the image intensities of each tissue type p_{wm}, p_{gm}, and p_{csf} have been integrated with the fuzzy spatial affinity of each tissue element to classify the WM, GM and CSF. Classification assigns voxels/regions in an image into one or more specified classes and can be a hard (binary) or fuzzy process. In the hard binary case, the voxels are assigned to classes with a value of 1 or 0, whereas in fuzzy classification, the process assigns the membership values for each tissue type in each voxel. Therefore, the membership values e.g. μ_{wm}, μ_{gm}, and μ_{csf} indicate the amount of tissue present in the voxel or the probability that that voxel belongs to the given tissue class. Alone the fuzzy process can not incorporate information about the spatial context making it sensitive to noise. In order to minimise this problem we calculate the connectedness between each group of tissues in the spatial domain.

The fuzzy classification process is designed to minimize the overall objective function F with respect to the membership functions μ_{ik} and the centroids v_k,

$$F = \sum_{i=1}^{w} \sum_{k=1}^{s} (\mu_{ik})^m \left(\|x_i - v_k\| \right)^2 \qquad (2)$$

where, x_i is the observation at voxel i, s is the number of clusters or classes, w is the image domain and the parameter m determines the amount of fuzziness of the resulting classification. The membership values of a voxel i to each class k are

$$\mu_{ik} \in [0,1] \text{ and } \sum_{k} \mu_{ik} = 1 \qquad (3)$$

and the cluster centres v_k are upgraded using the membership values

$$v_k = \sum_{i=1}^{w} (\mu_{ik})^m x_i \bigg/ \sum_{i=1}^{w} (\mu_{ik})^m \qquad (4)$$

The fuzzy digital topological and geometric concepts, initially developed by Rosenfield [11] are an extension of the crisp theory to the fuzzy set theory. In general, connectivity provides a useful tool for describing spatial relationships and region properties for image analysis. Rosenfield's degree of connectivity was further studied by Udupa [6], who showed how, a fuzzy object can be defined as a fuzzy connected component of spatial elements. Fuzzy connectedness is a fuzzy relation in the set of all spatial elements which combines together the notion of the fuzzy adjacency of spatial elements, which is independent of any image information, and fuzzy affinity between spatial elements which depends on image intensity values. A binary scene over a fuzzy digital space (Z^n, ρ) is a pair $\Re = (C, f)$, where ρ is a fuzzy spatial adjacency, Z is the digital space, n is the spatial elements (pixels or voxels), Z^n is the set of all spatial elements, and f is a function of the scene domain C, and the range of f is a subset of the closed interval $[0,1]$. *Fuzzy spatial adjacency* μ_ρ is a fuzzy relation ρ in Z^n if it is both reflexive and symmetric. $\Re$ would be a binary scene over (Z^n, ρ) if the range of f is $\{0,1\}$. When the result of segmentation is a fuzzy subset of the scene domain, this fuzzy subset can be equivalently represented by a scene wherein the scene intensity represents the fuzzy membership value μ_f in $[0,1]$ and such scenes are called *membership scenes* over (Z^n, ρ). The process that converts a scene to a membership scene is called *classification*.

Fuzzy spatial affinity μ_β is any reflexive and symmetric fuzzy relation β in C, that is,

$$\beta = \{((c,d), \mu_\beta(c,d)) | (c,d) \in C\}$$
$$\mu_\beta : C \times C \to [0,1]$$
$$\mu_\beta(c,c) = 1, \forall c \in C$$
$$\mu_\beta(c,d) = \mu_\beta(d,c), \forall (c,d) \in C$$

(5)

where, c, d are the image locations of the two voxels. The fuzzy spatial affinity between voxels has been taken into consideration in the classification process. Here, connectedness takes into account the adjacency of the voxels and the similarity of their intensity values. This affinity is then used to assign the strength of connectedness between the voxels and the tissue classes by using the strength of connectedness between the successive points in the connecting path. The final strength of connectivity within the same tissue class is the maximum strength along the path of minimum distance. The *fuzzy spatial affinity* μ_β can be explained as follows: for any $\forall (c,d) \in C$, $\mu_\beta(c,d)$ is a function of (i) the fuzzy adjacency between each voxel, (ii) the homogeneity of the voxel intensities along the connecting path, (iii) the closeness of the voxel intensities and of the intensity-based features to some expected intensity and feature values for the object, and (iv) the relative locations of the voxels.

Therefore, the general form of $\mu_\beta(c,d)$ can be expressed in equation (6)

$$\mu_\beta(c,d) = h(\mu_\rho(c,d), f(c), f(d), c, d)$$

(6)

where h is a scalar-valued function with range $[0,1]$, $\mu_\rho(c,d)$ is an adjacency function based on the distance of the two voxels, and $f(c), f(d)$ are the intensity of the voxels c and d, respectively.

Fuzzy connectedness is a fuzzy relationship in C, where $\mu_\beta(c,d)$ is the maximum strength of connectivity along the smallest path between c and d, which has the greatest affinity between them. In Udupa [6], a hard binary relationship is used in C based on the fuzzy connectedness: $\mu_\beta(c,d)=1, if\ \mu_\beta(c,d)\geq\theta\in[0,1]$, otherwise 0, where μ_β was chosen to be a hard adjacency relation and θ is a threshold that contains the spatial elements in an object when the strength of connectedness between the spatial elements c and d is highest at that threshold value. In our study, a modification was used in the fuzzy connectedness algorithm to take into account the spatial affinity relationship along with the fuzzy membership values. Therefore, in this study, we have used an affinity relationship based on μ_{wm}, μ_{gm}, and μ_{csf}, the adjacency of the tissue elements, and the intensities without any extra weighting parameter. With this modification, we are able to assign fuzzy values for each tissue class to each undefined voxel based upon their spatial affinity.

3 Results

3.1 Deformable Contour Model

The deformable contour model was applied to simulated MR volumes of different slice thicknesses (1mm – 5mm) with different noise levels ranging from 0% to 7%. Fig. 1 shows the resulting contours on a number of slices for T1-weighted simulated MR brain data of noise level 1%. A quantitative comparison has been carried out to investigate the percentage errors between the DCM results and the true anatomical volumes. The first row of Fig. 2 shows the percentage errors in a slice by slice comparison for noise levels 1% and 9% in 1mm slice thickness data. A comparison between the ICV in different slice thicknesses at different noise levels is given in the second row of Fig. 2.

3.2 Tissue Segmentation

The resulting ICV images from the DCM were then passed to the spatial affinity based fuzzy segmentation algorithm. The number of classes was set to three (CSF, GM and WM) in each case. The resultant fuzzy values assigned to the anatomical structures were used to calculate the mean and standard deviations for the image intensities associated with each tissue class. The algorithm results are assessed by comparing the results obtained on the simulated data with the true volumes provided with the data by calculating the number of mis-classified voxels. Fig. 1 shows the segmented results obtained from the fuzzy classification of CSF, GM and WM in the third, fourth and fifth rows, respectively. The algorithm was applied to simulated MR volumes of different slice thicknesses with different noise levels and a quantitative comparison was made between the 'true' classifications and the algorithm results (Fig. 2).

This algorithm was also applied to clinical MR data obtained from MGH website and the data from UCL volunteers. As the results were obtained as fuzzy values, the comparison was made between the class means obtained from the algorithm and the 'true' means of the corresponding data sets. Fig. 3 shows the performance of the spatial affinity based fuzzy segmentation on clinical MR data in terms of the percentage errors in means.

Fig. 4 shows a visual comparison between the segmented tissues obtained by the algorithms and the 'true' fuzzy tissues of the corresponding slices for the simulated brainweb. The results obtained from tissue classification are presented in Fig. 5 with the 'crisp' segmented tissue labels.

3.3 Accuracy

Deformable Contour Model. Fig. 2 illustrates the results of the extraction of the intracranial volume by applying the deformable contour model. The percentage errors were calculated from the difference between the segmented results and the 'true' values. We have observed that the DCM has successfully segmented ICV with percentage errors of 3.69% for the slice thickness of 1mm in the presence of 9% of noise. As shown in Fig. 2, the percentage errors are less in the middle of the brain because of less edge complexity. The errors are less than 4% in the case of 3mm slice thickness at every noise level. In the case of 5mm slice thickness, the percentage errors involved in assigning the voxels in the ICV are up to 5.32%. The likely explanation is that with thicker slices, the structural boundaries suffer greater from partial volume effects.

Spatial Affinity Based Fuzzy Segmentation. Fig. 2 shows the classification results after applying the proposed algorithm in terms of voxels assigned to each tissue class and the percentage errors with respect to the 'true' classifications. The errors associated with the number of voxels assigned tissue classes for WM and GM are less than 3% and 2%, respectively and the percentage errors for CSF are less than 4% for 1mm slice thickness simulated brain volume up to 5% of noise. Fig. 2 shows that this affinity based segmentation provides a good classification for GM (0.94% mis-classification at 3% noise of 1mm slice thickness). However, the errors in the number of mis-classified voxels are higher in the 7% of noise data with the slice thicknesses of 3mm and 5mm. Fig. 4 illustrates a visual comparison of the segmented tissues and the 'true' tissues, and revealed that the classification of brain tissues are well matched. The total brain volume (TBV) was calculated which is the volume of WM plus the volume of GM and it has been observed that the percentage errors varied from (-0.272 to 2.077) for 1mm slice thickness, (0.207 to 3.399) for 3mm and (0.063 to 4.527) for 5mm slice thickness at all different noise levels (0% to 7%). Similarly, the GM, WM and CSF volumes were calculated and the percentage errors varied from (-0.94 to 2.90), (2.23 to 5.20), and (3.00 to 4.2), respectively for 1mm slice thickness. For 3mm slice thickness, the percentage errors varied for GM (0.50 to 5.62), WM (3.0 to 7.21), CSF (4.00 to 6.50) and for 5mm slice thickness, GM (4.97 to 5.33), WM (4.00 to 7.20) and CSF (1.15 to 7.00) at different noise levels.

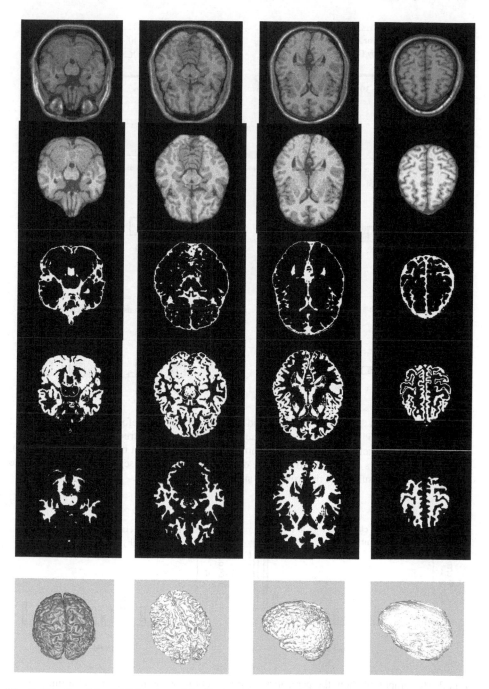

Fig. 1. Results of the DCM and spatial affinity based fuzzy segmentation applied to a simulated MR volume with 1% noise level. The first and second rows show the DCM around the ICV of the original slices and the extracted ICV. The third, fourth and fifth rows show the CSF, GM and WM tissues. The last row presents a 3D view of the extracted ICV, WM, GM and CSF.

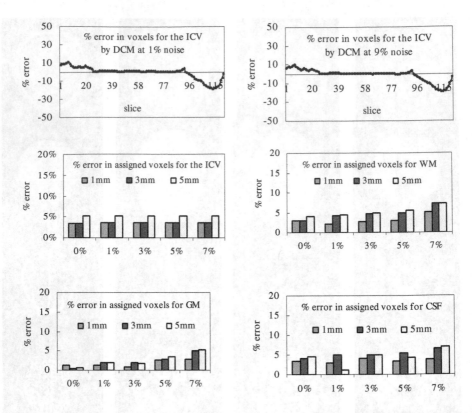

Fig. 2. Comparison between the segmented regions using the deformable contour model (DCM) and the spatial affinity based fuzzy segmentation with the 'true' values performed on the simulated brain volume of thicknesses 1mm to 5mm with different noise levels (0% to 7%). The percentage errors are calculated from the difference between the segmented results and the 'true' values. The result in the first row is for slice thickness of 1mm.

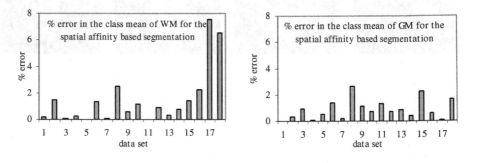

Fig. 3. Bar graphs to show the percentage errors in class means for the spatial affinity based fuzzy segmentation performed on the clinical MR brain volume in 18 data sets. The percentage errors are calculated from the difference between the class means result and the true mean values.

In the clinical MR volumes, the percentage errors in means were calculated for WM and GM and presented in Fig. 3 for 18 data sets from MGH where they have various levels of difficulty. It was observed that the percentage errors in WM were less than 0.5% in 8 cases, less than 2.5% in 8 cases and less than 7.5% in 2 cases. The percentage errors in means for GM are less than 0.5% for 7 cases and in between 0.5% to 2.6% for 11 case studies. The percentage errors in means of the remaining two data sets are more than 10%.

4 Discussion

The partial volume effect is a major obstacle to the accurate separation of GM, WM, and CSF in MR images. To counteract the partial volume effect, we have presented an algorithm to improve the segmentation and classification of MR T1-weighted brain tissues into WM, GM and CSF by using a spatial affinity based fuzzy classification. The classification of partial volume voxels were calculated from an affinity based fuzzy segmentation and the classification process has taken into account the spatial connectivity along with fuzzy labelling. The hypothesis is that a voxel will be labelled, with a fuzzy value, as containing a particular tissue, with the greatest affinity along the shortest path.

Table 1. Results of the spatial affinity based fuzzy segmentation performed on clinical MRI volume. The volume in voxels, means and standard deviations (std dev) of each tissue class of WM and GM are presented.

data	WM			GM			WM/TBV	GM/WM
	volume	Mean	Std dev	volume	mean	Std dev		
set 1	554289	1480.85	82	809599	1377.69	102	0.406	1.461
set 2	382564	186	32	483890	133.73	36	0.442	1.265
set 3	521230	1544.67	34.29	492555	1428.56	45.64	0.514	0.945
set 4	543570	1425.52	26.95	593586	1336.81	31.95	0.478	1.092
set 5	550276	1472.82	29.49	639256	1378.47	35.69	0.463	1.162
set 6	398789	90.04	7.71	414528	67.41	7.54	0.490	1.039
set 7	561102	1325.37	20.86	661508	1252.84	24.89	0.459	1.179
set 8	449231	88.9	8.54	509227	64.9	8.24	0.469	1.134
set 9	554631	1462.51	26.87	623667	1357.35	24.91	0.455	1.197
set 10	645368	1629.34	40.6	772561	1494.23	48.18	0.386	1.461
Set 11	381791	344.10	27.25	446989	254.37	30.80	0.461	1.170
Set 12	582219	1543.99	38.50	617945	1418.56	31.11	0.485	1.061
Set 13	608359	1579.71	39.45	603793	1444.71	48.46	0.501	0.992
Set 14	525237	1549.66	37.34	559475	1419.65	45.84	0.484	1.065
Set 15	425283	172.75	16.63	454384	124.52	15.65	0.483	1.068
Set 16	434186	393.46	35.2	494588	281.36	34.53	0.467	1.139
Set 17	312241	157.33	20.3	477474	107.13	15.45	0.395	1.529
Set 18	589909	104.56	38.22	1112127	71.26	35.26	0.347	1.885

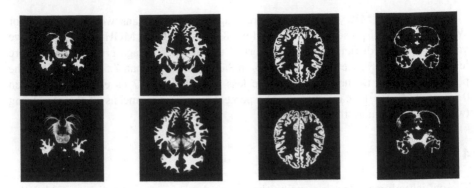

Fig. 4. Illustration of the CSF, GM and WM in the 'true' simulated brainweb volume with the results obtained from the fuzzy segmentation. The top and bottom rows present the result of the segmented tissues and the corresponding 'true' classification respectively.

This affinity based fuzzy segmentation along with the deformable contour model have been applied to the simulated brain web volume to make an investigation of the effects of noise and partial volume effects on tissue classification. The experimental results for GM, WM and CSF segmentation show promise. This segmentation algorithm was also applied to clinical MR brain volumes (MGH website) where the tissues are affected by various levels of difficulty. Even in the presence of this difficulty, it can be seen in Fig. 3, that the percentage errors in means of WM and GM are still small. The results of the clinical MR volume are presented in Table 1.

In order to make a comparison in this study, the ratio of WM to TBV was calculated and is presented in Table 1. Our values for this ratio are comparable with the values previously reported [1, 12]. In conclusion, we have demonstrated here a better segmentation algorithm to separate tissues from MR brain images with good accuracy and reproducibility. Both methods were extensively tested on well-established simulated brainweb data and with clinical datasets.

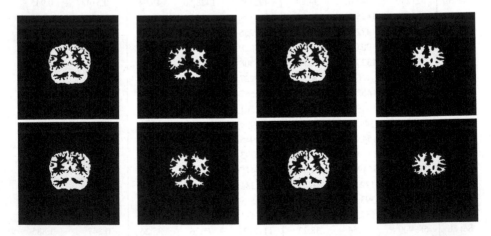

Fig. 5. A graphical comparison between the results of the spatial affinity based fuzzy algorithm performed on the clinical MR volume (upper row) with the corresponding 'true' crisp labelling

Acknowledgements

This work was partially funded by the fellowship of Bangladesh Atomic Energy Commission (BAEC) of the Government of Bangladesh.

References

1. Guttmann, C.R.G., Jolesz, F.A., Kikinis, R., Killiany, R.J., Moss, M.B., Sandor, T.: White Matter Changes with Normal Aging. Neurology. 50 (1998) 972-978
2. Bezdek, J.C., Hall, L.O., Clarke, L.P.: Review of MR image Segmentation Techniques Using Pattern Recognition. Med. Phys. 20 (1993) 1033-1047
3. Parveen, R., Todd-Pokropek, A.: Segmentation of MR Brain Images Using Region Growing Combined with an Active Contour Model. Conf. Proc. Comp. Aided Radiol. Surg. 2002
4. Niessen, W.J., Vincken, K.L., Weickert, J., ter Haar Romeny, B.M., Viergever, M.A.: Multiscale Segmentation of Three-Dimensional MR Brain Images. Int. J. Comput. Vis. 31 (1999) 185-202
5. Leemput, K.V., Maes, F., Vandermeulen, D., Suetens, P.: A Unifying Framework for Partial Volume Segmentation of Brain MR Images. IEEE Trans. Med. Imag. 22 (2003) 105-119
6. Udupa, J.K., Samarasekera, S.: Fuzzy Connectedness and Object Definition: Theory, Algorithms, and Applications in Image Segmentation. Graph. Models. Imag. Proces. 58 (1996) 246-261
7. Collins, D.L., Zijdenbos, A.P., Kollokian, V., Sled, J.G., Kabani, N.J., Holmes, C.J., Evans, A.C.: Design and Construction of a Realistic Digital Brain Phantom. IEEE Trans Med. Imag. 17 (1998) 463-468
8. Kass, M., Witkin, A., Terzopoulos, D.: Snakes: Active Contour Models. IEEE Proc. 1st International Conf. Comp. Vis. (1987) 259-268
9. Williams, D.J., Shah, M.: A Fast Algorithm for Active Contours and Curvature Estimation. Comp. Vis. Graph. Image Proc. (CVGIP): IU. 55 (1992) 14-26
10. Parveen, R., Ruff, C., Mcdonald, D., Lambrou, T., Todd-Pokropek, A.: Three-Dimensional Voxel Morphometry of MR Brain Images Using Deformable Models, Relative Fuzzy Clasification and Spatial Affinity. Proc. MIUA 2004, 117-120
11. Rosenfield, A.: Connectivity in Digital Pictures. J. Assoc. Comp. Mach. 17 (1970) 146-160
12. Alfano, B., Quarantelli, M., Brunetti, A., Larobina, M., Covelli, E.M., Tedeschi, E., Salvatore, M.: Reproducibility of Intracranial Volume Measurement by Unsupervised Multispectral Brain Segmentation. Magn. Reson. Med. 39 (1998) 497-499

3-D Ultrasound Probe Calibration
for Computer-Guided Diagnosis and Therapy

Michael Baumann[1,2], Vincent Daanen[1], Antoine Leroy[2], and Jocelyne Troccaz[1]

[1] TIMC Laboratory, GMCAO Department, Institut d'Ingénierie de l'Information de Santé
(IN3S), Faculty of Medecine - F-38706 La Tronche cedex, France
michael.baumann@imag.fr
[2] KOELIS, 4, Avenue de l'Obiou - F-38700 La Tronche cedex, France

Abstract. With the emergence of swept-volume ultrasound (US) probes, precise and almost real-time US volume imaging has become available. This offers many new opportunities for computer guided diagnosis and therapy, 3-D images containing significantly more information than 2-D slices. However, computer guidance often requires knowledge about the exact position of US voxels relative to a tracking reference, which can only be achieved through probe calibration. In this paper we present a 3-D US probe calibration system based on a membrane phantom. The calibration matrix is retrieved by detection of a membrane plane in a dozen of US acquisitions of the phantom. Plane detection is robustly performed with the 2-D Hough transformation. The feature extraction process is fully automated, calibration requires about 20 minutes and the calibration system can be used in a clinical context. The precision of the system was evaluated to a root mean square (RMS) distance error of 1.15mm and to an RMS angular error of $0.61°$. The point reconstruction accuracy was evaluated to 0.9mm and the angular reconstruction accuracy to $1.79°$.

1   Introduction

Until recently, 3-D ultrasound (US) volumes had to be manually reconstructed from a number of 2-D US slices acquired while slowly moving a 2-D probe over the target region. The so-called *3D freehand method* is time-consuming, imprecise and not usable for many clinical applications requiring real-time acquisition [1]. The emergence of 3-D swept-volume US probes solved most of the enumerated problems: a mechanical device capable of sweeping the 2-D crystal array of the probe over a target region makes it possible to acquire 3-D US volumes accurately and almost in real-time (1s to 4s per acquisition)[1].

These new capabilities open an entire new field of applications in the domain of computer guided medical interventions based on US imaging. One can imagine tool guidance systems that would operate with permanently updated US volumes, visualizing for instance slices at the tool tip position. More sophisticated applications could carry out

---

[1] However, most currently available systems don't yet provide a real-time data transfer interface for 3-D data. Nevertheless one can acquire so called "4-D" images of three orthogonal volume slices in real-time using a video-capture device. In the rest of this article we make abstraction of this restriction, hoping that it will disappear with the next generation of 3-D echographs.

R.R. Beichel and M. Sonka (Eds.): CVAMIA 2006, LNCS 4241, pp. 248–259, 2006.

target localization inside the volumes through real-time registration and segmentation techniques, thus allowing to match pre-operative planning with intra-operative data.

However, US-based guidance often requires knowledge about the position and orientation of the US volume in space. When using a tracking system this can be achieved by calibrating the US acquisition volume with a tracking reference fixed on the probe. Unfortunately it is virtually impossible to derive the calibration parameters directly from the geometry and parameterization of the probe. Almost all existing calibration systems rely therefore on statistical or segmentation-based object matching methods.

1.1 Calibration Methods Overview

A variety of techniques for 2-D US calibration was proposed in the literature; a comprehensive review being given in [2]. Calibration methods can be classified with respect to the target geometry they rely on. *Single-point target* methods identify a point, i.e. a bead, a calibrated pointer tip or a cross-wire, in the US image [3,4,5]. The difficulties consist in automatic geometry extraction in the US slice and US beam alignment with the phantom.

Multi-point target phantoms are extensions of the single-point bead or cross-wire phantoms. They consist of a number of point targets with precisely known coordinates in phantom space. Their geometric configuration makes it possible to derive the calibration parameters from the distances between the reconstructed intersection points visible in the 2-D US scan [6]. Compared to single-point phantoms they require less image acquisitions due to their more discriminative geometry, but share the phantom alignment and feature extraction problems.

Z-fiducial or *N-fiducial* phantoms address the alignment problem of point target methods. A calibration point is determined from the intersection points of a number of nylon strings with the US beam. This is possible due to a sufficiently discriminative wire geometry [7,8,9]. Fiducial methods are more robust than point target methods but the difficulties concerning fully automatic feature extraction subsist. Also, Z- or N-fiducial phantoms require a high manufacturing accuracy to achieve a satisfying calibration quality.

Wall phantom methods are based on detection of the intersecting line of a planar surface with the 2-D US beam. In [4], a water tank bottom is imaged for calibration. The authors of [10] address the reverberation and line thickness problems inherent of wall phantoms by using a membrane variant. Both phantoms have difficulties when confronted with steep angles between the US beam and the plane because they cause line intensity and line sharpness degradation [2]. The Cambridge phantom scans a rotating bar, thus creating a virtual plane, to solve these problems [4]. The advantage of plane phantoms lies in the robustness of the feature extraction process which can, as a consequence, be reliably and fully automated. The pitfall of this method lies in the non-discriminative phantom geometry which can result in underdetermined systems if the acquired calibration samples do not cover all degrees of freedom. This can be avoided by strictly respecting the acquisition protocols presented in [4,11].

Registration Phantoms: the last class of calibration methods relies on surface or intensity based registration techniques and therefore has the advantage of being independent of phantom geometry. The only requirement on phantom shape is that its US image is sufficiently discriminative with respect to rotations and translations, which is true for non-symmetric phantoms. The lack of precision of registration algorithms is the major drawback of this approach. To our knowledge, only one study examined registration-based 2-D probe calibration, registering US slices with an MRI image of the phantom [12]. A 3-D approach is discussed in the next paragraph.

1.2   3-D Probe Calibration

Until today, only few studies about calibration of 3-D probes were carried out. Poon and Rohling [13] compared 3-D calibration based on a IXI-fiducial wire phantom, a pointer tip phantom and a cube phantom. The IXI wire phantom and the cube phantom methods require only one volume acquisition for calibration. The presented feature detection is semi-automatic. The best results yielded the IXI phantom with a mean error in reproducibility of 1.5 mm, a RMS error of the point accuracy measure of 2.15 mm and a RMS error of the reconstruction accuracy by distance measure of 1.52 mm. Bouchet et al [14] examined Z-fiducial phantom and achieved a RMS point accuracy error of 1.1mm. Two variants of a surface registration based 3-D calibration method were presented by Lange and Eulenstein in [15]. The first one registers 3-D US images of the phantom with a geometric model derived from its CT scan. The second variant registers a number of US images of the phantom acquired from different positions. In both cases, surfaces are extracted manually. The authors claim that the latter approach could be fully automated. The CT variant performed best and yielded a RMS error in reproducibility precision of 1.8 mm and a RMS error in point accuracy of 2.0 mm. The ultrasound speed distortion problem is not addressed.

In this study we propose a 3-D US calibration method based on a single plane membrane phantom. A fast, precise and accurate 3-D feature extraction algorithm relying on the 2-D Hough transform is presented. In contrast to existing 3-D US calibration systems, the feature extraction process is fully automated. In the result section, precision and accuracy assessments are carried out using a specially designed validation phantom.

2   Materials and Methods

2.1   Acquisition Hardware

The acquisition hardware consists of a GE Voluson 730 Pro 3-D US scanner and a NDI Polaris optical tracker with a 0.25 mm RMS error (as communicated by NDI). The tracking system operates with wireless (passive) infrared-reflecting rigid bodies equipped with flat markers. The ultrasound volumes are acquired with a 5 to 9 Mhz two dimensional curved array probe (see Fig. 1a). The piezo array of the probe is mounted on a mechanical device which is capable of sweeping regularly around its rotation axis within a predefined angular range. During the continuous sweeping process the US hardware reconstructs 3-D volumes from the series of acquired 2-D slices. The 3-D acquisition time ranges from 1s to 4s, depending mainly on sweep angle and axial acquisition depth. Images are digitally transferred using a proprietary software from GE Medical Systems named 4D View. The US scanner also communicates the voxel size. The scan converter assumes the speed of sound (SoS) in tissue to be 1540 m/s.

2.2   The Membrane Phantom

The calibration phantom being dedicated to a clinical context, ergonomics considerations had an important impact on its design. We use a variation of the wall phantom presented in [4], which is based on imaging the bottom wall of a water tank. The geometric form of the wall, which is a line in 2-D and a plane in 3-D, can be very robustly extracted from the US data using statistical algorithms like the Hough transform. This makes it possible to fully automate the feature extraction process without significant loss in precision and accuracy. This represents a big advantage over semi-automatic point-detection based phantoms in terms of calibration speed and ease of use. To overcome the plane thickness and the reverberation problems observable in US images of rigid surfaces [4] a filigrane nylon mesh membrane, tightly spanned on a planar rigid support with a circular and about 20cm wide hole, is used as target (see Fig. 1b). Reverberation is further reduced by inclining the membrane plane with respect to the water tank bottom by 45°. A tracking reference (rigid body) is mounted on the membrane frame for phantom localization. The phantom is filled with water and equipped with a thermometer to measure water temperature.

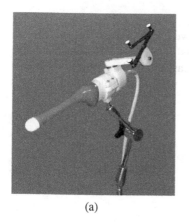
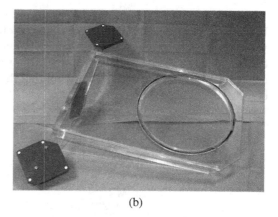

(a)   (b)

Fig. 1. Calibration hardware. Figure (a) shows an endorectal US probe mounted on an articulated arm. Figure (b) shows the membrane phantom. Both the probe and the membrane are equipped with infra-red reflecting passive rigid bodies for tracking.

2.3   3-D Calibration Mathematics

As illustrated in Fig. 2, four references are relevant for calibration: first of all, the membrane space **M** is defined as a reference in which the membrane lies in the origin and is parallel to e_x and e_y base vectors of **M**. In this space, every point with a zero z-ordinate is a membrane plane point. The phantom space **Ph** and the probe space **Pr** are defined by the rigid bodies that are attached on the phantom and on the probe. Finally, the US volume space **U** corresponds to the voxel space of the 3-D images acquired by the ultrasound device. $\mathbf{T_{Ph2M}}$, $\mathbf{T_{Pr2Ph}}$ and $\mathbf{T_{U2Pr}}$ are homogenous 4x4 transformation matrices.

Suppose that we identified a point $\mathbf{p} = (x, y, z)$ in a US volume **U** as a point belonging to the membrane. With $\mathbf{s} = (s_x, s_y, s_z)$ denoting the voxel scale factors, it is verified that

$$\begin{pmatrix} m_1 \\ m_2 \\ 0 \\ 1 \end{pmatrix} = \mathbf{T_{Ph2M}} \cdot \mathbf{T_{Pr2Ph}} \cdot \mathbf{T_{U2Pr}} \cdot \begin{pmatrix} s_x x \\ s_y y \\ s_z z \\ 1 \end{pmatrix}. \tag{1}$$

where $\mathbf{T_{Ph2M}}$ is known from membrane pre-calibration (see chap. 2.4) and $\mathbf{T_{Pr2Ph}}$ is given by the tracking system. Further, the scaling vector **s** is communicated by the US hardware. The remaining unknown element is the homogenous rigid transformation $\mathbf{T_{U2P}}$. For convenience we define the elements of $\mathbf{T_{Pr2Ph}} \cdot \mathbf{T_{Ph2M}}$ as a_{ij} and the elements of $\mathbf{T_{U2P}}$ as b_{ij} ($i, j \in 1..4$). The zero component of (1) yields then

$$\begin{aligned} 0 = \ & a_{31} \left(s_x x b_{11} + s_y y b_{12} + s_z z b_{13} + b_{14} \right) + \\ & a_{32} \left(s_x x b_{21} + s_y y b_{22} + s_z z b_{23} + b_{24} \right) + \\ & a_{33} \left(s_x x b_{31} + s_y y b_{32} + s_z z b_{33} + b_{34} \right) + \\ & a_{34} . \end{aligned} \tag{2}$$

Using Euler angles and a three-dimensional vector we can represent $\mathbf{T_{U2P}}$ with six variables, which leaves us in total with 6 unknowns to solve for. A detected plane can be added to the equation system by adding at least three plane points (Using of course the $\mathbf{T_{Pr2Ph}}$ measured while acquiring the US volume in which the plane was detected).

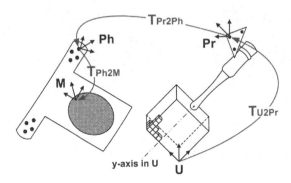

Fig. 2. Illustration of the transformations involved in the calibration process. Note that scaling is omitted from the scheme for simplification.

2.4   Membrane Pre-calibration

To reduce the number of degrees of freedom of the calibration process, the membrane space M is determined using a pointer equipped with a tracking reference. A large number of surface points of the membrane-supporting structure is acquired in order to compute the plane equation using a least square approximation combined with a simple M-estimator to increase robustness. Since the phantom rigid body is permanently fixed on the phantom, pre-calibration has to be carried out only once.

2.5   Acquisition Protocol

The major drawback of single-plane phantoms resides in their barely discriminative geometry. A plane can be described with only three variables, from which it follows that even with an optimal acquisition protocol, a minimum number of two acquisitions is necessary to cover all degrees of freedom. To obtain robust results the twelve-step acquisition protocol presented in [4] is used. The protocol improvement presented in [11] mainly addresses the z-axis imprecision problem inherent of most 2-D calibration systems. Since 3-D probes give as much information in z-direction as in x- or y- direction this modification yields no particular advantage in the 3-D domain but requires at least 18 steps. For that reason we stick to the original version.

Sweeping and volume reconstruction being a continuous process of 1 to 4 seconds, significant distortions can be observed in the US volume when the probe is moved rapidly. Also, no direct access to the digital data is available which prevented synchronization of probe position measurement with US image acquisition. Therefore an articulated arm for complete probe immobilization during acquisition is used, eliminating all motion-induced artifacts and time lags. Furthermore, immobilizing the probe makes it possible to perform high precision position measuring based on a large number of measures and outlier elimination.

2.6   Feature Extraction

The first step of the feature extraction process consists in correcting the distortion caused by the difference between US speed in water at room temperature and in human tissue at $37°$. To determine US speed in water in function of temperature the polynomial formula established by Bilaniuk and Wong was used [16,17]. A distortion geometry overview for all common probe types is given in [18]. The distortion geometry of a sectorial probe is given in Fig. 3a. With v_W^t being the US velocity in water for a given temperature t and v_T being the velocity in tissue, d_T is determined using the following formula:

$$d_T = \frac{v_T}{v_W} \cdot d_W. \tag{3}$$

Sectorial probe speed correction requires manual definition of the US origin and the scan head surface radius. A graphical user interface was developed for this purpose (see Fig. 3b). Origin and surface radius have to be defined only once during calibration. Plane detection can be carried out using the 3-D Hough transformation, but it would take several minutes to compute the result. Fortunately it is possible to determine the

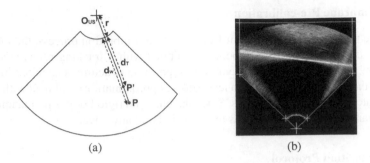

(a)   (b)

Fig. 3. US speed correction. Fig. (a) illustrates the correction geometry of a sectorial probe. O_{US} is the probe origin, r the probe surface radius, d_W the point's P distorted distance from the probe surface in water, d_T the corrected distance and P' the corrected point. Fig. (b) shows the probe mask used to determine US origin and probe surface radius.

plane with good precision by simply extracting its intersection with two arbitrary volume slices, using the 2-D Hough transform. To facilitate and to accelerate US speed correction the xy and zy planes passing through the scan head origin were used. The Hough transform implementation uses intensity accumulation and the following threshold s_H for an image $\mathbf{I}$:

$$s_H = \max\{i \in Hist(\mathbf{I})\} + (\max\{i \in \mathbf{I}\} - \min\{i \in \mathbf{I}\})/3 . \tag{4}$$

The purpose of s_H is to ignore the low-intensity water background, which represents the largest part of the image.

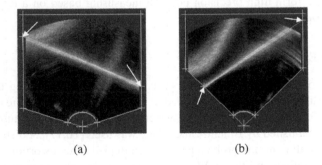

(a)   (b)

Fig. 4. Screenshot of a successful automatic plane extraction. Note that lines are correctly detected in spite of a degraded membrane image caused by a steep scan angle. The arrows point at the line intersections with the mask.

2.7 Optimization

Optimization of (2) is carried out with the non-linear Levenberg-Marquardt implementation given in [19]. A random restart scheme within a range of reasonable initialization values robustifies this process.

2.8   Visual Back-Tests

The plane coordinates as resulting from the optimization process are visualized as a line in the slices used for feature extraction, and distance plus rotational errors between the segmented and the calculated line are evaluated. This allows for manual replacement of evident outliers with new acquisitions and for recomputation of the calibration without requiring a complete restart.

3   Experimental Results

3.1   Test Configuration

Precision and accuracy assessments were carried out using a membrane plane pre-calibration with an RMS surface distance error of 0.43mm for the measured surface points. A total of ten calibrations were performed using the twelve-step protocol. The probe rigid body was not moved between calibrations. The probe was mounted on an articulated arm and immobilized during position and image acquisition. The water temperature was 23°. The acquired US volumes had a size of (199, 199, 199) isotropic voxels with 0.477mm side lengths.

3.2   Feature Extraction Quality

The Hough transform extracted lines correctly for 238 out of 240 acquired images. Line detection failed for images on which only a very small part of the membrane was visible. In these cases, lines had to be manually determined. Note that no manual outlier elimination was carried out. As detection failures were rare, calibration was in average carried out in about twenty minutes. To get a better idea about the quality of feature extraction and about the presence of distortions in the membrane images we measured the detection precision: using (2) we can calculate the distance error between a measured plane point and the computed plane as follows:

$$
\begin{aligned}
\epsilon(x, y, z) = & \, a_{31} \left(s_x x b_{11} + s_y y b_{12} + s_z z b_{13} + b_{14} \right) + \\
& \, a_{32} \left(s_x x b_{21} + s_y y b_{22} + s_z z b_{23} + b_{24} \right) + \\
& \, a_{33} \left(s_x x b_{31} + s_y y b_{32} + s_z z b_{33} + b_{34} \right) + \\
& \, a_{34} \, .
\end{aligned}
\tag{5}
$$

For each calibration, the average and the root mean square (RMS) distance of a set of points to the pre-calibration plane was computed using (5). For each line we computed ten equidistant points between the extreme points on the line segment inside the US volume. The angular feature extraction error is defined as the angle between the computed plane normal and the cross product of the directional vectors of the two extracted lines. Based on this definition the maximum and the RMS angular errors were computed for each acquired volume of the calibration. The aggregated errors for all calibrations can be found in Table 1.

Table 1. Aggregated Feature Extraction Precision

	Distance Error [mm]	Distance Error [vox]	Angular Error [deg]
RMS Error	0.37	0.77	0.26
Max Error	1.30	2.73	1.09

3.3 Calibration Precision

The calibration precision measures the reproducibility of calibration results. Again, both the translational and the angular errors were assessed. The translational error is defined as the standard deviation of the volume center after scaling and right-hand multiplication to the different calibration transformations T^i_{U2Pr}. The angular error is measured as the standard deviation of angular differences between the $(0, 0, 1)$ vector after scaling and right-hand multiplication to the different calibration transformations T^i_{U2Pr} (see Table 2).

Table 2. Calibration Precision

	Distance Error [mm]	Distance Error [vox]	Angular Error [deg]
Standard Deviation	1.15	2.41	0.61
Max Error	1.99	4.03	1.12

3.4 Reconstruction Accuracy

Reconstruction accuracy was assessed using the bead phantom illustrated in Fig. 5. Note that the beads are co-planar within a precision of 0.25mm (RMS). The left-hand three beads form the left triangle while the right-hand beads form the right triangle. The distance d_B of the triangle barycenters was evaluated with an estimated accuracy of about 0.5mm.

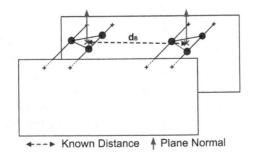

Fig. 5. Reconstruction Accuracy Measurement Phantom

Table 3. Reconstruction Accuracy Results

	Distance Error [mm]	Distance Error [vox]	Angular Error [deg]
RMS Error	0.90	1.90	1.79
Max Error	2.44	5.11	3.03

Twenty US images of the phantom were acquired, ten imaging the left triangle and ten the right triangle. Note that images of one triangle did not intersect with the second one. The bead centers were manually extracted from the images. The reconstructed triangle barycenters and normals were then projected into probe space for each calibration, which yielded 100 point and vector pairs. The distance error for a point pair is defined as the difference between their Euclidean distance and d_B. The angular error for a vector pair is defined as the angle between both vectors. The results are given in Table 3.

4 Discussion

Probe calibration for currently available swept-volume 3-D probes makes only sense for static applications. Real-time access to acquired 3D images is currently not provided by the Voluson hardware. Also, depending on scan parameters, the duration of the volume sweeping process ranges from 1s to 4s. Due to probe or tissue motion, the physical location of voxels can therefore be way off the position indicated by the calibration. The latter problem could be reduced by scan-heads equipped with high-frequency sweeping-devices, but it will disappear only with non-sweeping 2-D piezo array US probes. Until then, it is better to calibrate probes using an articulated arm for immobilization.

Passing from 2-D to 3-D calibration improves calibration results (for information on 2-D precision of the membrane phantom see [20]) because the z-axis-uncertainty inherent of 2-D calibration is eliminated: when giving a plane instead of a line as input to the optimizer the rotational degrees of freedom are significantly better covered. This allowed us to reduce the number of acquisitions for calibration while still achieving precise and accurate results.

Feature extraction from membrane phantom images showed both robust and precise results. On our set of test images the line blurring and intensity degradation effects occurring when scanning a wall phantom from an oblique angle were correctly handled by the Hough transform: lines were consistently placed in the center of the beam width. Note that the feature extraction precision RMS and maximum errors reported in Table 1 are relatively small, which indicates that the physical plane location corresponds indeed with the beam width center line. Membrane reverberation was not observable and did therefore not disturb the detection process. Also, the membrane phantom was not exposed to line thickness problems. Due to these characteristics, feature extraction could be fully automated (up to the manual US origin and probe radius determination required for US speed correction).

The user-independency resulting from automated feature extraction is partially coun-
ter-balanced by the necessity to follow a protocol for data acquisition, which can re-
introduce user bias. Nevertheless we believe that it is more convenient to follow a
simple acquisition protocol instead of extracting features semi-automatically from US
volumes. Further we preferred to correct for US speed errors instead of requiring 50°
water or phantom fill materials that have the same US characteristics than human tissue,
which makes it possible to use the phantom in a clinical context.

The overall calibration time of about 20 minutes is mostly due to manipulation of
the articulated arm, high precision probe position measurement and data transfer, which
requires several manual interventions. Feature extraction and optimization is computed
in several seconds. In cases where the feature extraction precision evaluation shows
poor results, a visual verification and eventually a correction have to be carried out,
which requires some additional minutes. Significant speed-up could be achieved by
automating the communication between the US scanner and the calibration computer.

The presented calibration system assumes that the SoS in human tissue is uniform
and that it corresponds to the SoS internally used by the US scanner, which is in general
the mean SoS in tissue of 1540m/s. However, SoS varies with different types of tissue:
The SoS in fat is approximately 1450m/s, in blood 1570m/s, in the brain 1541m/s and
in water 1480m/s. As the US generally crosses tissue layers of different thickness and
different types on its way through the body, and as the target tissue is often viewed from
various positions, the in vivo accuracy of the calibration may show fluctuations of more
than 5 per cents in extreme cases during an examination. Also, for some applications it
would be appropriate to use a different mean SoS than the 1540m/s for calibration, but
this is beyond the scope of this study.

Future work will address the twelve-step acquisition protocol which contains a lot of
redundancy. Also, our system does currently not provide a foolproof indicator for missing coverage of degrees of freedom. We therefore started experiments with an Eigenvalue system similar to the one presented in [21].

5   Conclusion

A robust 3-D US probe calibration method designed for clinical usage was presented.
Calibration can be carried out in about twenty minutes due to fully automatic 3-D Plane
extraction based on robust and efficient 2-D line detection. The point reconstruction
accuracy of our phantom can compete with previously presented 3-D phantoms: Lange
and Eulenstein communicated RMS errors between 2.0mm and 2.2mm [15], Bouchet
et al were confronted to 1.1mm RMS point accuracy [14] while Pohn and Rohling
published errors between 1.52mm for their IXI-wire, 1.59mm for the cube and 1.85mm
for their stylus approach. With 0.90mm RMS point accuracy (see Table 3) we achieved
slightly better results. Finally, the proposed method is temperature-independent and
uses water as transmission matter which facilitates its usage.

Acknowledgements. This project is supported by PRAXIM/KOELIS, ANRT and
PHRC 2003 "Prostate-echo" (from French Health Ministry) grants.

References

1. Rohling, R., Gee, A., Berman, L.: A comparison of freehand three-dimensional ultrasound reconstruction techniques. Medical Image Analysis 3(4) (1999) 339–359
2. Mercier, L., Langø, T., Lindseth, F., Collins, D.L.: A review of calibration techniques for freehand 3-D ultrasound systems. Ultrasound Med Biol 31(2) (2004) 143–165
3. State, A., Chen, D.T., Tektor, C., Brandt, A., Chen, H., Ohbuchi, R., Bajura, M., Fuchs, H.: Case study: Observing a volume rendered fetus within a pregnant patient. IEEE Visualization Proc (1994) 364–368
4. Prager, R.W., Rohling, R.N., Gee, A.H., Berman, L.: Rapid calibration for 3-D freehand ultrasound. Ultrasound Med Biol 24(6) (1998) 855–869
5. Muratore, D.M., Galloway, R.J.: Beam calibration without a phantom for creating a 3-D freehand ultrasound system. Ultrasound Med Biol 27(11) (2001) 1557–1566
6. Leotta, D.F.: An efficient calibration method for freehand 3-D ultrasound imaging systems. Ultrasound Med Biol 30 (2004) 999–1008
7. Comeau, R.M., Fenster, A., Peters, T.M.: Integrated mr and ultrasound imaging for improved image guidance in neurosurgery. SPIE Proc 3338 (1998) 747–754
8. Pagoulatos, N., Haynor, D.N., Kim, Y.: A fast calibration method for 3-D tracking of ultrasound images using a spatial localizer. Ultrasound Med Biol 27 (2001) 1219–1229
9. Linseth, F., Tangen, G.A., Langø, T.: Probe calibration for freehand 3-D ultrasound. Ultrasound Med Biol 29 (2003) 49–69
10. T., L.: Ultrasound guided surgery: Image processing and navigation. Ph.D. thesis. Norvegian University of Science and Technology, Trondheim (2000)
11. Treece, G.M., Gee, A.H., Prager, R.W., J., C.C., H., B.L.: High-definition freehand 3-D ultrasound. Ultrasound Med Biol 29(4) (2003) 529–46
12. Blackall, J.M., Rueckert, D., Maurer, C.R., Graeme, P.P., Hill, D.L.G., Hawkes, D.J.: An image registration approach to automated calibration for freehand 3-D ultrasound. MICCAI Proc 1935 (2000) 462–471
13. Poon, T.C., Rohling, R.N.: Comparison of calibration methods for spatial tracking of a 3-D ultrasound probe. Ultrasound Med Biol 31(8) (2005) 1095–1108
14. Bouchet, L.G., Meeks, S.L., Goodchield, G., Bova, F.J., Buatti, J.M., Friedmann, W.A.: Calibration of three-dimensional ultrasound images for image-guided radiation therapy. Physics Med Biol 46 (2001) 559–577
15. Lange, T., Eulenstein, S.: Calibration of swept-volume 3-D ultrasound. MIUA Proc 99(3) (2002) 29–32
16. Bilaniuk, N., Wong, G.S.K.: Speed of sound in pure water as a function of temperature. J. Acoust. Soc. Am. 93(3) (1993) 1609–1612
17. Bilaniuk, N., Wong, G.S.K.: Erratum: Speed of sound in pure water as a function of temperature [j. acoust. soc. am. 93, 1609-1612 (1993)]. J. Acoust. Soc. Am 99(5) (1996) 3257
18. Goldstein, A.: The effect of acoustic velocity on phantom measurements. Ultrasound Med Biol 26(7) (2000) 1133–1143
19. Press, W.H., Flannery, B.P., Teukolsky, S.A., T., V.W.: Numerical Recipies in C, 2nd edition. Cambridge University Press (1992)
20. Hook, I.: Probe calibration for 3-D ultrasound image localization. Internship report. TIMC laboratory, GMCAO (2003)
21. Hsu, P.W., Prager, R.W., Gee, A.H., Treece, G.M.: Rapid, easy and reliable calibration for freehand 3-D ultrasound. MIUA Proc (2005) 91–94

Author Index

Lecture Notes in Computer Science

For information about Vols. 1–4137

please contact your bookseller or Springer

Vol. 4187: J.J. Alferes, J. Bailey, W. May, U. Schwertel (Eds.), Principles and Practice of Semantic Web Reasoning. XI, 277 pages. 2006.

Vol. 4186: C. Jesshope, C. Egan (Eds.), Advances in Computer Systems Architecture. XIV, 605 pages. 2006.

Vol. 4185: R. Mizoguchi, Z. Shi, F. Giunchiglia (Eds.), The Semantic Web – ASWC 2006. XX, 778 pages. 2006.

Vol. 4184: M. Bravetti, M. Núñez, G. Zavattaro (Eds.), Web Services and Formal Methods. X, 289 pages. 2006.

Vol. 4183: J. Euzenat, J. Domingue (Eds.), Artificial Intelligence: Methodology, Systems, and Applications. XIII, 291 pages. 2006. (Sublibrary LNAI).

Vol. 4182: H.T. Ng, M.-K. Leong, M.-Y. Kan, D. Ji (Eds.), Information Retrieval Technology. XVI, 684 pages. 2006.

Vol. 4180: M. Kohlhase, OMDoc – An Open Markup Format for Mathematical Documents [version 1.2]. XIX, 428 pages. 2006. (Sublibrary LNAI).

Vol. 4179: J. Blanc-Talon, W. Philips, D. Popescu, P. Scheunders (Eds.), Advanced Concepts for Intelligent Vision Systems. XXIV, 1224 pages. 2006.

Vol. 4178: A. Corradini, H. Ehrig, U. Montanari, L. Ribeiro, G. Rozenberg (Eds.), Graph Transformations. XII, 473 pages. 2006.

Vol. 4177: R. Marín, E. Onaindía, A. Bugarín, J. Santos (Eds.), Current Topics in Aritficial Intelligence. XIII, 621 pages. 2006. (Sublibrary LNAI).

Vol. 4176: S.K. Katsikas, J. Lopez, M. Backes, S. Gritzalis, B. Preneel (Eds.), Information Security. XIV, 548 pages. 2006.

Vol. 4175: P. Bücher, B.M.E. Moret (Eds.), Algorithms in Bioinformatics. XII, 402 pages. 2006. (Sublibrary LNBI).

Vol. 4174: K. Franke, K.-R. Müller, B. Nickolay, R. Schäfer (Eds.), Pattern Recognition. XX, 773 pages. 2006.

Vol. 4173: S. El Yacoubi, B. Chopard, S. Bandini (Eds.), Cellular Automata. XV, 734 pages. 2006.

Vol. 4172: J. Gonzalo, C. Thanos, M. F. Verdejo, R.C. Carrasco (Eds.), Research and Advanced Technology for Digital Libraries. XVII, 569 pages. 2006.

Vol. 4169: H.L. Bodlaender, M.A. Langston (Eds.), Parameterized and Exact Computation. XI, 279 pages. 2006.

Vol. 4168: Y. Azar, T. Erlebach (Eds.), Algorithms – ESA 2006. XVIII, 843 pages. 2006.

Vol. 4167: S. Dolev (Ed.), Distributed Computing. XV, 576 pages. 2006.

Vol. 4166: J. Górski (Ed.), Computer Safety, Reliability, and Security. XIV, 440 pages. 2006.

Vol. 4165: W. Jonker, M. Petković (Eds.), Secure, Data Management. X, 185 pages. 2006.

Vol. 4163: H. Bersini, J. Carneiro (Eds.), Artificial Immune Systems. XII, 460 pages. 2006.

Vol. 4162: R. Královič, P. Urzyczyn (Eds.), Mathematical Foundations of Computer Science 2006. XV, 814 pages. 2006.

Vol. 4161: R. Harper, M. Rauterberg, M. Combetto (Eds.), Entertainment Computing - ICEC 2006. XXVII, 417 pages. 2006.

Vol. 4160: M. Fisher, W.v.d. Hoek, B. Konev, A. Lisitsa (Eds.), Logics in Artificial Intelligence. XII, 516 pages. 2006. (Sublibrary LNAI).

Vol. 4159: J. Ma, H. Jin, L.T. Yang, J.J.-P. Tsai (Eds.), Ubiquitous Intelligence and Computing. XXII, 1190 pages. 2006.

Vol. 4158: L.T. Yang, H. Jin, J. Ma, T. Ungerer (Eds.), Autonomic and Trusted Computing. XIV, 613 pages. 2006.

Vol. 4156: S. Amer-Yahia, Z. Bellahsène, E. Hunt, R. Unland, J.X. Yu (Eds.), Database and XML Technologies. IX, 123 pages. 2006.

Vol. 4155: O. Stock, M. Schaerf (Eds.), Reasoning, Action and Interaction in AI Theories and Systems. XVIII, 343 pages. 2006. (Sublibrary LNAI).

Vol. 4154: Y.A. Dimitriadis, I. Zigurs, E. Gómez-Sánchez (Eds.), Groupware: Design, Implementation, and Use. XIV, 438 pages. 2006.

Vol. 4153: N. Zheng, X. Jiang, X. Lan (Eds.), Advances in Machine Vision, Image Processing, and Pattern Analysis. XIII, 506 pages. 2006.

Vol. 4152: Y. Manolopoulos, J. Pokorný, T. Sellis (Eds.), Advances in Databases and Information Systems. XV, 448 pages. 2006.

Vol. 4151: A. Iglesias, N. Takayama (Eds.), Mathematical Software - ICMS 2006. XVII, 452 pages. 2006.

Vol. 4150: M. Dorigo, L.M. Gambardella, M. Birattari, A. Martinoli, R. Poli, T. Stützle (Eds.), Ant Colony Optimization and Swarm Intelligence. XVI, 526 pages. 2006.

Vol. 4149: M. Klusch, M. Rovatsos, T.R. Payne (Eds.), Cooperative Information Agents X. XII, 477 pages. 2006. (Sublibrary LNAI).

Vol. 4148: J. Vounckx, N. Azemard, P. Maurine (Eds.), Integrated Circuit and System Design. XVI, 677 pages. 2006.

Vol. 4147: M. Broy, I.H. Krüger, M. Meisinger (Eds.), Automotive Software – Connected Services in Mobile Networks. XIV, 155 pages. 2006.

Vol. 4146: J.C. Rajapakse, L. Wong, R. Acharya (Eds.), Pattern Recognition in Bioinformatics. XIV, 186 pages. 2006. (Sublibrary LNBI).

Vol. 4144: T. Ball, R.B. Jones (Eds.), Computer Aided Verification. XV, 564 pages. 2006.

Vol. 4143: R. Lämmel, J. Saraiva, J. Visser (Eds.), Generative and Transformational Techniques in Software Engineering. X, 471 pages. 2006.

Vol. 4142: A. Campilho, M. Kamel (Eds.), Image Analysis and Recognition, Part II. XXVII, 923 pages. 2006.

Vol. 4141: A. Campilho, M. Kamel (Eds.), Image Analysis and Recognition, Part I. XXVIII, 939 pages. 2006.

Vol. 4139: T. Salakoski, F. Ginter, S. Pyysalo, T. Pahikkala, Advances in Natural Language Processing. XVI, 771 pages. 2006. (Sublibrary LNAI).

Vol. 4138: X. Cheng, W. Li, T. Znati (Eds.), Wireless Algorithms, Systems, and Applications. XVI, 709 pages. 2006.